Preface

The Handbook of Pediatric Environmental Health was written for pediatricians and others who are interested in preventing children's exposure to environmental hazards during infancy, childhood, and adolescence.

In this handbook, we present concise summaries of the evidence that has been published in the scientific literature about environmental hazards to children, and provide guidance to pediatricians about how to diagnose, treat, and prevent childhood diseases linked to environmental exposures. Since this field is evolving rapidly, appropriate guidance may change as additional research findings become available.

The book is meant to be practical, containing information that is useful in the office setting, but that could also be helpful to a clinician preparing a talk for colleagues or for a school board meeting. Throughout the book, I have taken the liberty of combining the contributions of multiple authors in each chapter. I hope that the information presented in this handbook will foster an informed understanding of environmental health among those who care for children.

Parents of young children are intensely interested in the impact of the environment on their children's health. They may look to their pediatrician for guidance about how to evaluate news reports about potential hazards in the air, water, and food. Yet the history of such well-established hazards as the exposure of children to environmental tobacco smoke shows many years of epidemiologic and laboratory research before the weight of evidence compels a consensus. While the evidence is accumulating, what should a worried parent do? Prudently avoid exposure after the first study suggesting problems is published? At what point should the pediatrician advocate a specific action? Obviously, there are no easy answers to these questions. Issues of value, scientific understanding, and cost are involved. Each hazardous exposure must be considered in the context of other problems facing the child and the financial, emotional, and intellectual resources available to surmount them. After fully understanding the facts and the uncertainties, reasonable pediatricians may choose different ways to respond to the accumulating evidence.

I have many people to thank for their contributions to this work. Babasaheb (Bob) Sonawane, PhD, of the US Environmental Protection Agency and Wade Greene of Rockefeller Financial Services have provided support throughout the 4-year development process. Many committees and sections of the AAP reviewed and provided comments on each chapter of the handbook. I am very grateful to Lauri Hall for her outstanding work in keeping this book on track, and to Barbara Scotese, AAP senior medical copy editor for her help in its preparation. I am indebted to the Associate Editor, Sophie Balk, MD, for her expertise, tireless work, and immense contributions in her editorial and committee work. Members of the Committee on Environmental Health gave countless hours and deserve appropriate recognition for their dedication, revisions, and reviews. Shashikant Sane, MD, of Minneapolis Children's Medical Center kindly provided useful information to us. These individuals are only a few of the many contributors whose professional work and commitment have been integral to the committee's preparation of the *Handbook of Pediatric Environmental Health*.

Needless to say, there are many aspects of environmental health that could not be covered. We gave priority to those topics that appeared to have the greatest impact on child health, or to be of concern to parents. I hope that this handbook will help you in your practice and in counseling parents about preventing their children's exposure to environmental hazards.

Ruth A. Etzel, MD, PhD
Editor

Contributors

The American Academy of Pediatrics (AAP) gratefully acknowledges the invaluable assistance provided by the following individuals who served as contributors and reviewers in the preparation of the *Handbook of Pediatric Environmental Health*. Their expertise, critical review, and cooperation were essential to the committee's development of recommendations for the recognition, treatment, and prevention of diseases linked to environmental exposures.

Every attempt has been made to recognize all those who contributed to the *Handbook of Pediatric Environmental Health;* the AAP regrets any omissions that may have occurred.

Robert W. Amler, MD, Agency for Toxic Substances and Disease Registry, Atlanta, GA

Susan S. Aronson, MD, AAP Board of Directors, Narberth, PA

Lauren Ball, DO, MPH, Centers for Disease Control and Prevention, Atlanta, GA

Cynthia F. Bearer, MD, PhD, Dept of Pediatrics, Rainbow Babies and Childrens Hospital, Cleveland, OH

Jerome M. Blondell, PhD, MPH, United States Environmental Protection Agency, Washington, DC

John Carl, MD, Rainbow Babies and Childrens Hospital, Cleveland, OH

J. Milton Clark, PhD, United States Environmental Protection Agency, Chicago, IL

Deon Corkins, MPH, County Health Department, Salt Lake City, UT

Adolfo Correa, MD, PhD, Centers for Disease Control and Prevention, Atlanta, GA

Barbara J. Coven, MD, Westchester Medical Group, White Plains, NY

Karen M. Emmons, PhD, Dana-Farber Cancer Institute, Boston, MA

Henry Falk, MD, Centers for Disease Control and Prevention, Atlanta, GA

Laurence J. Fuortes, MD, MS, University of Iowa School of Medicine, Iowa City, IA

Lorne K. Garrettson, MD, Emory University School of Medicine, Atlanta, GA

Lynn R. Goldman, MD, Johns Hopkins School of Hygiene and Public Health, Baltimore, MD

Robin Goldman, MD, Montefiore Medical Center, Bronx, NY

Birt Harvey, MD, Palo Alto, CA

Jim G. Hendrick, MD, Jackson, MS

Richard Kreutzer, MD, California Department of Health Services, Emeryville, CA

Philip J. Landrigan, MD, MSc, Mt. Sinai School of Medicine, New York, NY

Susan W. Metcalf, MD, Agency for Toxic Substances and Disease Registry, Atlanta, GA

Mark D. Miller, MD, MPH, California Department of Public Health, Oakland, CA

Robert W. Miller, MD, PhD, National Cancer Institute, Bethesda, MD

Howard Mofenson, MD, Winthrop University Hospital, Mineola, NY

Mary Ellen Mortensen, MD, InHealth Health Care Corporation, Dublin, OH

Lawrie Mott, MS, Natural Resources Defense Council, San Francisco, CA

Herbert L. Needleman, MD, University of Pittsburgh School of Medicine, Pittsburgh, PA

Raymond Neutra, MD, PhD, California Department of Health Services, Emeryville, CA

Cynthia J. Osman, MD, Boston City Hospital, Boston, MA

Rossanne M. Philen, MD, Centers for Disease Control and Prevention, Atlanta, GA

Susan H. Pollack, MD, University of Kentucky, Lexington, KY

J. Routt Reigart, MD, Medical University of South Carolina, Charleston, SC

Walter J. Rogan, MD, National Institute of Environmental Health Sciences, Research Triangle Park, NC

Christine L. Rosheim, DDS, MPH, Agency for Toxic Substances and Disease Registry, Atlanta, GA

Lawrence M. Schell, PhD, School of Public Health, State University of New York, Albany, NY

Michael W. Shannon, MD, MPH, Children's Hospital, Boston, MA

Katherine M. Shea, MD, MPH, North Carolina State University, Raleigh, NC

Peter R. Simon, MD, MPH, Rhode Island Department of Health, Providence, RI

Catherine J. Staes, BSN, MPH, County Health Department, Salt Lake City, UT

Robert C. Thompson, United States Environmental Protection Agency, Washington, DC

Michael A. Wall, MD, Oregon Health Sciences University School of Medicine, Portland, OR

Mary C. White, ScD, Agency for Toxic Substances and Disease Registry, Atlanta, GA

Barry Zuckerman, MD, Boston City Hospital, Boston, MA

Table of Contents

I
Background

1 Introduction

nvironmental hazards are among the top health concerns many parents have for their children.[1,2] Little time is spent during medical school and residency training on environmental hazards and their relationship to illness.[3] General medical and pediatric textbooks devote scant attention to illness as a result of environmental factors. Information pertinent to pediatric environmental health is widely scattered in scientific, epidemiologic, and specialty journals not regularly read by clinicians.[4]

Forty-two years have passed since the formation of the American Academy of Pediatric's (AAP's) first committee on environmental health. In that time rapid progress has been made in understanding the role of the environment in the illnesses of childhood and adolescence. Consideration of illnesses traditionally associated with the environment, such as waterborne and food-borne diseases, has expanded to include study of toxic chemicals and other environmental hazards that derive from the rapid expansion of industry and technology in the developed world.

This book, written to be useful to practicing pediatricians, is organized into four sections. The first section gives background information. The second and third sections focus on specific pollutants and on specific environments. The fourth section addresses a variety of other complex environmental situations.

Most chapters on specific hazards are organized in sections that describe the pollutant, routes of exposure, systems affected, clinical effects, diagnostic methods, treatment, and prevention of exposure and include suggested responses to questions that parents may ask. Each chapter contains a list of pertinent resources. Appendix D refers readers to specific environmental agencies when further help is needed.

The Committee on Environmental Health recognizes that pediatric environmental health is a field in the early stages of development. Knowledge in some areas has evolved rapidly, whereas in other areas there are more questions than answers. The authors have attempted to make readers aware of the controversial areas and gaps in scientific data. Given the state of knowledge for any pollutant or situation, this handbook tries to provide the pediatrician with the most accurate and prudent information needed to advise parents and children.

■ History

In 1954, errant fallout from a nuclear weapons test on Bikini Island, an atoll of the Marshall Islands, caused acute burns from beta radiation to develop in neighboring islanders. Subsequently, severe hypothyroidism developed in two children exposed to fallout prior to 1 year of age. Of 18 children exposed before 10 years of age, 14 developed thyroid neoplasia (13 benign and 1 malignant), and one developed leukemia.[5] At about the same time, fallout in southwestern Utah from tests in Nevada apparently caused sickness in sheep, and people who were exposed worried about later effects. In 1956 expert committees of the National Academy of Sciences (NAS) and the British Medical Research Council reported on the biological effects of ionizing radiation in humans. These reports led to a marked reduction in unnecessary exposures from the use of radiotherapy for benign disorders and fluoroscopy. Therefore, in 1957, because of concerns about fallout from weapons testing and fears of nuclear war, the AAP, in keeping with its tradition of promoting research and advocacy for child health, established the Committee on Radiation Hazards and Congenital Malformations to develop policy on exposure of children to ionizing radiation. This was the forerunner of the present Committee on Environmental Health.

In 1961, as the interest of the Committee broadened, its name was changed to the Committee on Environmental Hazards. In 1966, an expert overview of the effects of radiation on children was organized by the Committee on Environmental Hazards—a Conference on the

Pediatric Significance of Peacetime Radioactive Fallout.[6] The participants included pediatricians, radiobiologists, scientists from relevant government health agencies, and Dr Benjamin Spock, who spoke about the psychological effects of radioactive fallout in children.

The Committee, recognizing that man-made chemicals were increasingly permeating the environment, organized a Conference on the Susceptibility of the Fetus and Child to Chemical Pollutants, held in 1973 at Brown's Lake, Wis.[7] Fresh thinking was sought by bringing together scientists knowledgeable about the effects of chemicals on the environment but not about child health and pediatricians who knew about child health but had not given much thought to environmental effects. This meeting led to more interaction between pediatric experts and federal agencies concerned with the environment to discuss the possible effects of the environment on the health of children.

By the early 1980s, the environment had become even more polluted. Areawide pollution occurred from polychlorinated biphenyls in Kyushu, Japan, and Taiwan; from polybrominated biphenyls throughout the Lower Peninsula of Michigan; from chemical dumps at the Love Canal (New York); from dioxin in Seveso, Italy; and from lead in Kellogg, Idaho, and El Paso, Texas.[8] In France, 224 children in diapers were poisoned and 36 died from an overdose of baby powder that contained hexachlorophene.[9] The public worried about the effects of Agent Orange, the near meltdown of a nuclear power reactor at Three Mile Island, the fallout from the Mount St Helen's volcanic eruption, nuclear waste, and the explosion of a Titan II missile in its silo. The Conference on Chemical and Radiation Hazards to Children, held in 1981 to enhance knowledge by expert consultation, enabled the exchange of concerns and information with the pediatric community[10] and led to further interactions between the Committee and federal environmental health agencies. The Council on Pediatric Research called for including pediatricians in meetings of government agencies and on other committees that make policy or deliberate on environmental matters of national importance. To foster relations with other groups, the Committee, which met twice a year, held every other meeting at an organization concerned with environmental research, such as the US Environmental Protection Agency (EPA), the National Institute of Environmental Health Sciences (NIEHS), the Kettering Laboratories in Cincinnati, and the National Institute of Child Health and Development.

In 1991, the name of the Committee on Environmental Hazards was changed to the Committee on Environmental Health to emphasize prevention.

Increasingly, academic and health organizations were studying the impact of the environment on infant and child health. In 1993, the publication of a report by the NAS entitled *Pesticides in the Diets of Infants and Children*[11] was instrumental in highlighting environmental hazards unique to children and the relative paucity of information relating environmental exposures and child health. In October 1995, EPA Administrator Carol Browner directed the agency to formulate a new national policy requiring, for the first time, that the health risks to children and infants from environmental hazards be considered when conducting environmental risk assessments.[12] A number of new initiatives, among them children's environmental health and disease prevention research programs funded by the EPA and the NIEHS, should stimulate more research into the impact of the environment on the health of children.

❚ References

1. Stickler GB, Simmons PS. Pediatricians' preferences for anticipatory guidance topics compared with parental anxieties. *Clin Pediatr.* 1995;34:384-387

2. United States Environmental Protection Agency. *Public Knowledge and Perceptions of Chemical Risks in Six Communities: Analysis of a Baseline Survey.* Washington, DC: USEPA 230-01-90-074. January 1990

3. Pope AM, Rall DP, eds. *Environmental Medicine: Integrating a Missing Element into Medical Education.* Washington, DC: National Academy Press; 1995

4. Etzel RA. Introduction. In: *Environmental Health: Report of the 27th Ross Roundtable on Critical Approaches to Common Pediatric Problems.* Columbus, Ohio: Ross Products Division, Abbott Laboratories; 1996:1

5. Merke DP, Miller RW. Age differences in the effects of ionizing radiation. In: Guzelian PS, Henry CJ, Olin SS, eds. *Similarities and Differences Between Children and Adults: Implications for Risk Assessment.* Washington, DC: International Life Sciences Institute; 1992:139-149

6. American Academy of Pediatrics, Committee on Environmental Hazards. Conference on the Pediatric Significance of Peacetime Radioactive Fallout. *Pediatrics.* 1968;41:165-378

7. American Academy of Pediatrics, Committee on Environmental Hazards. The susceptibility of the fetus and child to chemical pollutants. *Pediatrics.* 1974;53:777-862

8. Miller RW. Areawide chemical contamination. Lessons from case histories. JAMA, 1981;245:1848-1551.

9. Martin-Bouyer G, Lebreton R, Toga M, Stolley PD, Lockhart J. Outbreak of accidental hexachlorophene poisoning in France. *Lancet.* 1982;1:91-95

10. Finberg L. *Chemical and Radiation Hazards to Children: Report of the Eighty-fourth Ross Conference on Pediatric Research.* Columbus, Ohio: Ross Laboratories; 1982

11. National Research Council. *Pesticides in the Diets of Infants and Children.* Washington, DC: National Academy Press; 1993

12. United States Environmental Protection Agency. *Environmental Health Threats to Children.* Washington, DC: USEPA 175-F-96-001. September 1996

2 Special Considerations Based on Age and Developmental Stage

his chapter discusses the scientific basis for the unique vulnerability of children to environmental hazards. It describes the differences between adults and children in physical, biological, and social environments and why children should not be treated as "little adults." Six developmental stages are considered: the fetus (although there are multiple critical stages of development for the fetus), newborn (from birth to 2 months of age), infant/toddler (2 months to 2 years of age), preschool child (2 to 6 years of age), school-age child (6 to 12 years), and adolescent (12 to 18 years). There remains significant uncertainty in the estimates of environmental effects on children due to the lack of data.

■ Human Environments

A child's environment can be thought of as having three components: physical, biological, and social. The physical environment is anything that comes in contact with the body. Air, for example, which is in constant contact with our lungs and skin, is a large part of the physical environment. To define the physical environment more precisely, it may be necessary to divide a large environment into smaller units, called *micro environments*. Micro environments can differ enormously between adults and children. For example, in a room in which the air is contaminated with mercury, the mercury vapor may

9

not be evenly dispersed—air near the floor may have a higher concentration of mercury than air near the ceiling.[1] The environment of an infant lying on the floor therefore would be different from that of a standing adult. The biological environment consists of the internal physiologic interactions of the body with the chemicals it contacts. The absorption, distribution, metabolism, and the toxic action of chemicals may vary with the developmental stage of the child. The social environment includes the day-to-day circumstances of living as well as regulations that may affect day-to-day living.

■ Exposure: The Physical Environment

A child's exposure is the sum of the exposure in several environments during the course of a day, including the home, school, child care, and play areas. Estimates of exposure are often retrospective because it is difficult to monitor children. Even if the total duration of exposure to a toxicant* is the same for two children, different patterns of exposure may have different health effects. For example, ingestion of nitrates in well water may cause the hemoglobin to become reduced to methemoglobin.[3] However, if the nitrates are ingested at a slow enough rate for enzymes to oxidize the methemoglobin back to hemoglobin, no deleterious health effects occur. This is an example of a threshold effect; the health problem will not occur until the toxicant reaches a particular level in the body.

Exposure From Conception to Adolescence
In most instances, exposures to the fetus are from the pregnant woman. However, premature infants who spend months in the neonatal intensive care unit have very different exposures from healthy full-term infants (eg, exposure to noise, light, compressed gases, intravenous solutions, benzyl alcohol, etc).[4]

Exposures to newborns, infants, toddlers, preschool children, school-age children, and adolescents occur with changes in physical location, breathing zones, oxygen consumption, types of foods consumed, amount of food consumption, and normal behavioral development.[5]

---

*The term *toxicant* is used to refer to a chemical pollutant or hazard. The term *toxin* refers to a hazard that arises from a biological source, eg, mycotoxin or botulinum toxin.

Physical Location

Physical location changes with development. Newborn exposures are usually similar to those experienced by the mother. Moreover, the newborn frequently spends prolonged periods of time in a single environment, such as a crib. Because infants and toddlers are frequently placed on the floor, carpet, or grass, they have more exposure to chemicals associated with these surfaces, such as pesticide residues from flea sprays. Infants who are unable to walk or crawl may experience sustained exposure to some agents because they cannot remove themselves from their environment (eg, prolonged exposure to the sun).

Preschool children may spend part of their day in child care facilities with varied environments, including some time outdoors.

School-age children may be exposed to toxicants when schools are built near highways (resulting in exposure to motor vehicle emissions). Asbestos may be found in school buildings, and may become hazardous if it deteriorates or is disturbed. Adolescents not only have a school environment, but are beginning to select other physical environments, often misjudging or ignoring the risks to themselves. For example, listening to loud music may result in permanent hearing loss. Many adolescents work part-time in hazardous physical environments.[6]

Breathing Zones

The breathing zone for an adult is typically 4 to 6 ft above the floor. For a child, it is closer to the floor, depending on the height and mobility of the child. Within lower breathing zones, chemicals heavier than air, such as mercury, may concentrate.[7,8]

Oxygen Consumption

Children are smaller than adults and their metabolic rates are higher relative to their size. Thus, they consume more oxygen than do adults and produce more CO_2 per pound of body weight. This increased CO_2 production requires a higher minute ventilation. Minute ventilation for a newborn and adult are approximately 400 mL/min per kilogram and 150 mL/min per kilogram, respectively.[9] Thus, children's exposure to air pollutants may be greater than that of adults.

Quantity and Quality of Food Consumed

The amount of food that children consume per pound of body weight is higher than that of the adult because children not only need to maintain homeostasis, as adults do, but are growing. The average infant consumes 5 oz of formula per kilogram of body weight (for the average male adult, this is equivalent to drinking 30 12-oz cans of soda a day). If the food or liquid contains a contaminant, children may receive more of it relative to their size than adults.[3,10]

In addition, children consume different types of food. The diet of many newborns is limited to breast milk. The diet of children contains more milk products and certain fruits and vegetables than the typical adult diet.[4,5]

Normal Behavioral Development

Children pass through a developmental stage of intense oral exploratory behavior. Therefore, normal oral exploration may place children at risk, such as in environments with high levels of lead dust. Wood used in some playground equipment is treated with arsenic and creosote, thus exposing children when they place their mouths on these materials. Children also lack the cognitive ability to recognize hazardous situations.

Ambulatory children may be exposed to used drums containing potentially harmful chemicals while playing in abandoned areas. Adolescents, as they gain freedom from parental authority, may be less protected from some exposures. While at a stage of development where physical strength and stamina are at a peak, they are still acquiring abstract reasoning skills and often fail to consider cause and effect, particularly delayed effects. Thus adolescents may place themselves in situations with greater risk than would an adult.

▌Absorption, Distribution, Metabolism, and Target Organ Susceptibility: The Biological Environment

Absorption

Absorption generally occurs by one of four pathways: transplacental, percutaneous, respiratory, and gastrointestinal. The type of toxicant and the developmental stage of the child determine the pathway of absorption.

Transplacental

Several classes of compounds readily cross the placenta, including compounds with low molecular weight such as carbon monoxide, those that are fat-soluble, and other specific elements such as calcium and lead. Because carbon monoxide has a higher affinity for fetal hemoglobin than adult hemoglobin, the concentration of carboxyhemoglobin is higher in the fetus than in the pregnant woman.[11,12] Therefore, the infant may have a reduced level of oxygen delivered to tissues. Lipophilic compounds, such as polycyclic aromatic hydrocarbons (found in cigarette smoke) methyl mercury and ethanol, also readily gain access to the fetal circulation. Specific transport mechanisms in the placenta actively transport specific nutrients and metals such as lead, which is found in the same concentration in maternal and cord blood.[15]

Percutaneous

The skin undergoes enormous change with developmental stage, which changes the properties of absorption. Pathways of absorption through the skin are particularly important for fat-soluble compounds. Although chemicals such as nicotine and cotinine have been described in amniotic fluid, their absorption through the fetal skin has not been studied.[16] The dermis of a fetus lacks the exterior dead keratin layer, one of the major barriers of fully developed skin. The acquisition of keratin occurs over 3 to 5 days following birth. Therefore, the skin of a newborn remains particularly absorptive. Epidemics involving absorption of chemicals through the skin in newborns include hypothyroidism from iodine in Betadine scrub solutions,[17] neurotoxicity from hexachlorophene,[18] and hyperbilirubinemia from a phenolic disinfectant used to clean hospital equipment.[19]

An additional factor in percutaneous absorption is the larger surface-to-body mass ratio of newborns compared with older children and adults. The newborn has a three times larger surface to mass ratio, and the child has a two times larger surface to mass ratio than an adult. Thus, for the surface area of skin covered with a chemical, a newborn may absorb up to three times, and an older child up to two times, the amount absorbed by an adult.[20]

Respiratory

The fetus makes breathing motions. Although fluid flows from the lungs through the trachea into the amniotic fluid, some chemicals in the amniotic fluid may come in contact with the lining of the respiratory tract. Studies on this pathway of exposure to foreign chemicals are limited.

Lung development proceeds through proliferation of pulmonary alveoli and capillaries until the ages of 5 to 8 years. Thereafter, the lungs grow through alveolar expansion.[21] The surface absorptive properties of the lung do not change during development.

The brain attains four fifths of its adult size by the end of the second year of life.[21] By adolescence there are no gross changes in brain morphology.[21] Electroencephalographic studies demonstrate continued neurodevelopmental maturation.[21]

Gastrointestinal

The gastrointestinal tract undergoes numerous changes during development. Certain pesticides as well as chemicals from tobacco smoke are present in amniotic fluid,[16] but it is not known if the fetus, which actively swallows amniotic fluid, absorbs them. Following birth, stomach acid secretion is relatively low, but achieves adult levels by several months of age, markedly affecting absorption of chemicals from the stomach. If acidity levels are too low, bacterial overgrowth in the small bowel and stomach may result in formation of chemicals that can be absorbed. For example, several cases of methemoglobinemia in infants in Iowa were traced to well water contaminated with nitrate that was converted to nitrite by intestinal bacteria.[3]

The small intestine transports certain chemicals to the blood and may respond to increased nutritional needs by increasing absorption of that particular nutrient. For example, the bones of infants and children absorb more calcium from food sources than do adults. Lead, which may be absorbed in place of calcium, may also be absorbed to a greater extent: an adult absorbs 10% of ingested lead, whereas a 1- to 2-year-old absorbs 50%.[22]

Distribution

The distribution of chemicals within the body varies with developmental stage. For example, in animal models it has been shown that lead is retained to a larger degree in the infant animal brain than in the adult animal brain.[23] Lead may also accumulate more rapidly in children's bones.[24]

Metabolism

Metabolism of a chemical may result in its activation or deactivation. The activity in each step of these metabolic pathways is determined by development and genetics. Therefore, some children are genetically more susceptible to adverse effects from certain exposures. For example, children (and adults) with glucose 6-phosphate dehydrogenase (G6PD) deficiency are at risk of hemolytic anemia if exposed to certain chemicals such as naphthalene. Large differences also exist in the activity of enzymes in various developmental stages. The same enzyme may be more or less active depending on the age of the child. Two examples are the enzymes involved in the P450 cytochrome family, which metabolizes such xenobiotics as theophylline and caffeine,[25] and alcohol dehydrogenase, which converts ethanol to acetaldehyde.[26]

The differences between metabolism in children and adults may protect children from environmental hazards. Such is the case for acetaminophen. In the adult, high levels of acetaminophen are metabolized to products that may cause hepatic failure. Infants born to women with high blood acetaminophen levels have similar acetaminophen levels, but do not sustain liver damage because their metabolic pathways have not yet developed enough to break down acetaminophen into harmful metabolites.[27-30]

Target Organ Susceptibility

During growth and maturation the organs of children may be affected by exposure to harmful chemicals.[31] Following cellular proliferation, individual cells undergo two further processes to become the adult organism: differentiation and migration. Differentiation occurs when cells take on specific tasks within the body and lose the ability to divide. The trigger for differentiation may be hormonal, so chemicals that mimic hormones could alter the differentiation of some tissues. Because organ systems in children, including the reproductive system, are continuing to differentiate, chemicals that mimic hormones may have effects on the development of those organ systems. For example, chemicals referred to as endocrine disruptors have been linked to the increasing incidence of hypospadias.[32]

Cell migration is necessary for certain cells to reach their destination. Neurons, for example, originate in a structure near the center of the brain, then migrate to a predestined location in one of the many layers of the brain. Chemicals such as ethanol may have a profound effect on this process (eg, ethanol and fetal alcohol syndrome).

Synaptogenesis occurs rapidly during the first 2 years. Waves of specific synapses are then formed as learning occurs throughout life. Dendritic trimming is the active removal of synapses. A 2-year-old's brain contains more synapses than at any other age. These synapses are trimmed back to allow more specificity of the resulting neural network. There are some data to suggest that low-dose lead may interfere with this synapse trimming.[33]

Some organs continue developing for several years and development is not complete until adolescence, increasing the vulnerability of these organs. For example, brain tumors are frequently treated by radiation therapy in adults with uncomfortable but reversible side effects. However, in infants, radiation therapy is generally avoided because of the profound and permanent effects on the developing central nervous system. Similarly, lead affects the brain and nervous system of children. The current blood lead concentration of concern for children is 10 μg/dL.[34] The occupational limit for adults is 2.5 times higher than the concentration of concern for children.[35]

Exposure to environmental tobacco smoke (ETS) compromises lung development. The rate of growth of lung function in children exposed to ETS is slower than that of nonexposed children. The forced expiratory volumes in 1 second of children exposed to ETS are measurably lower than those of children without exposure.[36]

Tissues undergoing growth and differentiation are particularly susceptible to cancer due to the shortened time period for DNA repair and the changes occurring within the DNA during cell growth. The epidemic of scrotal cancer among adolescent chimney sweeps of Victorian England illustrates the likelihood that the scrotum at this stage of development has increased susceptibility to the chemicals in soot.[37] Although occupational exposure at that time to cancer-causing chemicals such as soot was common in many occupations, scrotal tumors were uncommon except in young male chimney sweeps.

∎ Regulations and Laws: The Social Environment

Regulatory policies usually do not take into account the unique combinations of developmental characteristics, physical environment, and biological environment that place children at risk. Most laws and regulations are based on studies using adult men weighing an average of 70 kg. However, recent advances have been made to change regulations to protect children. For example, the Food Quality Protection Act of 1996 states that pesticide tolerances need to be set to protect the health of infants and children. New rules on cigarette vending machines make cigarettes less available to children. The EPA enacted more stringent regulations on outdoor air quality to protect children. How can a clinician integrate information about children's developmental susceptibility into practice? The roles of educator, investigator, and advocate are extremely important. The most important intervention is the education of parents and children about exposures. Prevention efforts have the most impact when developmentally appropriate. Parents, children, teachers, community leaders, and policy makers need to be educated about the unique vulnerability of children to environmental pollution. The role of the clinician as investigator is also very important. Most diseases caused by environmental factors have been diagnosed by an alert clinician, and publication of case studies has enabled further description of these illnesses. Finally, clinicians must advocate for children, working to ensure that regulatory policies take into account their unique vulnerability.

▌ References

1. Agocs MM, Etzel RA, Parrish RG, et al. Mercury exposure from interior latex paint. *N Engl J Med.* 1990;323:1096-1101

2. Bearer CF. How are children different from adults? *Environ Health Perspect.* 1995;103(suppl 6):7-12

3. Luyens JN. The legacy of well-water methemoglobinemia. *JAMA.* 1987;257:2793-2795

4. Bearer CF. Occupational and environmental risks to the fetus. In: Fanaroff AA, Martin RM. *Neonatal-Perinatal Medicine: Diseases of the Fetus and Infant.* 6th ed. St Louis, Mo: Mosby-Year Book; 1997:188-199

5. Guzelian PS, Henry CJ, Olin SS, ed. *Similarities and Differences Between Children and Adults: Implications for Risk Assessment.* Washington, DC: ILSI Press; 1992

6. Pollack SH, Landrigan PH, Mallino DL. Child labor in 1990: prevalence and health hazards. *Ann Rev Public Health.* 1990;11:359-375

7. Leaderer BP. Assessing exposures to environmental tobacco smoke. *Risk Analysis.* 1990;10:19-26

8. Blot WJ, Xu ZY, Boice JD Jr, et al. Indoor radon and lung cancer in China. *J Natl Cancer Inst.* 1990;82:1025-1030

9. Snodgrasss WR. Physiological and biochemical differences between children and adults as determinants of toxic response to environmental pollutants. In: Guzelian PS, Henry CJ, Olin SS, eds. *Similarities and Differences Between Children and Adults: Implications for Risk Assessment.* Washington, DC: ILSI Press; 1992;35-42

10. Shannon MW, Graef JW. Lead intoxication in infancy. *Pediatrics.* 1992;89:87-90

11. Longo LD, Hill EP. Carbon monoxide uptake and elimination in fetal and maternal sheep. *Am J Physiol.* 1977;232:H324-H330

12. Longo LD. Carbon monoxide in the pregnant mother and fetus and its exchange across the placenta. *Ann NY Acad Sci.* 1970;174:312-341

13. Bush B, Snow J, Koblintz R. Polychlorobiphenyl (PCB) congeners, p,p¹-DDE, and hexachlorobenzene in maternal and fetal cord blood from mothers in upstate New York. *Arch Environ Contam Toxicol.* 1984;13:517-527

14. Clarke DW, Smith GN, Patrick J, Richardson B, Brien JF. Activity of alcohol dehydrogenase and aldehyde dehydrogenase in maternal liver, fetal liver and placenta of the near-term pregnant ewe. *Dev Pharmacol Ther.* 1989;12:35-41

15. Goyer RA. Transplacental transport of lead. *Environ Health Perspect.* 1990;89:101-105

16. Van Vunakis H, Langone JJ, Milunsky A. Nicotine and cotinine in the amniotic fluid of smokers in the second trimester of pregnancy. *Am J Obstet Gynecol.* 1974;20:64-66

17. Clemens PC, Neumann RS. The Wolff-Chaikoff effect: hypothyroidism due to iodine application. *Arch Dermatol.* 1989;125:705

18. Shuman RM, Leech RW, Alvord EC. Neurotoxicity of hexachlorophene in the human: I. A clinicopathologic study of 248 children. *Pediatrics.* 1974; 54:689-695

19. Wysowski DK, Flynt JW Jr, Goldfield M, Altman R, Davis AT. Epidemic neonatal hyperbilirubinemia and use of a phenolic disinfectant detergent. *Pediatrics.* 1978;61:165-170

20. Plunkett LM, Turnbull D, Rodricks JV. Differences between adults and children affecting exposure assessment. In: Buzelian PS, Henry CJ, Olin SS, eds. *Similarities and Differences Between Children and Adults: Implications for Risk Assessment.* Washington, DC: ILSI Press; 1992: 79-94

21. Behrman RE. *Nelson Texbook of Pediatrics.* 15th ed. Philadelphia, Pa: W.B. Saunders Co; 1996

22. US Environmental Protection Agency. *Review of the National Ambient Air Quality Standards for Lead: Exposure Analysis Methodology and Validation.* Air Quality Management Division, Office of Air Quality Planning and Standards, US EPA; 1989

23. Momcilovic B, Kostial K. Kinetics of lead retention and distribution in suckling and adult rats. *Environ Res.* 1974;8:214-220

24. Barry PS. A comparison of concentrations of lead in human tissues. *Br J Ind Med.* 1975;32:119-139

25. Nebert DW, Gonzalez FJ. P450 genes: structure, evolution, and regulation. *Annu Rev Biochem.* 1987;56:945-993

26. Card SE, Tompkins SF, Brien JF. Ontogeny of the activity of alcohol dehydrogenase and aldehyde dehydrogenases in the liver and placenta of the guinea pig. *Biochem Pharmacol.* 1989;38:2535-2541

27. Byer A, Traylor TR, Semmer JR. Acetaminophen overdose in the third trimester of pregnancy. *JAMA.* 1982;247:3114-3115

28. Kurzel RB. Can acetaminophen excess result in maternal and fetal toxicity? *South Med J.* 1990;83:953-955

29. Rosevear SK, Hope PL. Favourable neonatal outcome following maternal paracetamol overdose and severe fetal distress: case report. *Br J Obstet Gynaecol.* 1989;96:491-493

30. Stokes IM. Paracetamol overdose in the second trimester of pregnancy: case report. *Br J Obstet Gynaecol.* 1984;91:286-288

31. WHO: Environmental Health Criteria 59. *Principles for Evaluating Health Risks From Chemicals During Infancy and Early Childhood: The Need for a Special Approach.* Geneva, Switzerland: World Health Organization; 1986

32. Kelce WR, Wilson EM. Environmental antiandrogens: developmental effects, molecular mechanisms, and clinical implications. *J Mol Med.* 1997;75:198-207

33. Goldstein GW. Developmental neurobiology of lead toxicity. In: Needleman HL, ed. *Human Lead Exposure.* Boca Raton, Fla: CRC Press; 1992:125-135

34. American Academy of Pediatrics, Committee on Environmental Health. Screening for elevated blood lead levels. *Pediatrics.* 1998;101:1072-1078

35. Sussell A, ed. *Protecting Workers Exposed to Lead-Based Paint Hazards: A Report to Congress.* US Dept of Health and Human Services, Public Health Service, CDCP, NIOSH; January 1997

36. Tager IB, Weiss ST, Munoz A, Rosner B, Speizer FE. Longitudinal study of the effects of maternal smoking on pulmonary function in children. *N Engl J Med.* 1983;309:699-703

37. Nethercott JR. Occupational skin disorders. In: LaDou J, ed. *Occupational Medicine.* Norwalk, CT: Appleton and Lange; 1990

3 How To Do a Home Inventory*

lthough the utility of home audit questionnaires has not been scientifically tested, some pediatricians find them helpful in obtaining an environmental history. Parents can fill out a questionnaire in the waiting room or at home after the visit. Answers that indicate possible exposure to environmental hazards can be followed up with appropriate actions such as (1) testing the child for lead poisoning, (2) testing the home for radon, (3) advising family members about prevention, or (4) advising parents about eliminating the hazard.

The following questionnaire can be used or adapted to include environmental issues specific to a community. Basic questions are included. Information for parents can be found in the brochure, *Your Child and the Environment,* by the American Academy of Pediatrics.

---

*This questionnaire is adapted from Sophie J. Balk, MD. The original material appeared in the manual, *Kids and the Environment—Toxic Hazards,* edited by the Children's Environmental Health Network, California Public Health Foundation. The sponsors for this project were the Agency for Toxic Substances and Disease Registry and the California Department of Health Services.

The material was presented in 1994 in *Raising Children Toxic-Free,* by Philip J. Landrigan and Herbert Needleman; Farrar, Strauss, Giroux, New York.

Home Audit or Home Inventory Questionnaire*

Where does the child live or spend time?	*Further information found in chapter(s) on*
1. What is the age and condition of the home?	Lead
2. Are the windowsills peeling? Do the window wells contain solid material?	Lead
3. Are you renovating a room or planning to?	Lead, Asbestos
4. Do you have a basement?	Asbestos, Radon
5. Are there sleeping or playing areas in the basement?	Asbestos, Radon
6. Do you have water damage or visible mold in any part of your home?	Asthma, Indoor Air Pollutants
7. Do you live in a mobile home?	Indoor Air Pollutants
8. Do you have a wood stove or fireplace? Does smoke enter the room when you use it?	Indoor Air Pollutants, Carbon Monoxide
9. Do you have a gas stove? Does it have a pilot light? Do you use the stove for additional heat?	Indoor Air Pollutants, Carbon Monoxide
10. Do you use pesticides on your lawn, or use a proprietary lawn service? Do you use pesticides in your home?	Pesticides
11. Is your home located near a polluted lake or stream, industrial area, highway, dumpsite, farm, etc.?	Water Pollutants, Outdoor Air Pollutants, Waste Sites, Pesticides

Smoking
12. Does anyone in the home smoke? How many people? Is smoking allowed by visitors to your home, or in the car? ....

Diet—water and food
13. Is your baby breastfeeding? ....

14. Do you use well water? ....

15. Do you use tap water?....................
16. Do you wash fresh fruits and vegetables? ....
17. Do you use dietary supplements or ethnic remedies? ....

Job-Related Hazards
18. What do you and your spouse do for a living? Does your job or your spouse's job involve contact with metals, dust, chemicals, or fibers?

19. Do teenagers in the home work?

Hobbies
20. Are you or your child involved in a hobby at home? ....

Further information found in chapter(s) on

Environmental Tobacco Smoke

Human Milk

Nitrates, Pesticides, Water Pollutants

Lead

Food Contaminants

Dietary Supplements and Ethnic Remedies

Workplaces

Workplaces

Workplaces; Arts and Crafts; Lead

4 | Taking an Environmental History

Questions about a child's environment are basic to a comprehensive pediatric health history. The answers can help the pediatrician to understand the child's physical surroundings and offer appropriate suggestions to promote a healthy environment. Questions can be incorporated during visits for health supervision and illnesses or complaints that may have environmental causes. Further information about toxicants and abatement measures can be found elsewhere in the text.

∎ Health Supervision Visits

The following questions can be integrated into health supervision visits; parents' answers can guide pediatricians in providing anticipatory guidance about preventing or abating exposures.

1. Where does the child live or spend time?
2. Does anyone in the home smoke?
3. Do you use well water? Tap water?
4. Is the child protected from excessive sun exposure?
5. What do parents/teenagers do for a living?

Additional questions can be added to determine whether particular environmental health risks in the community may be affecting the child. The patient's developmental stage is an important consideration during evaluation; Table 4.1 suggests when to introduce environmental questions.

Table 4.1. When to Introduce Environmental Questions*

Topic	Suggested Time
Home environment, smoking, environmental tobacco smoke (ETS), mold, occupational exposures, breast-feeding and bottle-feeding issues	Prenatal period
ETS, sun exposure, mold	When the child is 2 months old
Poison exposures, including household pesticides; lead poisoning	When the child is 6 months old
Arts and crafts exposures	Preschool period
Occupational exposures, exposures from hobbies	When the patient is a teenager
Lawn and garden products, lawn services, scheduled chemical applications	Spring and summer
Wood stoves and fireplaces, gas stoves	Fall and winter

* This table is adapted from reference 9.

Where Does the Child Live or Spend Time?

At home: Infants and toddlers spend most of their time indoors in their own home or in child care settings. Important features of these settings are:

Type of dwelling: Private homes or apartments may have high levels of radon in basements or lower floors, or friable asbestos. Parents may need advice about testing for either or both toxicants. Building materials commonly used in mobile homes (eg, particle board and pressed wood products) may contain formaldehyde, a respiratory and dermal irritant.

Age and condition: Buildings constructed before 1950 are likely to have leaded paint, which may peel, chip, or chalk. Lead dust can be released from poorly maintained surfaces that encounter friction, such as windows. Homes that have flooded or that have plumbing or roof leaks may have problems with mold growth. A "tight" home, built to conserve energy, may have inadequate ventilation, which may result in trapping of pollutants indoors. When asked about whether hazards exist for the child, parents may be able to provide some information (eg, the condition of the window wells) but not other information (the year the home was built).

Ongoing or planned renovation: Renovation of a bedroom is common to prepare for the birth of a baby or to update the room decor as the child grows. Improper renovation procedures may expose a pregnant woman, her fetus, infant, or toddler to lead or other dusts, asbestos, and molds. Newly installed carpets may release irritating or toxic vapors.

Heating sources: Wood stoves and fireplaces emit respiratory irritants (nitrogen dioxide) [NO_2], respirable particulates, and polycyclic aromatic hydrocarbons), especially when they are not properly vented and maintained. Gas stoves, which may produce NO_2, are used in more than half of US homes. Respiratory symptoms may occur when gas stoves are used as supplemental heat.

Indoor and outdoor pesticides: Children may inhale and absorb pesticides as they crawl or play on freshly sprayed surfaces indoors or outdoors. The hazards of spraying pesticides while children are young should be explained to parents.

Proximity to sites of potential hazardous exposure: Exposures include polluted lakes and streams, industrial plants, highways, and dump sites. Children can be exposed to lead if they live downwind from a lead smelter, or have agricultural exposures to pesticides or other chemicals if they live on farms or at the urban-rural interface. Low-income families are more likely to live in contaminated areas.

At school: Many hazards found in school environments are similar to those in homes.[1] In addition, children engaging in arts and crafts activities may encounter potential hazards such as felt-tip markers (containing aromatic hydrocarbons) and oil-based paints, which are legally allowed to contain lead, cadmium, or chromium.

Participation in arts and crafts activities carries the potential for toxic exposure, especially for certain children. Visually impaired children working close to a project or children with asthma may be affected by fumes. Children with disabilities who are unable to follow safety precautions may contaminate their skin or place art materials in their mouths. Emotionally disturbed children may abuse art materials, endangering themselves and others.

Hobbies: Hobby activity may pose a risk to school-age children and adolescents. Shooting at an indoor firing range may result in lead exposure. Toluene and other solvents may be encountered in glues used in model-building.

Does Anyone in the Home Smoke?

Exposure to environmental tobacco smoke (ETS) places children at risk for significant morbidity and mortality. If parents smoke, the pediatrician should advise them to quit. Educating parents about the associations between ETS and their child's illness may help them to quit. Parents can also be informed that their children are more likely to begin smoking if the parents smoke. The National Cancer Institute recommends that physicians enter into verbal agreements with parents who express the desire to quit, and that the issue be reinforced at every visit. Pamphlets, posters, and information about programs that may help parents to quit may assist educational efforts. Parents should avoid exposing their children to environments that contain tobacco smoke.

Pediatricians should discuss the hazards of cigarette smoking with school-age children and teenagers.

Do You Use Well Water? Tap Water?

Tap water is often used to reconstitute infant formula. To avoid possible contamination from leaded pipes and solder, water which has been standing in pipes overnight should be run for 2 minutes, or until cold, before it is used. Parents can also choose to test their water for lead.

Because well water used to reconstitute infant formula may be contaminated with nitrates, possibly resulting in methemoglobinemia and death, it should be tested before being offered to an infant.

Overboiling water for infant formula preparation concentrates lead and nitrates.[2] Water brought to a rolling boil for 1 minute kills microorganisms such as *Cryptosporidium* without concentrating lead or nitrates.

Is the Child Protected from Excessive Sun Exposure?

About 80% of a person's exposure to the sun occurs before the age of 18. Advice about sun protection includes covering up with clothing and hats, timing children's activities to avoid peak sun exposure, consulting the Ultraviolet Index, using sunscreen and reapplying frequently as needed, and wearing sunglasses.

What Do Parents/Teenagers Do for a Living?

Parental occupations: Parental occupations may produce hazards for a child. Workplace contaminants may be transported to the home on clothes, shoes, and skin surfaces.[3] Lead poisoning has been described in children of lead storage battery workers,[4] asbestos-related lung diseases have been found in families of shipyard workers,[5] and elevated mercury levels have been reported in children whose parents worked in a mercury thermometer plant.[6] Parents who work with art materials at home may expose children to toxicants such as lead used in solder, pottery glazes, or stained glass.

An occupational history can be obtained when information about family composition and the family history is obtained. Workers exposed to toxic substances are legally entitled to be notified of this exposure under federal "right-to-know" and "hazard communication" laws. Parents who work with toxic substances should shower, if possible, and change clothes and shoes before leaving work. At home, children should not be allowed in rooms where parents work with toxic substances.

Adolescent employment: Although employment may help teenagers become more responsible, develop skills, and earn money, work activities may carry the risk of toxic exposure or injury. Work may also interfere with an adolescent's education, sleep, and social behavior. Federal and state child labor laws regulate employment of children under 18 years of age. These laws address the minimum ages for general and specific types of employment, maximum daily and weekly number of hours of work permitted, prohibition of work during night hours, prohibition of certain types of employment, and the registration of minors for employment.[7]

▮ Visits for Illness: Considering Environmental Etiologies in the Differential Diagnosis

Environmental tobacco smoke is the most common toxicant associated with respiratory diseases such as asthma, recurrent lower and upper airway disease, and persistent middle ear effusion. Lead poisoning may present with symptoms of recurrent abdominal pain, constipation, irritability, developmental delay, seizures, or unexplained coma. Headaches may be caused by acute and chronic exposure to carbon monoxide from improperly vented heating sources, formaldehyde, and chemicals used on the job. Pediatricians should ask about mold and water damage in the home when they treat infants with acute pulmonary hemorrhage.

Environmental causes of illness may not always be apparent. As most environmental or occupational illnesses present as common medical problems or have nonspecific symptoms, the diagnosis may be missed unless a history of exposure is obtained, which is especially important if the illness is atypical or unresponsive to treatment.[8] The following questions may provide information about whether an illness is related to the environment.

1. Do symptoms subside or worsen in a particular location (eg, home, child care, school, or room)?
2. Do symptoms subside or worsen on weekdays or weekends? At a particular time of day?
3. Do symptoms worsen during hobby activites, such as working with arts and crafts?
4. Are children your child spends time with experiencing similar symptoms to your child's?

∎ References

1. Common teaching, hobby materials could pose significant health risks. *Environmental Health Letter.* 1996;35:153

2. United States Environmental Protection Agency. Office of Ground Water and Drinking Water. Guidance for people with severely weakened immune systems. Internet: HYPERLINK http://www.epa.gov/safewater/crypto.html. June 1999

3. Chisolm JJ. Fouling one's own nest. *Pediatrics.* 1978;62:614-617

4. Watson WN, Witherell LE, Giguere GC. Increased lead absorption in children of workers in a lead storage battery plant. *J Occup Med* 1978;20:759-761

5. Kilburn KH, Lilis R, Anderson HA, et al. Asbestos disease in family contacts of shipyard workers. *Am J Public Health.* 1985;75:615-617

6. Hudson PJ, Vogt RL, Brondum J, Witherell L, Myers G, Pascal DC. Elemental mercury exposure among children of thermometer plant workers. *Pediatrics.* 1987;79:935-938

7. Rose KL, Fraser BS, Chavner I. *Minor Laws of Major Importance.* Dubuque, Iowa: Kendall/Hunt Publishing Co; January 1994

8. Frank AL, guest contributor. Balk SJ, guest editor. Taking an Exposure History. In: *Case Studies in Environmental Medicine.* Agency for Toxic Substances and Disease Registry, Dept of Health and Human Services; October 1992

9. Balk SJ. The environmental history: asking the right questions. *Contemp Pediatr.* 1996;13:19-36

II
Specific Contaminants and Diseases

5 Asbestos

A sbestos includes a group of six fibrous minerals (amosite, chrysotile, crocidolite, and the fibrous varieties of tremolite, actinolite, and anthophyllite). Asbestos occurs naturally in rock formations in certain areas of the world and is mined. Asbestos fibers vary in length; may be straight or curled; can be carded, woven, and spun into cloth; and can be used in bulk or mixed with materials such as asphalt or cement.

Asbestos fibers are virtually indestructible. They resist heat, fire, and acid. Because of these properties, asbestos has been used for a wide range of manufactured goods, including roofing shingles, ceiling and floor tiles, paper products, asbestos cement, clutches, brakes and transmission parts, textiles, packaging, gaskets, coatings, and insulation. Between the 1920s and the early 1970s, millions of tons of asbestos were used in the construction of homes, schools, and public buildings in the United States, mainly for insulation.

Today in the United States, use of asbestos in new construction is limited. However, large amounts of asbestos remain in place in buildings, especially in schools, posing a hazard now and in the future. A major challenge to pediatricians, public health officials, and school authorities has been to develop a systematic and rational approach to dealing with asbestos in schools and other buildings in order to protect the health of children.

In 1980 (the last time that national statistics were compiled) the US Environmental Protection Agency (EPA) estimated that more than 8500 schools nationwide contained deteriorated asbestos, and that approximately 3 million students (and also more than 250 000 teachers, personnel, and others) were at risk of exposure.[1] Subsequent field studies have found that about 10% of the asbestos in schools is deteriorating and/or accessible to children and thus poses a threat to health. The remaining 90% is not deteriorating or accessible to children and therefore does not pose an immediate hazard.[2]

■ Routes of Exposure

Inhalation of microscopic airborne asbestos fibers is the major route of exposure. Asbestos becomes a health hazard when the fibers become airborne.[3] Asbestos that is tightly contained within building materials (such as in insulation or ceiling tiles) poses no immediate health hazard. However, when asbestos fibers are liberated into the air through deterioration or destruction of asbestos-containing materials, children and adults are at risk of inhaling these fibers into the pulmonary alveoli.

Gastrointestinal exposure to asbestos rarely occurs, usually in circumstances in which drinking water is transferred through deteriorating concrete-asbestos pipes. Asbestos fibers can also enter drinking water if the water passes through rock formations that naturally contain asbestiform fibers.

■ Systems Affected

The lung, throat, larynx, and gastrointestinal tract are affected.

■ Clinical Effects

Asbestos produces no acute toxicity. Employees who have been heavily exposed to asbestos in industry may develop fibrotic disease of the lungs and/or pleura termed *asbestosis*; in its earlier stages, asbestosis neither causes symptoms nor impairs lung function. Asbestosis is not seen in children because of their much lower levels of exposure.

The main risk of asbestos lies in its capacity to cause cancer in adults.[4] The two most important cancers caused by asbestos are

(1) lung cancer and (2) malignant mesothelioma, a rapidly growing malignancy that can arise from the pleura, the pericardium, and peritoneum. Asbestos can also cause cancer of the throat, larynx, and gastrointestinal tract in adults.

The relationship between asbestos and cancer was first recognized among employees exposed occupationally as miners, shipbuilders, and insulation workers. Thousands of cases of mesothelioma and lung cancer have occurred and cases resulting from past exposures will continue to develop into the 21st century. An estimated 300 000 US workers will eventually die of asbestos-related diseases.[5]

Lung Cancer

A strong synergistic interaction has been found between asbestos and cigarette smoking and lung cancer.[6] Adults who are exposed to asbestos, but who do not smoke, have five times the background rate of lung cancer. In contrast, adults who are exposed to asbestos and who also smoke have more than 50 times the background rate of lung cancer.[6] This powerful association is one more reason why children and adolescents should not smoke.

Mesothelioma

Malignant mesothelioma appears to arise solely as a result of exposure to asbestos. No interaction is known between asbestos and smoking in the causation of mesothelioma. This form of cancer is of greatest concern to children through exposure to asbestos in homes and schools. The disease can appear as long as 5 decades after exposure.

Dose-Response

The degree of cancer risk associated with asbestos is dose-related.[7] Any exposure to asbestos involves some risk of cancer; no safe threshold level of exposure has been established. For example, mesotheliomas have been observed in the spouses and children of asbestos workers who regularly brought home fibers on their work clothing. The risk associated with low levels of exposure or with brief encounters lasting a few days or weeks is, however, much less than from continuing exposure, such as in adults who have been exposed for many years in industry.

Some scientists and industry personnel have argued that the form of asbestos used most commonly in buildings in North America (Canadian chrysotile) is harmless. However, extensive clinical, epidemiologic, and toxicologic data have consistently documented its carcinogenicity in humans and all can cause lung cancer and mesothelioma. All forms of asbestos are hazardous and carcinogenic. Exposure to asbestos needs to be kept to a minimum.

∎ Diagnostic Methods

There is no method of detecting asbestos exposure other than the patient's history of exposure. Chest roentgenograms are not indicated for children exposed to asbestos. To determine whether children are at risk of asbestos exposure, an environmental inspection should be undertaken in schools and other buildings where children live, work, and play. Children may be at risk if the asbestos is deteriorating, if it is within reach, or if renovations are taking place.

∎ Treatment

Because asbestos produces no acute symptoms, there is no treatment for acute exposure. There is no known treatment to remove asbestos fibers from the lungs once they are inhaled. Discussion of the meaning of risk with patients and parents is very important (see Chapter 33).

∎ Prevention of Exposure

The most effective approach to prevention of exposure to asbestos is the use of alternative, less toxic materials. This approach is now followed almost universally in the United States, where use of asbestos in new construction is restricted.[10]

Prevention of exposure to asbestos in the home is most efficiently achieved by wrapping any small areas of fraying asbestos with duct tape. If more than minor repairs are needed or if asbestos is to be removed, a certified asbestos contractor should always be recruited. "Do-it-yourself" removal of asbestos is not recommended.

Prevention of asbestos exposure in schools is discussed more fully in Chapter 28.

∎ Frequently Asked Questions

Q *How will I know if there are asbestos materials in my house?*

A Asbestos is not found as commonly in private homes in the United States as it is in schools, apartment buildings, and public buildings. Nevertheless, asbestos is present in many homes, especially those built prior to the 1970s.

The following are locations in homes where asbestos may be found:

- insulation around pipes, stoves, and furnaces (the most common locations)
- insulation in walls and ceilings, especially as sprayed-on or troweled-on material
- patching and spackling compounds and textured paint
- roofing shingles and siding
- older appliances such as washers and dryers

To determine if your home contains asbestos, you can take the following steps:

- To evaluate appliances and other consumer products, examine the label or the invoices to obtain the product name, model number, and year of manufacture. If this information is available, the manufacturer can supply information about asbestos content.

- To evaluate building materials, a professional Asbestos Manager with qualifications similar to those of managers employed in school districts may be hired. This person can inspect your home to determine whether asbestos is present and to give advice on its proper management.

- State and local health departments as well as regional offices of the EPA have lists of individuals and laboratories certified to analyze a home for asbestos.

Q *If there is asbestos in my home, what should I do?*

A If asbestos-containing materials are found in your home, the same options exist for dealing with these materials as in the schools. In most cases, asbestos-containing materials in a home are best left alone. If materials such as insulation, tiling, and flooring are in good condition, there is no need to worry. However, if materials containing asbestos are deteriorating, or if you are planning renovations and the materials will be disturbed, it is best to find out if they contain asbestos and, if necessary, to have them properly removed. Improper removal of asbestos may cause serious contamination by dispersing fibers throughout the area. Any asbestos removal in a home should be performed only by properly accredited and certified contractors. Information on certified contractors in your area may be obtained from state or local health departments or from the regional office of the EPA. Many contractors who advertise as asbestos experts have not been trained properly. Only contractors who have been certified by the EPA or by a state-approved training school should be hired. The contractor should be able to provide written proof of up-to-date certification.

Children should not be permitted to play in areas where there are friable asbestos-containing materials.

To obtain additional information about asbestos in the home, you can write for the booklet "Asbestos in Your Home," which can be obtained from the EPA Public Information Center, 401 M Street SW, Washington, DC 20460. State or local health departments will have additional information about asbestos (see the Resources section).

Q Is *there asbestos in hair dryers?*
A In the past, asbestos was used in electrical appliances, including hair dryers. However, hair dryers containing asbestos were recalled by the Consumer Product Safety Commission more than a decade ago, and currently manufacturers of household appliances in the United States are not allowed to utilize asbestos. If your hair dryer is more than 10 years old, it should be discarded. Hair dryers should not be opened and inspected.

Q *My spouse works with asbestos. Is there danger to my child?*
A Any family member who works in an occupation potentially involving contact with asbestos (or similar fibers such as fiberglass or reactive ceramic fibers) is at risk of bringing asbestos or similar fibers home on clothing, shoes, hair, and skin and in the car. These fibers can contaminate your home and become a source of exposure to children.

Studies conducted in the homes of asbestos workers have shown that the dust in these homes can be heavily contaminated by asbestos fibers.[11] Mesothelioma, lung cancer, and asbestosis have all been observed in the family members of asbestos workers. In many cases, these diseases have occurred years or even decades after the exposure.

Prevention of household exposure is essential in this situation. Persons who work with asbestos must scrupulously shower, change clothing, and change shoes before getting into a car and returning home. These procedures are mandated by federal Occupational Safety and Health Administration law, but are often not enforced. Also, employees are often not aware of their exposure. Exposure is prevented only if employees leave their contaminated shoes and clothing at the workplace.

Many jobs involve potential occupational exposure to asbestos. These include:
• asbestos mining and milling
• asbestos product manufacture
• construction trades, including sheet metal work, carpentry, plumbing, insulation work, air-conditioning, rewiring, cable installation, spackling, and drywall work
• demolition work
• shipyard work
• asbestos removal
• fire fighting
• custodial and janitorial work

▮ Resources

The principal resource for information on asbestos in buildings is in the ten Regional Offices of the US EPA. Each office has an Asbestos Coordinator. Regional offices are located in Boston, New York City, Philadelphia, Atlanta, Chicago, Dallas, Kansas City, Denver, San Francisco, and Seattle.

Another important resource is the US Public Health Service Agency for Toxic Substances and Disease Registry (ATSDR) in Atlanta at 404/639-6000; fax 404/639-6315.

The EPA National Asbestos Information Line is 800/368-5888.

State and local health departments also can provide information on asbestos.

EPA Regional Asbestos Coordinators

For information on asbestos identification, health effects, abatement options, analytic techniques, asbestos in schools, and contract documents.

Region 1 (CT, ME, MA, NH, RI, VT)
Regional Asbestos Coordinator
USEPA
JFK Federal Building
1 Congress St; Suite 1100
Boston, MA 02204
617/918-1505

Region 2 (NY, NJ, PR, VI)
Regional Asbestos Coordinator
USEPA
290 Broadway, 21st Fl
New York, NY 10007
212/637-4042

Region 3 (DE, DC, MD, PA, VA, WV)
Regional Asbestos Coordinator
USEPA
1650 Arch St.
Philadelphia, PA 19103
215/814-5797

Region 4 (AL, FL, GA, KY, MS, NC, SC, TN)
Regional Asbestos Coordinator
USEPA
61 Forsyth St, SW
Atlanta, GA 30303
404/562-8977

Region 5 (IL, IN, MI, MN, OH, WI)
Regional Asbestos Coordinator
USEPA
77 W Jackson St
Chicago, IL 60604
312/353-9062

Region 6 (AR, LA, NM, OK, TX)
Regional Asbestos Coordinator
USEPA
1445 Ross Ave
Dallas, TX 75202-2733
214/665-2295

Region 7 (IA, KS, MO, NE)
Regional Asbestos Coordinator
USEPA
726 Minnesota Ave
Kansas City, KS 66101
913/551-7602

Region 8 (CO, MT, ND, SD, UT, WY)
Regional Asbestos Coordinator
USEPA
999 18th St, Suite 500
Denver, CO 80202-2466
303/312-6021

Region 9 (AZ, CA, HI, NV, AS, GU)
Regional Asbestos Coordinator
USEPA
75 Hawthorne St
San Francisco, CA 94105
415/744-1122

Region 10 (AK, ID, OR, WA)
Regional Asbestos Coordinator
USEPA
1200 Sixth Ave
Seattle, WA 98101
206/553-4762

∎ References

1. American Academy of Pediatrics, Committee on Environmental Hazards. Asbestos exposure in schools. *Pediatrics.* 1987;79:301-305

2. US Environmental Protection Agency. Asbestos-containing materials in schools: final rule and notice. *Federal Register.* 1987;52:41826-41903

3. American Academy of Pediatrics, Committee on Injury and Poison Prevention. *Handbook of Common Poisonings in Children.* 3rd ed. Elk Grove Village, Ill: American Academy of Pediatrics; 1994

4. Selikoff IJ, Churg J, Hammond EC. Asbestos exposure and neoplasia. *JAMA.* 1964;188:22-26

5. Nicholson WJ, Perkel G, Selikoff IJ. Occupational exposure to asbestos: population at risk and projected mortality—1980-2030. *Am J Ind Med.* 1982;3:259-311

6. Selikoff IJ, Hammond EC, Churg J. Asbestos exposure, smoking and neoplasia. *JAMA.* 1968;204:106-112

7. *Toxicological Profile on Asbestos.* Atlanta, Ga: US Dept of Health and Human Services, Public Health Service, Agency for Toxic Substances and Disease Registry; August 1995

8. IARC monographs on the evaluation of carcinogenic risks to humans. Lyon, France: International Agency for Research on Cancer; 1987;suppl 7:106-116

9. Landrigan PJ. Asbestos—still a carcinogen. *N Engl J Med.* 1998;338:1618-1619

10. Needleman HL, Landrigan PJ. Asbestos. In: *Raising Children Toxic Free: How to Keep Your Child Safe From Lead, Asbestos, Pesticides, and Other Environmental Hazards.* New York, NY: Farrar, Straus and Giroux; 1994

11. Chisolm JJ. Fouling one's own nest. *Pediatrics.* 1978;62:614-617

6 | Environmental Precipitants of Asthma

A sthma is characterized by intermittent reversible airway obstruction, occurring as a result of chronic airway inflammation and hyperresponsiveness to a variety of stimuli. The precise pathogenic mechanisms for both the bronchospastic and inflammatory components that characterize asthma remain poorly understood. A variety of environmental exposures have been linked to increased risk of developing asthma and/or the exacerbation of asthma.[1] Since children living in temperate climates spend an estimated 90% of their time indoors, that environment may play an important role.

Major indoor triggers of asthma include environmental tobacco smoke (ETS); irritants such as commercial products (paints, cleaning agents, pesticides, perfumes); components of building structures (sealants, plastics, adhesives, insulation materials); animal and insect allergens (such as dander and cockroach antigen); and molds (Table 6.1). Although most agents that exacerbate asthma in children are inhaled, asthma may be exacerbated in some atopic individuals who touch (eg, latex) or ingest (eg, peanuts) certain products.

Outdoor air pollution has also been associated with asthma exacerbations. Motor vehicle emissions contribute significantly to nitrogen oxides, hydrocarbons, diesel particles, and other airborne particulate matter. Health effects from these sources are discussed in Chapter 19.

Table 6.1. Indoor and Outdoor Agents Precipitating Asthma

Agent	Major Sources
Indoor	
Allergens	
Dust mite	Carpeting, mattresses, bed linens, toys, feathers
Animal allergens (dander, saliva, urine)	Cats, dogs, rodents
Cockroaches	Kitchens, bathrooms (moisture, organic materials)
Environmental tobacco smoke	Cigarettes, cigars, other tobacco products
Molds	Air conditioning units, plumbing leaks, floods, damp basements
Nitrogen Oxides	Space heaters, gas-fueled cooking stoves
Odors	Sprays, deodorizers, pesticides
Volatile organic compounds	Pesticides, sealants, adhesives, insulation materials, combustion products, molds
Outdoor	
Ozone (O_3)	Hydrocarbon combustion (motor vehicles, power plants)
Sulfur dioxide (SO_2)	Fossil fuels (power plants), industrial sources

■ Indoor Environmental Precipitants

Environmental Tobacco Smoke

Forty-three percent of children in the United States live with at least one smoking parent.[2] Children whose mothers smoke have more wheezing symptoms and a higher incidence of lower respiratory tract illnesses.[3] The greatest effect seems to be related to maternal smoking during pregnancy and/or early infancy,[4] perhaps due to inflammatory stimuli on lung parenchyma during a period of rapid lung development and prolonged close exposure to the mother. Exposure to ETS is associated with an increase in asthma attacks, earlier symptom onset, increased medication use, and a more prolonged recovery from acute attacks.[5,6] Maternal smoking of half a pack or more per day has been associated with a 2.5-fold increase in asthma in children prior to age 12 years.[7] Acute short-term ETS exposure has been demonstrated to increase bronchial hyperreactivity, with baseline pulmonary function returning to normal 3 weeks following the exposure.[8,9]

Other Indoor Irritants

In the modern home, natural gas-fueled home appliances, including furnaces, cooking stoves, clothes dryers, and water heaters, are the most common potential sources of pollution. However, if these appliances are properly vented and used, they seldom cause adverse health effects. Other major sources of indoor pollution include wood fireplaces and gas space heaters. Nitrogen dioxide (NO_2) is generated by improperly or unvented gas-fueled cooking stoves and space heaters. Average NO_2 levels in the majority of enclosed ice rinks greatly exceed the National Ambient Air Quality Standards (recommended by the US Environmental Protection Agency) due to the exhaust of diesel- and propane-fueled ice resurfacing machines. Such levels have been associated with respiratory symptoms. Although NO_2 concentrations found in most homes and workplaces are unlikely to reach toxic levels, higher exposures may be experienced by individuals living in deteriorating homes with poor or no ventilation for cooking stoves or ancillary heat sources.

Wood smoke is a complex mixture of particulates and a number of pollutants, including NO_2, and organic compounds. Fireplaces and woodburning stoves are the primary sources, with great variability between emissions from airtight and nonairtight stoves. Measurement of indoor concentrations of total and respirable suspended particles reveals several-fold increases when woodburning stoves are used.

Numerous strong-smelling agents may induce acute asthma episodes in susceptible individuals. Perfumes, paint, cosmetic sprays (hair spray, deodorant), pesticides, and scented cleaning solutions have been reported to precipitate an acute asthma attack.[10] The mechanism of action is unknown, but presumed to be nonspecific irritation. Because it is difficult to identify high-risk children, exposure to these agents should be minimized in the homes of children with asthma. Use of nonaerosol, unscented cleaners and cosmetics should be encouraged.

Allergenic Precipitants

Animal Allergens

Animal allergens are acidic glycoproteins with molecular weights of 15 000 to 30 000 kD. They are in highest concentrations on the skin of the animal and in secretions, including saliva, sebaceous glands, and urine. The allergen-containing secretions dry on fur, bedding, and other household objects (including clothing) and become airborne, easily remaining in the air because they are so lightweight. Therefore animal allergens are often found in homes that have never had pets; once inhaled they are easily deposited in distal airways. Clinical manifestations of animal allergy range from mild cutaneous urticaria to rhinoconjunctivitis to life-threatening bronchospasm and anaphylaxis. Although symptoms may occur instantly following exposure, it is more common for upper and lower respiratory tract symptoms to develop within 30 minutes. Low-level chronic exposures may not trigger clinically significant symptoms for several days.

Cats. The severity of allergic reactions to cats is stronger than those to other common domestic pets and is about twice as common as reactions to dogs. Over 6 million US residents have allergies to cats and up to 40% of atopic patients demonstrated skin test sensitivity.[11] The major allergen, *Fel d I*, is present in high concentration in skin, with saliva, sebaceous glands, and urine containing lesser amounts. The grooming habits of cats result in a large amount of saliva on the fur. *Fel d I* remains airborne for prolonged periods and adheres to clothing and other objects. These characteristics frequently allow antigen to be transmitted between environments, resulting in clinically relevant levels even in households without pets. Once a cat is removed from an indoor environment, the allergen may persist for months, unless vigorous efforts are made to remove the antigen.

Dogs. Dogs are the most common domesticated animal species found in US homes. Five percent to 30% of atopic patients have a positive skin test to the major allergen, *Can f I*, although many do not demonstrate clinical symptoms or have positive bronchoprovocation tests.[12] It seems that more variations in clinical sensitivity exist between dog breeds, and breed-specific allergens have been suggested.[13] Nevertheless, no dog breed is considered nonallergenic. As with cat allergen, the highest concentrations of *Can f I* are found in canine fur and dander.[14]

Other domestic animal species. Various species of rodents are kept as domestic pets, although most literature about allergy to these animals is derived from evaluation of occupational settings. High domestic levels of mouse and rat antigen have been reported in some central urban residences. Rodent allergy affects 10% to 15% of exposed laboratory workers. The two primary rat allergens, *Rat n Ia* and *IB*, are mainly found in urine, with the highest levels produced by sexually mature males. Mouse antigen *Mus m I* is primarily found in urine.

Birds. Allergic symptoms have long been associated with exposure to bird feathers. Although data demonstrating specific feather allergens are sparse, large quantities of dust mites have been documented in feathers, and mite allergen is the likely source of the allergic stimulus from feather-containing items in the home, including pillows, comforters, bedding, and down-filled clothes. Immunologic responses in poultry industry employees or bird fanciers are not IgE-mediated and are often represented by hypersensitivity pneumonitis rather than immediate-type hypersensitivity reactions; however, concomitant immediate hypersensitivity reactions in these populations occur at a higher rate than those in the general population.

Cockroaches

The incidence of cockroach hypersensitivity is related to the degree of infestation found in the living environment, although nonresidential exposures may cause allergy in an individual whose residence is not infested. Cockroach allergen can be found in numerous areas of infested houses, with the highest accumulation in the kitchen, where allergen levels are up to 54-fold higher than levels found in bedrooms or on upholstered furniture. Numerous species of cockroaches have been described in the United States, and three predominant species have been associated with IgE-antibody production. The German roach, *Blattella germanica*, is the source of two primary antigens, *Bla g 1* and *Bla g 2*; however, significant cross-reactivity exists between cockroach antigens. Roach allergens have been described as principal triggers of allergic rhinitis and asthma. Positive skin tests to cockroach antigen can be found in up to 60% of urban residents with asthma. Although several parts of the cockroach are allergenic, the whole body and feces seem to be more potent. Inner-city asthmatic children with cockroach allergy and exposure to elevated allergen levels in the home had more days wheezing, more missed school days, and more emergency department visits and hospitalizations than nonsensitized and/or nonexposed asthmatic children. In this inner-city population, cockroach allergen was more important when compared with dust mite and cat allergens.[15] Hospitalization rates for children who were sensitized and exposed to excessive levels of cockroach allergen were nearly three times as high as for those with low exposure and sensitivity.

Cockroach infestations are more common in warm, moist environments with readily accessible food sources. Although the highest allergen levels are typically found in the kitchen, significantly elevated concentrations of roach allergen are also found in bedrooms or television-watching areas, particularly if food is consumed in these places.

House-Dust Mites (*Dermatophagoides*)
House-dust mites probably play a major role in inducing the asthmatic phenotype and triggering asthma exacerbations in sensitized children. Mite antigen is commonly found where human dander is found, and the principal allergen—*Der p1*—is found in the outer membrane of mite fecal particles. Indoor environments that provide optimal growth conditions for *Dermatophagoides* species have high relative humidity (up to 80%) and temperatures (25°C). Mites proliferate on mattress surfaces, carpeting, and upholstered furniture, each of which also contains a large amount of human dander, its primary food source. A gram of dust may contain 1000 mites and 250 000 fecal pellets. Pellet diameters range from 10 to 40 μm and therefore are not easily transported into the lower airway passages. Exposure occurs either by proximity of the nasopharyngeal mucosa to mite reservoirs (especially mattresses, pillows, carpets, bed linens, clothes, and soft toys) or to airborne antigen during housecleaning activities.

Mold Allergens
Molds are most prominent in climates with increased ambient humidity, although some can grow in relatively dry areas. For instance, *Alternaria* spp is a common indoor mold in the arid climate of Arizona. Other species of common indoor mold—including *Aspergillus*, *Penicillium*, and *Cladosporium*—also require sufficient moisture for growth, and household areas with high humidity (eg, basements, crawlspaces, ground floors, bathrooms, and areas with standing water such as air conditioner condensers) are where mold growth is most commonly found. Carpeting, ceilings, and paneled or

hollow walls are also common reservoirs. Epidemiologic studies have suggested an association between damp, moldy homes and asthma symptoms.[16]

Miscellaneous Allergens

Latex. Latex may cause an allergic response either by direct contact or by inhalation of latex particles. The more widespread use of latex gloves and revised processing procedures making the allergen more potent may have contributed to the increase in reported cases. Most sensitivities occur in medical personnel, food service workers, or environmental service workers, although household exposures to balloons, gloves, condoms, and certain sporting equipment may also trigger allergic responses. Symptoms range from cutaneous eruption, sneezing, and bronchospasm to anaphylaxis. More than 110 reactions have been reported in the past 5 years, of which 15 were fatal.[17] Certain subgroups are at increased risk of developing latex allergy, including children with urogenital abnormalities, cerebral palsy, and preterm infants. Up to one third of children with spina bifida have been reported to have positive skin tests to latex, possibly related to repeated exposure.

Food. Many foods contain allergenic proteins that can trigger asthma, anaphylaxis, or anaphylactoid reactions in sensitized individuals. Nuts, fish, shellfish, and milk are the most common associated foods. Although oral ingestion is typically needed to elicit symptoms, contact with aerosolized particulates and oils that contain the offending antigens can induce symptoms in highly allergic individuals. Food additives, including sulfites and food coloring (especially tartrazine), can also be highly allergenic.

∎ Outdoor Environmental Precipitants

Ozone

Ozone (O_3) is generated by photochemical reactions of ultraviolet light with nitrogen oxides and volatile organic compounds from hydrocarbon combustion, especially from automobiles, power plants, and natural sources such as trees. Warm season ambient O_3 concentrations exceeding the National Ambient Air Quality Standards occur in many urban and rural areas of the United States, with highest levels often being reached in suburban regions of major metropolitan areas. Levels typically rise in mid-morning and peak in late afternoon.

Studies of hospitalization and acute visit rates suggest that children with asthma may be adversely affected by O_3 exposure.[18] However, studies of single short-term exposures have not conclusively demonstrated greater lung function decrements than those experienced by children without asthma.[19-21] Because children with asthma and those with other obstructive pulmonary diseases may start at lower baseline pulmonary function, the clinical effect of O_3 exposure may be significant. The role of exposure to chronically elevated ambient O_3 concentrations in the development of irreversible lung damage is still unclear.

Sulfur Dioxide
Sulfur dioxide (SO_2) is highly soluble in water and thus hydration occurs in the mucous layer of the respiratory epithelium. Outdoor SO_2 concentrations of up to 1.0 ppm have not been demonstrated to alter lung mechanics in healthy persons, while persons with asthma experience an early response at concentrations greater than or equal to 0.25 ppm.

Outdoor Allergens
Outdoor air contains a variety of allergens, most of which arise from plant pollen, and mold spores. Seasonal exposures to high concentrations of tree, grass, and ragweed pollens that occur in the spring and late summer, respectively, can induce respiratory symptoms, such as sneezing, rhinitis, and bronchospasm in sensitized children. Spores from mold, such as *Alternaria* and *Aspergillus*, are commonly found in damp, wooded areas, including the wood chips often used as ground cover in playgrounds. These allergens can also cause acute and recurrent asthma exacerbations.[22] Exposure to outdoor fungal spores has been implicated in fatal exacerbations of asthma.[23,24]

■ Diagnosis

The diagnosis of asthma is suggested by a clinical history of wheezing and/or cough that is episodic, nocturnal or exertional, and occurs apart from acute respiratory infections.[25] Atopy, as well as a family history of asthma and/or atopy, is strongly correlated as a predictor of persistent asthma. Pulmonary function testing in children younger than 5 years is seldom reproducible, and response to a therapeutic trial of bronchodilator or anti-inflammatory medications is frequently helpful in confirming the diagnosis. Chest roentgenography helps determine the presence of peribronchial thickening and hyperinflation, which may help determine chronicity of illness and also help rule out other diagnostic possibilities such as congenital anomaly or foreign body. Baseline pulmonary function testing may demonstrate a decreased forced expiratory volume in 1 second (FEV_1) or forced expiratory flow, midexpiratory phase compared with predicted norms, although prebronchodilator and postbronchodilator spirometry (>15% FEV_1 improvement) or methacholine, exercise, or cold air bronchoprovocation (≥20% FEV_1 decrease) may be of more help in diagnosing the patient with mild symptoms. Daily or diurnal variability in peak flow measurements may also be of help.

Determination of the degree of atopy is also helpful in diagnosing asthma. Elevation of the peripheral blood eosinophil count and serum IgE levels and skin prick test responses to inhaled antigens or specific foods may help confirm suspected triggers. The radioallergosorbent test (RAST) is generally less sensitive than skin prick tests, although it may be more readily available and easily tolerated (but more expensive) when screening a patient for numerous potential sensitivities.

∎ Treatment Goals

Goals of asthma therapy include preventing chronic and troublesome symptoms, maintaining normal pulmonary function, maintaining normal activity levels, preventing recurrent exacerbations, and minimizing emergency department visits and hospitalizations. Medications are categorized into the following two general classes: (1) long-term preventive medications that achieve and maintain control of persistent asthma, and (2) quick-relief medications that treat acute symptoms and exacerbations. The "step care" approach to asthma therapy emphasizes initiating higher level therapy at the onset of treatment in order to control symptoms, and then "stepping down" the use of quick-relief medications followed by control medications. Preventive medications include inhaled corticosteroids and non-steroid medications, such as leukotriene receptor antagonists.

Relief medications are largely inhaled rapid-acting β-adrenergic agonists.

▌ Control Measures for Allergens and Irritants

Environmental Tobacco Smoke

Smoking has been banned in many public places. Pediatricians' efforts should be to help parents eliminate sources of smoke in the child's environment.

Indoor Allergens

Animal Allergens

The preferred treatment for animal allergy is to avoid animals that provoke reaction. This may not be possible in all situations, particularly if the pet owner is unwilling to remove the pet from the home. Control of the major cat allergen, *Fel d I*, is often complicated because of its properties. Unlike dust mite allergen, *Fel d I* remains suspended in the air for hours indoors, saturating carpeting, clothing, upholstery, and walls. Even if the cat is removed from the home, it may take more than 3 months to reduce the levels of allergen. Aggressive cleaning (eg, removing carpets and washing of walls and furniture) may accelerate the process. If the cat cannot be removed from the home, allergen abatement methods include removing carpeting, using high-efficiency filter (HEPA) vacuuming and filters, regular damp mopping, and weekly cat bathing. These methods have experimentally been found to reduce airborne cat allergen levels by about 90%. HEPA filters are effective for cat allergen only when used in conjunction with the other measures, however.

Dog allergens provoke significant bronchial hyperresponsiveness in persons less often than do cat allergens. The decrease in response may be due to antigens that vary between breed and source (dander, hair, saliva, and serum extracts), and because more dogs reside outside and better tolerate regular bathing. This allergen may be controlled by avoiding dogs, but the other methods used for minimizing cat allergen should also be employed.

Levels of airborne rodent urinary allergens have been reduced in most laboratory environments by regulations that mandate rapid room air exchanges and high-efficiency filters. No such controls exist for populations exposed by infestations in housing. Even after successful rodent extermination, indoor rodent allergen may persist for months at levels that trigger clinical symptoms, particularly when vigorous cleaning measures are not followed.

Dust Mites

Eliminating mite exposure reduces symptoms and the degree of nonspecific bronchial hyperreactivity.[26] Lowering humidity below 50% can result in a tenfold reduction in mite numbers and allergen burden.[27] Continuous air conditioning is effective during summer months when the mite population peaks in temperate climates. Enclosing mattresses and pillows in plastic or zippered vinyl-lined covers also greatly reduces mite exposure.[28] Where possible, bed linens should be washed in hot water (>130°F, 55°C) weekly. This is higher than the temperature of 120°F recommended by the American Academy of Pediatrics; significant skin burns can be sustained within seconds of exposure to water at this temperature. However, washing at cooler temperatures does not kill or remove mites.[29] Ideally, when children are at school, water temperature should be elevated during linen washing and can be returned to a lower temperature once laundering is complete.

Carpeting, a major source of mite antigen and proliferation, should be removed. A single vacuuming may decrease mite burden by only 35% for a carpeted surface but by 80% for a solid surface. Acaricides (chemicals which kill mites) containing benzyl benzoate or tannic acid used every 3 months on carpeting and upholstery may reduce antigen levels. Using acaricides is far less effective than removing carpet followed by regular damp mopping of hardwood or vinyl flooring. Information about acaricides can be obtained from the state EPA. Upholstered furniture should be replaced with washable vinyl, leather, or wood. Window shades are preferable to curtains or venetian blinds. If curtains are used, they should be made of washable fabric. Blinds should be made of vinyl.

Cockroaches

Cockroaches may be found wherever water, heat, and organic material are present.[30] It is essential to minimize organic material on open surfaces to reduce infestation. Other measures are storing all foodstuffs in sealed containers, eliminating water sources, eating only in the kitchen, caulking all cracks around faucets and pipe fittings, and placing roach "stick traps" in kitchens and bathrooms. Boric acid can be used in areas that are not accessible to children. If primary avoidance measures, stick traps, and boric acid are ineffective in controlling cockroach infestation, a professional exterminator should be consulted. Families should avoid using over-the-counter "bug sprays" because they may cause toxic reactions.

Molds

Dehumidifiers can be considered for areas with consistently elevated humidity levels, with a target humidity range of less than 50%. Dehumidifiers reduce ambient humidity, but do not significantly reduce growth on surfaces in contact with ground water. Mold growth on wet surfaces may be controlled by treatment with a bleach solution (add 1 part bleach to 4 parts water). To effectively control further growth on these surfaces, the water source must be eliminated. Eliminating indoor organic sources, such as plants, wood, or paper products, also helps to control the growth of mold. Less obvious sources of water include damage due to prior flooding or rainwater and condensation on pipes and ductwork within interior or exterior structure walls.

Outdoor Sources of Allergens

It is important to identify seasonal allergens that trigger a patient's asthma. This will allow the practitioner to initiate prophylactic antihistamine or anti-inflammatory therapies and/or to recommend the use of air conditioning, if available. Staying indoors during the afternoon hours may help symptoms. Outdoor molds, especially *Alternaria,* may be present in moderate climates, but are greatly reduced following the onset of frost or recurrent freezing temperatures. Affected individuals should be instructed to follow pollution alerts for high pollen counts, especially during summer months.

▮ Frequently Asked Questions

Q *Do you recommend any special air filtration system for patients with asthma?*

A Avoid room humidifiers, and keep central furnace system humidification below 45% to 50% during winter months. Electrostatic filters/precipitators are beneficial for central furnace and air conditioning systems. Room HEPA filters are also of benefit, but only work in a single room. Preferably, they should be used in the child's bedroom, but are of little benefit in reducing exposure to environmental tobacco smoke. Avoid the use of air cleaners that generate ozone.

Q *How can we better prepare the house to prevent asthma attacks from occurring?*

A Eliminate all sources of ETS. Reduce or eliminate dust mites, cockroaches, and molds. Remove pets to which the child demonstrates specific allergy. If removal of the pet is not possible, routinely perform allergen reduction measures. Consider the use of a vacuum cleaner equipped with an HEPA filter.

Q *Can odors of cooking foods cause an allergic reaction (eg, asthma) in susceptible patients?*

A Although rare, odors from foods may cause reactions in some patients. For example, a patient with known anaphylactic/anaphylactoid response to peanuts may react to aerosolized peanut oil used for cooking. The presence of a positive skin-prick test or RAST or an elevated IgE level to a given food should not necessarily lead to an elimination diet, however, because only one third of individuals have an asthmatic response when challenged orally with the specific food.

Q *Should I use a humidifier?*

A Humidifiers should be avoided, if possible. If used, the humidifier must be cleaned frequently to prevent growth of mold.

Q *Are foam pillows safe to use in children or can they also be allergenic?*

A Foam pillows are generally hypoallergenic, although occasionally they may produce allergic responses. Polyester pillows are preferred over those made with animal down or foam.

Q *What can be done when a family lives in a multi-unit building where there are barriers to asthma control due to pest infestation and cigarette smoking in common areas?*

A If families share concerns about issues such as pest control and cigarette smoking, they may want to organize as a group to alert management to their concerns for their children's health.

■ Resources

American Lung Association 800/LUNG-USA
Asthma and Allergy Foundation of America 202/466-7643
Centers for Disease Control and Prevention 770/488-7320
National Institutes of Health 301/594-7430
Mothers of Asthmatics, Inc 800/878-4403

■ References

1. Becklake MR, Ernst P. Environmental factors. *Lancet.* 1997;350(suppl II):10-13

2. Pirkle JL, Flegal KM, Bernert JT, Brody DJ, Etzel RA, Maurer KR. Exposure of the US population to environmental tobacco smoke: the Third National Health and Nutrition Examination Survey, 1988 to 1991. *JAMA.* 1996;275:1233-1240

3. Erlich RI, Du Toit D, Jordaan E, et al. Risk factors for childhood asthma and wheezing: importance of maternal and household smoking. *Am J Respir Crit Care Med.* 1996;154:681-688

4. Martinez FD, Cline M, Burrows B. Increased incidence of asthma in children of smoking mothers. *Pediatrics.* 1992;89:21-26

5. Weitzman M, Gortmaker S, Walker DK, Sobol A. Maternal smoking and childhood asthma. *Pediatrics.* 1990;85:505-511

6. Abulhosn RS, Moray BH, Llewellyn CE, Reading GJ. Passive smoke exposure impairs recovery after hospitalization for acute asthma. *Arch Pediatr Adolesc Med.* 1997;151:135-139

7. Sherrill DL, Martinez FD, Lebowitz MD, et al. Longitudinal effects of passive smoking on pulmonary function in New Zealand children. *Am Rev Respir Dis.* 1992;145:1136-1141

8. Menon P, Rando RJ, Stankus RP, Salvaggio JE, Lehrer SB. Passive cigarette smoke challenge studies: increase in bronchial hyperreactivity. *J Allergy Clin Immunol.* 1992;89:560-566

9. Committee of the Environmental and Occupational Health Assembly of the American Thoracic Society. Health effects of outdoor air pollution. *Am J Respir Crit Care Med.* 1996;153:3-50

10. Shim C, Williams MH Jr. Effect of odors in asthma. *Am J Med.* 1986;80:18-22

11. Wood RA, Eggleston PA. Management of allergy to animal danders. *Pediatr Asthma, Allergy Immunol.* 1993;7:13-22

12. Luczynska CM, Li Y, Chapman MD, Platts-Mills TA. Airborne concentrations and particle size distribution of allergen derived from domestic cats (*Felis*

domesticus): measurements using cascade impactor, liquid impinger, and a two-site monoclonal antibody assay for *Fel d I. Am Rev Respir Dis.* 1990;141:361-367

13. deGroot H, Goei KG, van Sweiten P, Aalberse RC. Affinity purification of a major and minor allergen from dog extract: serologic activity of affinity-purified *Can f I* and *Can f I*-depleted extract. *J Allergy Clin Immunol.* 1991;87: 1056-1065

14. Lindgren S, Belin L, Dreborg S. Breed-specific dog-dandruff allergens. *J Allergy Clin Immunol.* 1988;82:196-204

15. Rosenstreich DL, Eggleston P, Kattan M, et al. The role of cockroach allergy and exposure to cockroach allergen in causing morbidity among inner-city children with asthma. *N Engl J Med.* 1997;336:1356-1363

16. Strachan DP, Flannigan B, McCabe EM, McGarry F. Quantification of airborne moulds in the homes of children with and without wheeze. *Thorax.* 1990;45:382-287

17. Landwehr LP, Boguniewicz M. Current perspectives on latex allergy. *J Pediatr.* 1996;128:305-312

18. White MC, Etzel RA, Wilcox WD, Lloyd C. Exacerbations of childhood asthma and ozone pollution in Atlanta. *Environ Res.* 1994;65:56-68

19. Avol EL, Linn WS, Shamoo DA, et al. Respiratory effects of photochemical oxidant air pollution in exercising adolescents. *Am Rev Respir Dis.* 1985;132: 619-622

20. Avol EL, Linn WS, Shamoo DA, et al. Short-term respiratory effects of photochemical oxidant exposure in exercising children. *JAPCA.* 1987;37:158-162

21. Spektor DM, Thurston GD, Mao J. He D, Hayes C, Lippmann M. Effects of single- and multiday ozone exposures on respiratory function in active normal children. *Environ Res.* 1991;55:107-122

22. Licorish K, Novey HS, Kozak P, Fairshter RD, Wilson AF. Role of *Alternaria* and *Penicillium* spores in the pathogenesis of asthma. *J Allergy Clin Immunol.* 1985;76:819-825

23. O'Hollaren MT, Yunginger JW, Offord KP, et al. Exposure to an aeroallergen as a possible precipitating factor in respiratory arrest in young patients with asthma. *N Engl J Med.* 1991;324:359-363

24. Targonski PV, Persky VW, Ramekrishnan V. Effect of environmental molds on risk of death from asthma during the pollen season. *J Allergy Clin Immunol.* 1995;95:955-961

25. National Institutes of Health. *Highlights of the Expert Panel Report 2: Guidelines for the Diagnosis and Management of Asthma; 1997.* Bethesda, MD: National Heart, Lung, and Blood Institute. Publication NIH 97-4051A

26. Von Mutius E. Towards prevention. *Lancet.* 1997;350(suppl II):14-17

27. Lintner TJ, Brame KA. The effects of season, climate, and air-conditioning on the prevalence of *Dermatophagoides* mite allergens in house dust. *J Allergy Clin Immunol.* 1993;91(4):862-867

28. Etzel RA. Indoor air pollution and childhood asthma: effective environmental interventions. *Environ Health Perspect.* 1995;103(suppl):55-58

29. Katzman GH. Scalding, dust mites and lice, and your washing machine. *Pediatrics.* 1998;101:1094

30. Call RS, Smith TF, Morris E. Chapman MD, Platts-Mills TA. Risk factors for asthma in inner city children. *J Pediatr.* 1992;121:862-866

7 Carbon Monoxide

C arbon monoxide (CO) is a colorless, odorless, tasteless toxic gas that is a product of the incomplete combustion of carbon-based fuels. Carbon monoxide has a vapor density slightly less than that of air. The health effects from CO exposure range from nonspecific flu-like symptoms such as headache, weakness, dizziness, nausea, and vomiting to coma and death from prolonged or intense exposure. Carbon monoxide accounts for the most poisoning deaths attributed to a single agent in the United States.[1] Unintentional CO poisonings account for hundreds of deaths annually. Death rates from fire-related CO intoxication are higher for children younger than 15 years and for the elderly than for other age groups.[1] In a study of 3034 poisoning deaths among 10- to 19-year-olds, 38.2% were due to CO inhalation, of which 65.1% were categorized as suicide and 34.9% as unintentional. Motor vehicle exhaust accounted for 84.4% of the CO-related suicides and 65.6% of the unintentional fatal CO poisonings.[2] The prevalence of unintentional nonfatal CO poisonings is difficult to estimate because early symptoms of intoxication are often nonspecific.[3-5]

■ Routes of Exposure

Unintentional exposure to CO can be largely attributed to smoke inhalation from fires, motor vehicle exhaust, faulty or improperly vented combustion appliances, and tobacco smoke. Confined, poorly ventilated spaces such as garages, campers, tents, and boats are also susceptible to elevated levels of CO.[6] Common sources of CO exposure are listed in Table 7.1. Exposure to CO may occur in and around automobiles when there is inadequate combustion resulting from substandard vehicle maintenance and poor ventilation. Exposure may also occur when gasoline-powered equipment such as generators, lawn mowers, snow blowers, leaf blowers, and ice rink resurfacing machines are used in poorly ventilated spaces.[1,6,7]

Table 7.1. Sources of Carbon Monoxide

Motor vehicle exhaust

Unvented kerosene and propane gas space heaters

Leaking chimneys and furnaces

Backdrafting from furnaces

Wood stoves and fireplaces

Charcoal grills

Gas appliances: stoves, dryers, water heaters

Gasoline powered generators

Gasoline powered equipment: ice rink resurfacers, lawnmowers, leaf blowers, floor polishers, snowblowers, pressure washers

Tobacco smoke

■ Systems Affected

Carbon monoxide is inhaled, diffuses across the alveolar-capillary membrane, and is measurable in the bloodstream as carboxyhemoglobin (COHb). The relative affinity of CO for hemoglobin is approximately 240 to 270 times greater than that of oxygen, resulting in decreased oxygen-carrying capacity of the blood when CO levels are elevated. Carbon monoxide in the bloodstream also results in a leftward shift of the oxyhemoglobin dissociation curve, causing decreased oxygen delivery to the tissues. Removal from the source of CO exposure leads to dissociation of the COHb complex, resulting in excretion of CO by the lungs.[6,8-10]

Infants and children have an increased susceptibility to CO toxicity because of their higher metabolic rates. Fetuses are especially vulnerable. Maternal CO diffuses across the placenta and increases the levels of CO in the fetus. Fetal blood has a higher affinity for CO than does adult blood, and the elimination half-life of carboxyhemoglobin is longer in the fetus than in the adult. Both CO and fetal hemoglobin cause a leftward shift in the normal oxyhemoglobin, resulting in a substantial decrease in oxygen delivery to the placenta and ultimately to fetal tissues.[11-13]

Intoxication from exposure to CO and the resultant tissue hypoxia affects multiple organ systems. Systems with high metabolic rates and high oxygen demand are preferentially affected. Neurologic and cardiovascular and pulmonary manifestations of CO intoxication are reported most frequently.[3-6,8-10] Typical pathologic changes revealed in neuroimaging studies have shown bilateral necrosis in the globus pallidus and diffuse homogenous demyelination of the white matter of the cerebral hemispheres.[14]

∎ Clinical Effects

The clinical presentation of CO intoxication is highly variable and the severity of the symptoms may not correlate to COHb blood levels. Low levels of COHb may be present in cases of severe poisoning.[3,5,8,9] Symptoms of CO intoxication include headache, dizziness, fatigue, lethargy, weakness, drowsiness, nausea, vomiting, loss of consciousness, skin pallor, dyspnea on exertion, palpitations, confusion, irritability, irrational behavior, coma, and death.

Symptoms from acute CO poisoning commonly found in adults with varying COHb levels are reported in Table 7.2. In a series of pediatric patients treated for CO poisoning, lethargy and syncope were reported more frequently than in adult series. These symptoms also occurred at lower COHb levels than usually reported for adults.[5]

Delayed neuropsychologic sequelae following CO exposure have been reported in both adults and children.[5,6,8-10,15] The frequency of delayed neuropsychiatric sequelae is unknown as there is no standardized neuropsychometric testing battery and testing is only completed on a small proportion of patients being treated for CO intoxication.[15]

Table 7.2. Symptoms Commonly Found in Adults With Different COHb Levels*

Blood Level of COHb (%)	Symptoms
0-10	Usually none in healthy individuals; reduced exercise tolerance in patients with pulmonary disease; decreased threshold for angina in patients with coronary artery disease
10-20	Headache; dyspnea on mild exertion; angina in patients with coronary heart disease; dilation of cutaneous vessels
20-30	Throbbing headache; nausea or vomiting (or both); easy fatigability and irritability; difficulty with concentration
30-40	Severe headache; dizziness; fatigue and weakness; syncope on exertion; impaired thought processes
40-50	Tachypnea; tachycardia; syncope; confusion
50-60	Respiratory failure; collapse; intermittent convulsions or seizures; coma
60-70	Respiratory failure; severe hypotension; coma; frequently fatal
> 70	Coma, rapidly fatal

*The clinical presentation of carbon monoxide poisoning is highly variable and the severity of symptoms may not correlate to carboxyhemoglobin (COHb) levels in the blood.[3,5,8,9,16]

■ Diagnosis

A thorough history and physical examination as well as a high index of clinical suspicion are necessary to diagnose CO poisoning. Physicians should consider CO exposure when cohabitants present with similar nonspecific symptoms as previously mentioned. Clinical examination is often without findings suggestive of CO intoxication, as the characteristic signs (cherry red mucosal membranes and retinal hemorrhages) are late findings and rarely observed. Initial laboratory findings may be misleading. Oxygen saturation via pulse oximetry will be falsely normal, since spectrophotometric determinations cannot differentiate oxyhemoglobin from COHb. Arterial blood gas analysis is also misleading because the arterial oxygen tension (PaO_2) is a measure of dissolved oxygen in the plasma and is not affected by changes in hemoglobin saturation. Because this PaO_2 value is commonly used to calculate total oxygen content and hemoglobin saturation in blood gas samples, these values may also appear deceptively normal.[8,10,16]

The measurement of COHb blood levels establishes that exposure to CO has occurred. An elevated level may confirm the diagnosis of CO intoxication. Low and moderately increased levels must be interpreted with caution as the COHb level does not indicate severity of illness. Delay between exposure and laboratory measurement, treatment with oxygen, and complicating factors such as exposure to tobacco smoke should be considered when interpreting COHb results. Background levels of COHb from endogenous production are typically 0.3% to 0.7% in nonsmokers. Baseline COHb levels in smokers typically range from 3% to 8%, although higher values have been reported.[6]

▮ Treatment

Patients who have been exposed to CO should be removed from the source immediately. Therapy consists of supplemental oxygen, ventilatory support, and monitoring for cardiac dysrhythmias. Administration of 100% oxygen is required to improve the oxygen content of the blood. The elimination half-life of COHb is approximately 4 hours in room air and approximately 1 hour with the administration of 100% oxygen. Administration of hyperbaric oxygen decreases the half-life to approximately 20 to 30 minutes.[6,8,9]

The use of hyperbaric oxygen (HBO) has been the subject of recent debate. Absolute criteria have not been determined. There is no agreement among physicians that HBO is of benefit,[17] nor is there agreement on selection criteria for HBO therapy.[9,15,18] There is also lack of consensus regarding HBO treatment protocols for the CO poisoned patient.[18] Lack of consensus and lack of standardized treatment protocols for CO poisoning reflect the variability in the presentation of symptoms, the choice of treatment modalities, and variable patient outcomes.[17] When the CO poisoned patient is cared for, consultation with a critical care specialist familiar with treatment options, including HBO therapy, is recommended.

Prevention

Primary prevention of CO poisoning requires limiting exposure to known sources. Proper installation, maintenance, and use of combustion appliances can help to reduce excessive CO emissions. Table 7.3 provides suggestions to prevent CO poisoning.[7]

Smoke and CO detectors, when used properly, may provide early detection and warning and prevent unintentional CO-related deaths. Carbon monoxide detectors measure the amount of CO that has accumulated and are set to alarm when CO in the air corresponds to 10% COHb level in the blood. This is based on relationships between CO levels measured in air and corresponding blood levels. Underwriters Laboratories (UL) has implemented a standard (UL2034) for certifying detectors for home use.[19]

Frequently Asked Questions

Q *Should I purchase a CO detector for my home? If so, how many and where should they be placed? When is it more appropriate to use a battery powered CO detector?*

A Recommendations are to use a detector meeting the most recent version of the UL standard referenced above. *Consumer Reports* (November 1996) published a review of some available detectors. At least one detector should be placed in a hallway or outside sleeping areas. Because electric heating and cooking appliances shut down during a power failure, battery-operated detectors are recommended when gas appliances or auxiliary heating sources (eg, fireplaces) are used during periods when electrical service is disrupted. Carbon monoxide detector technology is still evolving and detectors should not substitute for the proper use and maintenance of fuel-burning devices. All fuel-burning appliances, furnaces, venting, and chimney systems should be checked professionally once a year or as recommended by the manufacturer.

Q *What sort of things should I have a professional look for when checking my furnace and appliances?*

A Table 7.3 lists recommendations for preventing CO problems in the home.[7]

Table 7.3. Preventing Problems With Carbon Monoxide (CO) in the Home

Fuel-Burning Appliances

Forced-air furnaces should be checked by a professional once a year or as recommended by the manufacturer. Pilot lights can produce CO and should be kept in good working order.

All fuel-burning appliances (eg, gas water heaters, gas stoves, gas clothes dryers) should be checked professionally once a year or as recommended by the manufacturer.

Gas cooking stove tops and ovens should not be used for supplemental heat.

Fireplaces and Woodstoves

Fireplaces and woodstoves should be checked professionally once a year or as recommended by the manufacturer. Check to ensure the flue is open during operation. Proper use, inspection, and maintenance of vent-free fireplaces (and space heaters) are recommended as well.

Space Heaters

Fuel-burning space heaters should be checked professionally once a year or as recommended by the manufacturer.

Space heaters should be properly vented during use according to the manufacturer's specifications.

Barbecue Grills/Hibachis

Barbecue grills and hibachis should never be used indoors.

Barbecue grills and hibachis should never be used in poorly ventilated spaces such as garages, campers, and tents.

Automobiles/Other Motor Vehicles

Regular inspection and maintenance of the vehicle exhaust system are recommended. Many states have vehicle inspection programs to ensure this practice.

Never leave an automobile running in the garage or other enclosed space; CO can accumulate even when a garage door is open.

Generators/Other Fuel-Powered Equipment

Follow the manufacturer's recommendations when operating generators and other fuel-powered equipment.

Never operate a generator indoors.

∎ Resources

Consumer Product Safety Commission; Washington, DC 20207; telephone, 800/638-2772

Indoor Air Quality Information Clearinghouse (A service of the US Environmental Protection Agency); telephone, 800/438-4318

National Fire Protection Association; 1 Batterymarch Park, Quincy, MA 02269-9101; telephone, 617/770-3000

Undersea and Hyperbaric Medical Society; 10531 Metropolitan Avenue, Kensington, MD 20895-2627; telephone, 301/942-2980

Centers for Disease Control and Prevention; 1600 Clifton Road, Atlanta, GA 30333. Public Inquiries, telephone 800/311-3435

Carbon Monoxide Headquarters
http://www.phymac.med.wayne.edu/FacultyProfile/penney/COHQ/co1.htm

∎ References

1. Cobb N, Etzel R. Unintentional carbon monoxide-related deaths in the United States, 1979 through 1988. *JAMA.* 1991;266:659-663

2. Shepherd G, Klein-Schwartz W. Accidental and suicidal adolescent poisoning deaths in the United States, 1979-1994. *Arch Pediatr Adolesc Med.* 1998;152:1181-1185

3. Baker MD, Henretig FM, Ludwig S. Carboxyhemoglobin levels in children with nonspecific flu-like symptoms. *J Pediatr.* 1988;113:501-504

4. Heckerling PS, Leikin JB, Terzian CG, Maturen A. Occult carbon monoxide poisoning in patients with neurologic illness. *Clin Toxicol.* 1990;28:29-44

5. Crocker PJ, Walker JS. Pediatric carbon monoxide toxicity. *J Emerg Med.* 1985;3:443-448

6. US Environmental Protection Agency. Air Quality Criteria for Carbon Monoxide. Research Triangle Park, NC: Office of Health and Environmental Assessment, Office of Research and Development, 1991 (EPA/600/8-90/045F)

7. Samet J. Environmental controls and lung disease. Report of the ATS Workshop on Environmental Controls and Lung Disease. *Am Rev Respir Dis.* 1990;142:915-939

8. Vreman HJ, Mahoney JJ, Stevenson DK. Carbon monoxide and carboxyhemoglobin. *Adv Pediatr.* 1995;42:303-325

9. Varon J, Marik PE, Fromm RE, Gueler A. Carbon monoxide poisoning: a review for clinicians. *J Emerg Med.* 1999;17:87-93

10. Thom SR, Keim LW. Carbon monoxide poisoning: a review of epidemiology, pathology, clinical findings, and treatment options including hyperbaric oxygen therapy. *J Toxicol Clin Toxicol.* 1989;27:141-156

11. Koren G, Sharav T, Pastuszak A, et al. A multicenter prospective study of fetal outcome following accidental carbon monoxide poisoning in pregnancy. *Reprod Toxicol.* 1991;5:397-403

12. Longo LD. The biological effects of carbon monoxide on the pregnant woman, fetus, and newborn infant. *Am J Obstet Gynecol.* 1977;129:69-103

13. Kopelman AE, Plaut TA. Fetal compromise caused by maternal carbon monoxide poisoning. *J Perinatol.* 1998;18:74-77

14. Bianco F, Floris R. MRI appearances consistent with haemorrhagic infarction as an early manifestation of carbon monoxide poisoning. *Neuroradiology.* 1996;38(suppl):S70-S72

15. Seger D, Welch L. Carbon monoxide controversies: neuropsychologic testing, mechanism of toxicity, and hyperbaric oxygen. *Ann Emerg Med.* 1994;24:242-248

16. Ilano AL, Raffin TA. Management of carbon monoxide poisoning. *Chest.* 1990;97:165-169

17. Tibbles PM, Perrotta PL. Treatment of carbon monoxide poisoning: a critical review of human outcome studies comparing normobaric oxygen with hyperbaric oxygen. *Ann Emerg Med.* 1994;24:269-276

18. Hampson NB, Dunford RG, Kramer CC, Norkool DM. Selection criteria utilized for hyperbaric oxygen treatment of carbon monoxide poisoning. *J Emerg Med.* 1995;13:227-231

19. Underwriters Laboratories. UL2034: *Standard for Single and Multiple Station Carbon Monoxide Detectors.* Northbrook, IL: Underwriters Laboratories, Inc, April 30, 1992

8 Dietary Supplements and Ethnic Remedies

A dietary supplement is legally defined as a product (other than tobacco) intended to supplement the diet that bears or contains one or more of the following dietary ingredients: a vitamin, a mineral, an herb or other botanical, an amino acid, or a dietary substance for use by humans to supplement the diet by increasing the total dietary intake, or a concentrate, metabolite, constituent, extract, or combination of the above ingredients.

Greater consumer interest in alternative and "natural" medicines increases the likelihood that infants and children may be given a variety of dietary supplements, some of which are clearly or potentially toxic.

Clinicians can play an important role in identification, reporting, and prevention of adverse effects from dietary supplements.

Pediatricians should be aware that:

- Pharmacologically active substances such as melatonin, ephedrine, and dehydroepiandrosterone (DHEA) can be marketed as dietary supplements provided no therapeutic claims are made for them.
- Dietary supplements can be consumed in large doses (megavitamin doses).
- Effects in children (and often in adults) are not known for many dietary supplements; frequency and patterns of use in children are also not well known.
- No requirements exist for child-resistant packaging.
- A 1993 survey of adults showed that at least one third of respon-

dents had used "unconventional therapies" in the past year.[1] Most (72%) did not inform their physicians of these therapies. Similar surveys for children would be helpful.

- Dietary supplements lack standards for manufacture and purity.
- A survey of dietary supplements advertised in popular health and bodybuilding magazines showed that no human toxicology data were available in the peer-reviewed scientific literature for approximately 60% of ingredients in the products advertised.[2] Adolescents may be a target of such advertising.
- Labels and promotional material for dietary supplements often lack information regarding potential adverse side effects or contraindications.
- Dietary supplements are often promoted for health-related benefits. Many consumers may be using these products for various health conditions or for pharmacologic effects.
- Consumers frequently assume that "natural" means "safe." Products that are natural are frequently promoted to consumers as having no side effects; however, many potent drugs are derived from natural products (ie, opiates, digitalis, estrogen), and other natural substances and plants are poisonous (ie, certain types of mushrooms, snake venom, and hemlock).

■ Routes of Exposure

Children may be exposed to dietary supplements in many of the same ways they are exposed to pharmaceutical products: ingestion as a liquid (see Table 8.1), tablet, or capsule. Although dietary supplements include only orally ingested products, many of the same ingredients are available in topical or suppository form, subject to different regulations than orally ingested products. Ingestion as a liquid can be in the form of an extract, tincture, decoction, or tea, all made from herbs, or as an elixir or suspension. Most supplement products are available in capsule or tablet form, and could possibly be consumed by children. Although few products are available as rectal suppositories, a wide variety of substances, in particular herbal products, are used in solutions for "therapeutic enemas."

Table 8.1. Types of Solutions

Decoction	A dilute aqueous extract prepared by boiling an herb in water and straining and filtering the liquid. May be the same as an infusion. Not available commercially in the United States but can be prepared by the consumer.
Elixir	A clear sweetened hydroalcoholic for oral use.
Suspension	The dispersion through a liquid of a solid in finely divided particles.
Extract	A concentrated form of a natural substance, which can be a powder, liquid, or tincture. The concentration varies from 1:1 in a fluid extract to 1:0.1 in a tincture.
"Natural" product	The term natural defies accurate definition because, strictly speaking, everything is derived from nature. In common usage it is often intended to imply a substance that is not synthetic.

▮ Systems Affected and Clinical Effects of Dietary Supplements

Adverse effects resulting from consumption of dietary supplements may involve one or more organ systems. In some cases a single ingredient can have multiple adverse effects. More than one dietary supplement product may be consumed concurrently, and many products may contain more than one physiologically active ingredient. Some ingredients known to cause adverse effects are listed in Table 8.2.

Hepatotoxicity
Many herbal products contain pyrrolizidine alkaloids, which can be extremely hepatotoxic, causing hepatic veno-occlusive disease, hepatomegaly, and with some alkaloids, liver cancers.[3] Comfrey, which has been banned in Germany and restricted in Canada, may still be purchased and consumed in the United States, at times with

Table 8.2. Some Known Hazardous Dietary Supplements

Common Name	Latin Name (for Herbs) or Toxic Ingredient	Primary Toxic Effect
Azarcon, greta	Lead	Lead poisoning
Barberry	*Berberis vulgaris*	Stupor, daze, diarrhea, nephritis
Bee pollen		Allergic reactions in sensitive people
Blue cohosh	*Caulophyllum thalictroides*	Increased blood pressure, stimulation of small intestine and hyperglycemia, uterine and cardiac stimulation; severe stomach pain
Bracken fern	*Pteridium aquillium*	Bone marrow depression; cancer
Broom	*Cytisus scoparius*	Tachycardia, cardiovascular collapse, nausea, diarrhea, vertigo, stupor
Butterbur	*Petasites hybridus*	Hepatic veno-occlusive disease (HVOD)
Chamomile	*Matricaria chamomilla* *Anthemis nobilis*	Contact dermatitis, anaphylaxis, hypersensitivity reactions in people allergic to asters, chrysanthemums and other *compositae*
Chaparral	*Larrea tridentata*	Hepatotoxicity
Coltsfoot	*Tussilago farfara*	HVOD
Comfrey	*Symphytum officinale*	HVOD
Germander	*Teucrium chamaedrys*	Hepatotoxicity
Ghasard, bala goli, kandu	Lead	Lead poisoning
Golden ragwort	*Senecio aureus* *Echium* species	HVOD HVOD
Gum asafoetida	*Ferula asa-foetida*	Methemoglobinemia when Hb-F present
Heliotrope, turnsole	*Heliotropium* species *Crotolaria fulva* *Cynoglossum officinale*	HVOD HVOD HVOD
Hound tongue Iron supplements or iron-containing multivitamins	Iron	Gastrointestinal symptoms, shock, coma, seizures, hepatic and renal failure, cardiovascular collapse

Common Name	Latin Name (for Herbs) or Toxic Ingredient	Primary Toxic Effect
Jin Bu Huan (product name)	*Stephania* species	CNS and respiratory depression
L-tryptophan	Contaminants in the product	Eosinophilia, myalgia, sclerodermiform skin changes
Lobelia (Indian tobacco)	*Lobelia inflata*	Autonomic nervous system stimulation or depression
Mistletoe	*Phoradendron* species *Viscum* species	Hepatotoxicity Gastrointestinal bleeding, cardiotoxicity, hepatotoxicity
Monkshood	*Acotinum napellus* *A columbianum*	Respiratory center or cardiac muscle paralysis leading to death
Pay-loo-ah	Arsenic	*Arsenic poisoning:* chronic—myalgias, peripheral neuropathies; acute—nausea, vomiting, diarrhea, severe abdominal pain, circulatory collapse, death
	Lead	*Lead poisoning:* headache, irritability, learning problems, vomiting, abdominal pain, weight loss, encephalopathy, coma, death
Pennyroyal oil	*Hedeoma pulegoides*	Internal bleeding, shock, hepatitis, multiple organ failure, seizures, death
Ragwort	*Senecio jacobaea*	HVOD
Senna	*Casia acutifolia*	Hepatotoxicity
Shield fern, Aspidium	*Dryopterix filix-mas*	Muscle weakness, coma, blindness, seizures, cardiac and respiratory failure
Skullcap	*Scutellaria laterifolia*	Hepatotoxicity
Thread-leafed groundsel or groundsel	*Senecio longilobus*	HVOD
Wolf's bane, leopard's bane, mountain tobacco	*Arnica montana*	Vomiting, drowsiness, coma, cardiotoxicity
Wormwood	*Artemisia absinthium*	Neurologic symptoms often leading to convulsions

disastrous results.[4] Pediatric veno-occlusive disease has occurred in near epidemic proportions in Jamaica, where the condition was first described, after ingestion of "bush tea" brewed from pyrrolizidine containing plants. In particular, *Crotolaria fulva* is used by Jamaicans to treat common ailments. Other ethnic groups consume potentially hepatotoxic herbs, and the practice of herbal medicine is rapidly entering the American mainstream.[5] While alert clinicians should be aware of the cultural heritage and practices of patients, lack of a unique cultural identity should not dissuade them from inquiring into the use of these products.

Exposure to pyrrolizidine alkaloids in herbal teas has led to acute liver failure and death in infants and toddlers, as well as in newborns whose mothers consumed the tea during pregnancy.[6] In older children, the effects may be less dramatic, presenting as mild elevations in liver enzyme,[5] which may lead to cirrhosis with chronic use. Chronic exposure to low levels of pyrrolizidine alkaloids in experimental animals causes lung lesions that can progress to pulmonary arterial hypertension and right ventricular hypertrophy. No analytical method is available to analyze body fluids or tissue samples to detect pyrrolizidine alkaloids.

Other Adverse Effects

A number of ethnic groups use toxic remedies, including *azarcón*, a lead-containing orange powder, and *greta*, a lead-containing yellow powder used by Mexican Hispanics[7]; *pay-loo-ah*, a lead- and arsenic-containing orange powder used by Hmong[8]; and *ghasard*, *bala goli*, and *kandu*, lead-containing brown, black, or red powders used by Asian Indians.[9] Acute and chronic intoxication has occurred from use of these remedies, and deaths have been reported.[9]

Differences in metabolism may make some products more toxic in children. Gum asafetida, *Ferula* species, can be consumed by adults with no apparent adverse effects, but infants may demonstrate a severe methemoglobinemia due to the oxidizing effect on fetal hemoglobin.[10]

Adulterated Chinese "herbal" medications have caused adverse effects in both adults and children. These medications may contain prescription drugs, including nonsteroidal anti-inflammatory drugs, diazepam, and phenylbutazone, and heavy metals such as lead, mercury, and cadmium. In one case, a 12-year-old child developed aplastic anemia from ingesting a Chinese "herbal" medication that was later found to contain phenylbutazone. Ingestion by three children of another product labeled as containing the herb *Polygala chinensis* resulted in life-threatening bradycardia and central nervous system and respiratory depression.[11] Subsequent analyses showed the tablets contained 36% levo-tetrahydropalmatine, which is derived from the genus *Stephania*, and is known to cause sedation, neuromuscular blockade, and dopamine receptor antagonism.

∎ Trends in Supplement Use

The use of supplements often appears faddish. Currently, popular products include melatonin,[12] ephedrine,[13] dehydroepiandros–terone (DHEA),[14] and blue-green algae.[15] Melatonin is used by adults to induce sleep and combat the effects of jet lag. While it may be tempting to use this product in children who have difficulty sleeping, there are few data about benefits and risks of the long-term use of melatonin in adults and none in children. Few clinical trials have been conducted. Ephedrine has been promoted for weight loss and as an "energy booster," and as a safe and "legal" substitute for recreational street drugs. Nationwide, a large number of adverse events, including several deaths, have been attributed to ephedrine.[13] While DHEA has not been promoted for use in children, it has been promoted as a weight-loss aid and as a muscle builder. These purported effects could be attractive to adolescents who are concerned with physical training and muscle building. Although DHEA is a naturally occurring hormone in humans, the potential adverse effects of increased doses or prolonged supplementation are unknown.[14] Microcystins, toxic compounds produced by some species of blue-green algae, have been responsible for fish kills and some incidents of poisoning in people. Supplements containing blue-green algae are now available, but consumers will not know whether particular algae are toxic.

∎ Prevention of Exposure

Scientific evidence to support the benefits of supplement products in adults is often lacking, and there is a critical lack of evidence of safety in children. Physicians and other health professionals routinely ask questions about use of dietary supplements, minerals, vitamins, or herbs, as well as the reasons or health conditions for which these products are used. A careful history is crucial because some symptoms of adverse effects may be too nonspecific to make a diagnosis.

Most dietary supplement products do not have child-resistant packaging, and unintentional ingestion by children resulting in serious adverse effects has been reported. All supplements should be kept out of the reach of the children. Iron, ingested alone or in combination with vitamins, is one of the most common causes of poisoning in children in the United States. Aggressive public information campaigns, combined with attempts to restrict access to iron-containing preparations, have led to a dramatic drop in the number of deaths in children from iron overdose; nonetheless, 23 170 cases of intoxication and 3 deaths occurred in the United States in 1995.†

In addition to unintentional exposure, children have experienced adverse effects from a variety of supplement products. In 1989, eosinophilia-myalgia syndrome resulted from nationwide uncontrolled use of heavily promoted L-tryptophan. Adults used L-tryptophan primarily to enhance sleep, for premenstrual syndrome, or for stress; in children, it was apparently given to treat "hyperactivity." Use of this product led to a disorder that affected the hematopoietic, immunologic, pulmonary, and integumentary systems, among others. The eosinophilia-myalgia syndrome epidemic affected approximately 6000 persons, many of whom are still disabled, and led to at least 38 deaths in the United States.[16] Similar "experiments" are going on nationwide today as people consume other dietary supplements that contain untested ingredients. Secondary prevention of unintentional exposure consists of detailed history taking that includes documentation of supplement use.[17]

Some parents administer herbs and dietary supplements to their children despite medical advice to the contrary. Any adverse effects should be reported to the FDA.

---

† In the October 6, 1994 *Federal Register* (59 FR 51030), the FDA proposed regulations to require label warning statements and unit-dose packaging requirements for iron-containing products, including dietary supplements, to reduce the risk of unintentional overdoses of iron in young children.

∎ Frequently Asked Questions

Q *Conventional medications have many side effects; shouldn't I worry more about the known side effects?*

A Conventional pharmaceutical products have been through extensive testing for both safety and efficacy by manufacturers and through Food and Drug Administration (FDA) approval processes. Many of the known side effects in adults have been documented and studied. None of this is true for dietary supplements.

Q *Does my child need extra vitamins/food supplements? Won't they help my child grow, eat, and study better?*

A A diet that provides enough calories and is balanced in all the major food groups should provide adequate nutrition for an otherwise healthy growing child. However, since many children do not consume a balanced diet, and may consume extensive amounts of junk food, a multiple vitamin may be appropriate. Additional supplements are rarely necessary for children. Certain kinds of birth defects are known to occur more frequently when the diet is deficient in folic acid. Therefore, women in their reproductive years, including teenagers who may become pregnant, should consume 0.4 mg of folic acid daily.

Q *Doesn't the FDA approve food additives and dietary supplements?*

A No. Legislation enacted in 1994 made dietary ingredients exempt from the FDA's premarket approval for a food additive. Manufacturers no longer must prove that an ingredient is safe; the FDA needs to prove the ingredient is hazardous if it believes there is a risk. The 1994 law also allows companies to make medical claims for dietary supplements that in the past would have been regulated as a drug.

∎ Resources

Health professionals should report adverse effects to the FDA's MedWatch Program at 800/322-1088 or to the Centers for Disease Control and Prevention at 770/488-7350.

Consumers can report adverse events to the FDA Consumer Hotline at 800/322-4010. Local or regional poison control centers are also a valuable resource for information on the adverse effects of dietary supplements. The Office of Dietary Supplements at the National Institute of Health has information about dietary supplements online at http://dietary-supplements.info.nih.gov.

■ References

1. Eisenberg DM, Kessler RC, Foster C, Norlock FE, Calkins DR, Delblanco TL. Unconventional medicine in the United States. *N Engl J Med.* 1993;328: 246-252

2. Philen RM, Ortiz DI, Auerbach S, Falk H. Survey of advertising for nutritional supplements in health and bodybuilding magazines. *JAMA.* 1992;268: 1008-1011

3. Huxtable RJ. Herbal teas and toxins: novel aspects of pyrrolizidine poisoning in the United States. *Perspect Biol Med.* 1980;24:1-14

4. Ridker PM, McDermott WV. Comfrey herb tea and hepatic veno-occlusive disease. *Lancet.* 1989:1;657-658

5. Centers for Disease Control and Prevention. Self-treatment with herbal and other plant derived remedies - rural Mississippi, 1993. *MMWR Morb Mortal Wkly Rep.* 1995;44:204-207

6. Roulet M, Laurini R, Rivier L, Calame A. Hepatic veno-occlusive disease in the newborn infant of a woman drinking herbal tea. *J Pediatr.* 1988;112:433-436

7. Risser A, Mazur LJ. Use of folk remedies in a Hispanic population. *Arch Pediatr Adolesc Med.* 1995;149:978-981

8. Centers for Disease Control and Prevention. Folk remedy-associated lead poisoning in Hmong children–Minnesota. *MMWR Morb Mortal Wkly Rep.* 1983;32:555-556

9. Centers for Disease Control and Prevention. Lead poisoning-associated death from Asian Indian folk remedies – Florida. *MMWR Morb Mortal Wkly Rep.* 1984;33:638-645

10. Kelly KJ, Neu J, Camitta BM, Honig GR. Methemoglobinemia in an infant treated with the folk remedy glycerated asafetida. *Pediatrics.* 1984:73:717-719

11. Centers for Disease Control and Prevention. Jin bu huan toxicity in children – Colorado, 1993. *MMWR Morb Mortal Wkly Rep.* 1993;42:633-636

12. Lamberg L. Melatonin potentially useful but safety, efficacy remain uncertain. *JAMA.* 1996;276:1011-1014

13. Centers for Disease Control and Prevention. Adverse events associated with ephedrine-containing products - Texas, December 1993 - September 1995. *MMWR Morb Mortal Wkly Rep.* 1996:45;689-693

14. Skolnick AA. Scientific verdict still out on DHEA. *JAMA*. 1996;276:1365-1367

15. Carmichael WW. Cyanobacteria secondary metabolites - the cyanotoxins. *J Appl Bacteriol*. 1992;72:445-459

16. Philen RM, Posada M. Toxic oil syndrome and eosinophilia-myalgia syndrome: May 8-10, 1991, World Health Organization meeting report. *Semin Arthritis Rheum*. 1993;23:104-124

17. Huxtable RJ. The myth of beneficent nature: the risks of herbal preparations. *Ann Intern Med*. 1992;117:165-166

9   Endocrine Disruptors

Endocrine disruptors are chemicals that may mimic or disrupt the action of naturally occurring hormones. Many of these substances have estrogenic effects.

The notion that certain pesticides could interfere with hormonal, especially estrogenic, processes in vertebrates probably goes back to the observation that dichlorodiphenyltrichloroethane (DDT) decreased the hatchability of the eggs of pelagic birds.[1] The mechanism of this effect was likely a combination of induction of enzymes that metabolized endogenous estrogens and occupancy of the estrogen receptor by very weak but persistent compounds. Some forms of DDT, other pesticides, such as methoxychlor and chlordecone,[2] and industrial chemicals, such as some polychlorinated biphenyls (PCBs), increase the wet weight of a virgin mouse uterus, which is the classic bioassay for estrogenicity. Compounds of diverse structures can be potent estrogens; the best example of this structural heterogeneity is the stilbene diethylstilbestrol, which looks nothing like a 17-ketosteroid. Clear examples of human-made environmental chemicals acting as estrogens, or more generally, disrupting hormonal events, have been documented in wildlife. Male alligators in Florida were feminized by exposure to a spill of the pesticide dicofol,[3] and Great Lakes birds have failed to reproduce because of high body burdens of DDT.[1]

Besides the synthetic chemicals, there are also many naturally occurring phytoestrogens in plants, mostly isoflavones that are less potent than estradiol and more readily cleared than the pesticides, but that can occur at sufficiently high concentrations or be consumed in sufficiently large quantities to show biological activity. Ecologists believe that phytoestrogens may have evolved to protect the plants by interfering with reproduction in grazing animals. Endogenous and pharmaceutical estrogens are excreted in urine in amounts similar to the administered or produced amounts. Human sewage or runoff from lots in which the animals are fed can contain substantial amounts of estrogen.

■ Route of Exposure

The primary route of exposure is ingestion.

■ Systems Affected and Clinical Effects

Although estrogenicity is the most familiar of the hormone-like activity of exogenous chemicals, one form of dichlorodiphenyldichloroethane (DDE) is an antiandrogen,[4] some pesticides and congeners of PCBs can occupy the thyroid hormone receptor, and other agents produce symptoms (such as infertility in workers in contact with chlordecone and dibromochloropropane) that are plausibly the result of interference with normal endocrine function, even if a hormonal basis is not established.

Secular trends in sperm counts and rates of testicular cancer, undescended testicles, and hypospadias have all been attributed to endocrine disruption by synthetic environmental agents, although no studies are available in which the outcome and the responsible chemical have been measured in the same people. There are such studies in breast cancer, and these show no consistent relationship between body stores of DDT or PCBs and the risk of breast cancer.[5] An estrogen-like effect of DDE, ie, shortened duration of lactation, was seen in two studies, one in North Carolina, the other in Mexico.[6]

In studies of background exposures to PCBs,[7,8] hypotonia at birth was related to prenatal exposure to PCBs, which was accompanied by higher levels of thyrotropin in one study[9]; PCBs are toxic to the developing thyroid gland and also occupy the thyroid hormone receptor. Whether the hypotonia is due to a hypothyroid mechanism is unknown.

In Taiwan, adolescent males who were exposed in utero to high levels of PCBs and polychlorinated dibenzofuran had normal progression through the Tanner stages but smaller penises than control subjects. Puberty in girls was unaffected, as far as could be determined. This is a complicated effect, not obviously an estrogenic one, and its mechanism is unknown.

Soybeans contain very large amounts of estrogenic isoflavones. In a clinical trial in which postmenopausal women ate soy foods or their regular diets, vaginal smears showed some estrogen effect, but all other physiologic measures, including sex hormone binding globulin, were unaffected.[10] In a clinical trial in which infants were fed cow's milk or soy-based formulas, the infants absorbed and excreted the estrogenic isoflavones, and their cholesterol synthesis patterns were modified in association with isoflavone excretion.[11] Foods high in phytoestrogen, such as soybeans, are a major source of protein for some people, and soy formula can be very useful in the milk-intolerant infant. The significance of the changes in cholesterol metabolism are unclear.

What role, if any, environmental chemicals have in morbidity due to endocrine disruption is unclear. Many studies are underway of breast cancer, endometriosis, testicular cancer, and other plausible end points. Currently, environmental endocrine disruption of humans is mainly speculation.

■ Regulation

In 1996, Congress enacted legislation to be implemented in 1998, requiring the Environmental Protection Agency to screen and test chemicals in food and water for estrogenic and possibly other hormonal activity. Most likely, such testing would serve to select agents for more intense study. It would not replace more traditional tests for general toxicity and carcinogenicity.

■ Frequently Asked Questions

Q *Could my child's undescended testicle or hypospadias be due to my exposure to something during pregnancy?*

A No studies show such associations. Some evidence exists that these conditions have been increasing, but if they are increasing, the cause of such an increase is unclear.

Q *Is breast cancer due to estrogen-like chemicals stored in women's bodies?*

A Several studies have found that one or another environmental chemical has been higher in women with breast cancer than in a comparison group, but so far, these studies have not consistently shown any specific chemical to be higher. More studies are underway.

Q *My daughter started her menstrual period when she was 10 years old. Could this be because of chemical exposure?*

A Since about 1840, menarche has been starting earlier among white, northern European girls, perhaps due to better nutrition. However, the average age of menarche has been stable at 12.7 years or so in white girls for about 50 years.

■ References

1. Fry DM. Reproductive effects in birds exposed to pesticides and industrial chemicals. *Environ Health Perspect.* 1995;103(suppl 7):165-171

2. Boylan JJ, Egle JL, Guzelian PS. Cholestyramine: use as a new therapeutic approach for chlordecone (Kepone) poisoning. *Science.* 1978;199:893-895

3. Guilette LJ Jr, Gross TS, Masson GR, Matter JM, Percival HF, Woodward AR. Developmental abnormalities of the gonad and abnormal sex hormone concentrations in juvenile alligators from contaminated and control lakes in Florida. *Environ Health Perspect.* 1994;102:680-688

4. Kelce WR, Stone CR, Laws SC, Gray LE, Kemppainen JA, Wilson EM. Persistent DDT metabolite p,p1-DDE is a potent androgen receptor agonist. *Nature.* 1995;375:581-585

5. Key T, Reeves G. Organochlorines in the environment and breast cancer [editorial]. *BMJ.* 1994;308:1520-1521

6. Gladen BC, Rogan WJ. DDE and shortened duration of lactation in a northern Mexican town. *Am J Public Health.* 1995;85:504-508

7. Jacobson JL, Jacobson SW, Fein GG, Schwartz PM, Dowler JK. Prenatal exposure to environmental toxin: a test of the multiple effects model. *Dev Psychol.* 1984;20:523-532

8. Rogan WJ, Gladen BC, McKinney JD, et al. Neonatal effects of transplacental exposure to PCBs and DDE. *J Pediatr.* 1986;109:335-341

9. Koopman-Esseboom C, Morse DC, Weisglas-Kuperus N, et al. Effects of dioxins and polychlorinated biphenyls on thyroid hormone status of pregnant women and their infants. *Pediatr Res.* 1994;36:468-473

10. Baird DD, Umbach DM, Lansdell L, et al. Dietary intervention study to assess estrogenicity of dietary soy among postmenopausal women. *J Clin Endocrinol Metab.* 1995;80:1685-1690

11. Cruz ML, Wong WW, Mimouni F, et al. Effects of infant nutrition on cholesterol synthesis rates. *Pediatr Res.* 1994;35:135-140

10 Electric and Magnetic Fields

T he most commonly used type of electricity in the home and workplace is alternating current (AC), in which the current does not flow steadily in one direction but moves back and forth. In the United States, it reverses direction 60 times per second. The unit that denotes the frequency of alternation is called a Hertz (Hz). Wherever there is electric current, there are also electric and magnetic fields, which are invisible lines of force created by the electric charges. The forces of attraction, when standing still, create electric fields with a strength related to the voltage or "electrical pressure" in the circuit. Electric fields are measured in volts per meter. When the charges are in motion, they create "magnetic fields." The magnetic field depends on the motion of the charges, and its strength is proportional to the current flow in the circuit. The current is measured in amperes. Both types of fields alternate with the electric current, so a 60-Hz electric power system has 60-Hz electric and magnetic fields. If two power lines have current that runs in opposite directions, the lines create magnetic fields with opposite directions. If the lines are in proximity, the two fields cancel each other. Electric fields may be blocked by earth, trees, or buildings, whereas magnetic fields are generally not blocked by objects. The strength or intensity of magnetic fields is commonly measured in units called gauss or tesla. A milligauss (mG) equals 0.001 G. Another unit often used is the micro Tesla (μT). One milligauss is the same as 0.1 micro Tesla. The 60-Hz component at the middle of the typical living room would measure about 0.7 milligauss (mG) or 0.07 micro Tesla.

■ Sources of Exposure

Alternating current fields come from many sources, such as high-voltage, long-distance transmission lines (usually on metal towers), from the distribution lines (on wooden poles) that bring electricity to homes, schools, and workplaces, and from electric appliances of all sorts, including TV monitors, arcade games, radios, hair dryers, and electric blankets. The strengths of electromagnetic fields (EMFs) are reduced dramatically by movement away from the source. The field strength falls off more rapidly with distance from point sources, such as appliances or the canister transformers on power poles, compared with line sources, such as transmission lines. The magnetic field is down to background level at 3 or 4 feet from an appliance, while it reaches background level around 100 feet from a distribution line and 300 to 500 feet from a transmission line. The point sources in an outdoor substation with its many transformers actually do not produce magnetic fields much beyond the fence line, but the many power lines running in and out of the station may. Studies of adults who carried computerized meters taking measurements every few seconds suggest that the average of all these measurements over the course of 24 hours is about 1 mG. About 40% of the population's EMF exposure comes from power lines near their homes and 60% from other sources. Prominent among these would be fields created by the method of internal wiring in the home, stray currents running back to the electrical system through the grounding on plumbing and cables, and from brief high exposure to appliances and outdoor power lines.

■ Controversy About Possible Health Effects

The controversy about the health effects of EMFs derives from the statement by many physicists that the magnetic fields of power lines are too weak to be detected by the cell, the inconclusive nature of cellular and animal experiments, and the inconsistent and weak epidemiological associations.

The 60-Hz fields differ in important ways from other types of electromagnetic energy, such as x-rays and microwaves. X-rays, for example, deliver "packets" of energy strong enough to ionize and break up molecules, such as DNA. The packets from microwaves cannot break up DNA, but the electric charges on water molecules "wiggle" in response to the oscillations of the microwaves. The friction generated by the wiggling generates heat by the same basic principle that allows microwave ovens to heat food. Radiofrequency fields from radio and TV transmitters are another step weaker than microwaves. Although they alternate millions of times per second, compared with fields that alternate only 60 times per second, radiofrequency fields lack the energy to ionize molecules and can only heat body tissues or create electric currents that might interfere with a cardiac pacemaker or the normal cardiac conduction system when a person is very near the source. Occupational standards have been derived to avoid these well-understood effects. With their relatively slow oscillations, 60-Hz fields do not have enough energy to break chemical bonds or to heat body tissues (beyond a trivial amount compared with natural body heat). Because the 60-Hz and radiofrequency fields usually present in the environment do not ionize molecules or heat tissues, it was believed that they have no effect on biological systems. Indeed, physicists have indicated that the weak electric currents produced in the human body by 60-Hz AC magnetic fields in a typical living room are thousands of times weaker than the physiological currents running in nerve cells. Even fields 10 to 50 times stronger than that would deposit energies equivalent to a whisper in the "hurricane of Brownian molecular movement" in the body. For this reason, many physicists have argued that physiological or pathological effects of AC magnetic fields below 100 mG are theoretically impossible.[1] Other physicists have argued that there may be an array of molecules or interconnected cells that could sort out the weak "signal" from the "noise."

▮ Inconsistent Laboratory Results

During the mid-1970s, a variety of laboratory studies on cell cultures and animals demonstrated that biological changes can be produced by these fields when applied in intensities of hundreds or thousands of mG. These studies are continuing in an effort to determine whether and how 60-Hz fields affect living tissue. Laboratory scientists have found that fields above 100 mG can produce changes in the levels of ornithine decarboxylase, which has a role in intracellular signal transduction.[2] However, whether these types of changes can lead to any increase in risk to human health is unclear. The preponderance of the evidence suggests that EMFs are not genotoxic.

■ Whole Animal Experiments

Experiments on 60-Hz AC fields as initiators and as copromoters of cancer in laboratory animals have been recently completed or are still underway. So far, independent laboratories have been unable to confirm an effect.

■ Epidemiology Results

Although there is epidemiologic evidence consistent with a modest association between occupational exposures to magnetic fields and breast cancer in men (a very rare condition),[3,4] adult leukemia, and adult brain cancer, the greatest public concern has arisen because of epidemiologic studies showing a statistical association between childhood cancer and proximity to power lines. The November 1996 report by a special committee of the National Research Council[5] provided a careful review of this literature with a particular focus on 11 epidemiologic studies of the relationship between childhood leukemia and residential proximity to power lines (earlier studies had suggested an association with childhood brain cancer as well, but the larger more recent studies have not confirmed this association). The studies estimated exposure in a variety of ways: (1) distance from the lines; (2) "wire codes," a system of classification based on type of power line (transmission lines or distribution lines) and distance from the lines; (3) measurements of the magnetic field many years after diagnosis; and (4) estimates of the magnetic field around the time of diagnosis based on historic records of current flows and the distance of the lines from the home.

The Committee concluded that living in homes classified as being in the high wire-code category is associated with about a 1.5-fold excess of childhood leukemia. In other words, children living in homes which were classified as having high magnetic fields were about 50% more likely to be diagnosed with leukemia than children living in homes which were classified as having lower magnetic fields. They suggested that research be undertaken to identify the source of the association between wire codes and childhood leukemia, even if the source has nothing to do with magnetic fields.

In July 1997, the National Cancer Institute published the results of a large epidemiologic study of EMF and childhood leukemia. This study found no association between living near a power line and leukemia. When this study was added to the National Research Council's analysis, the estimate of risk fell from 1.5 to 1.3 (suggesting that children living in homes with higher magnetic fields were about 30% more likely to be diagnosed with leukemia than children living in homes with lower magnetic fields).[6,7]

▮ Frequently Asked Questions

Q I *am about to buy a house, but there is a power line (or transformer) near the home. Should I buy it?*

A This is a decision only a parent can make. Reasonable people, when they think of the uncertainty of the hazard, the low individual risk, the comparable environmental risks (eg, traffic hazards) in other locations, may make the purchase. Obtaining magnetic field measurements in the home will sometimes show that field levels are at about the average level despite proximity to the power line.

Q *Our child has leukemia and was exposed to power lines or an electric appliance. Could this have caused the leukemia?*

A It is important to find out why the parents suspect the power lines as the cause of leukemia and whether they are blaming themselves for the exposure or considering litigation. Be attentive to the feelings related to the question and deal with those. From an objective viewpoint, pinpointing the cause of a particular case of childhood leukemia is currently beyond the ability of science. Even when there is scientific consensus that a factor such as ionizing radiation can cause childhood leukemia, it is impossible to be certain whether a particular case was due to radiation. It is even more problematic for an agent such as EMFs, which are so scientifically controversial.

Q *Have any states or countries set standards for EMFs?*
A Lack of knowledge has constrained scientists from recommending any health-based regulations. Despite this, several states have adopted regulations governing transmission line-generated 60-Hz fields. The initial concern was the risk of electric shock from strong electric fields (measured in kilovolts per meter [kV/m]). More recently, some states, such as Florida and New York, have adopted regulations that preclude new lines from exceeding the fields at the edge of the current right of way. These standards are in the hundreds of mG. The California Department of Education requires that new schools be built at certain distances from transmission lines. These distances, 100 feet for 100 kV lines and 250 feet for 345 kV lines, were chosen based on the estimate that electric fields would have reached the background level at these distances. All of the current regulations relate to transmission lines, and no state has adopted regulations that govern distribution lines, substations, appliances, or other sources of EMFs.

Q *I understand the uncertainty in the science, but I believe that it is prudent to avoid magnetic fields when possible. What low- and no-cost measures of avoidance can I take?*
A The easily avoidable exposures would come from appliances. Cathode ray video monitors (but not liquid crystal monitors) that emit fields from the front, side, and back fall to near background beyond 3 feet. Place the monitor so maintaining that distance is easy. If the monitor is adjacent to a wall, consider maintaining the distance on the other side of the wall as well. Hair dryers, electric blankets, electric waterbeds, clock radios, computer printers, disk drives, arcade computer games, and other appliances with small electric motors emit fields that fall off sharply with distance. See the documents in the Resources section for more detail.

∎ Resources

Possible Health Effects of Exposure to Residential Electric and Magnetic Fields, National Research Council, National Academy Press, November 1996, 2101 Constitution Ave, NW, Box 285, Washington, DC 20055; 800/624-6242.

Questions and Answers About EMF: National Institute of Environmental Health Sciences and US Department of Energy, January 1995, US Government Printing Office. A free copy can be obtained by calling 800/363-2383. Order from Superintendent of Documents, US Government Printing Office, Washington, DC 20402; 202/512-1800.

Fields From Electric Power: What Are They? What Do We Know About Possible Health Risks? What Can Be Done?" Order from Department of Engineering and Public Policy, Carnegie Mellon University, Pittsburgh, PA 15213-3890; 412/268-2670.

∎ References

1. American Physical Society's Statement. Approved by APS governing body on April 22, 1995. *APS News Online.* July 1995. Available at: http://aps.org/apsnews/july95.html

2. Byus CV, Pieper SE, Adey WR. The effects of low-energy 60-Hz environmental electromagnetic fields upon growth-related enzyme ornithine decarboxylase. *Carcinogenesis.* 1987;8:1385-1389

3. Liburdy RP, Sloma TR, Sokolic R, Yawsen P. ELF magnetic fields, breast cancer, and melatonin. *J Pineal Res.* 1993;14:89-97

4. Erren TC. Epidemiologic studies of EMF and breast cancer risk: a biologically based overview. In: Stevens RG, Wilson BW, Anderson LE, eds. *The Melatonin Hypothesis: Breast Cancer and Use of Electric Power.* Columbus, Ohio: Battelle Press; 1997:701–735

5. Committee on the Possible Effects of Electromagnetic Fields on Biologic Systems, Board on Radiation Effects Research, National Research Council. *Possible Health Effects of Exposure to Residential Electric and Magnetic Fields.* Washington, DC: National Academy Press; 1997

6. Linet MS, Hatch EE, Kleinerman RA, et al. Residential exposure to magnetic fields and acute lymphoblastic leukemia in children. *N Engl J Med.* 1997;337:1-7

7. Campion EW. Power lines, cancer, and fear. *N Engl J Med.* 1997;337:44-46

11 Environmental Tobacco Smoke and Smoking Cessation

nvironmental tobacco smoke (ETS), or second-hand smoke, is exhaled smoke or smoke released from the smoldering end of cigarettes, cigars, and pipes. Environmental tobacco smoke is composed of more than 3800 different chemical compounds. Concentrations of particulates less than 2.5 μm (a size that reaches the lower airways) can be two to three times higher in homes with smokers than in homes without smokers. Cigarette smoking is the most important factor determining the level of particulate matter in the indoor air.

■ Routes of Exposure

In 1995, 47 million US adults (24.7%) were cigarette smokers.[1] Forty-three percent of children aged 2 months to 11 years lived in a home with at least one person who smoked.[2] Because many young children spend a large proportion of their time indoors, they may have significant exposures to ETS. These exposures may occur in a variety of environments, such as in their home, child care settings, relatives' homes, and motor vehicles.

■ Systems Affected

In children, ETS affects the upper and lower respiratory tract. The mechanism of its action may be due, in part, to its ciliostatic effect.

Environmental tobacco smoke may also affect the hematopoetic system.[3]

■ Clinical Effects

Exposure to ETS and Lower Respiratory Tract Illness Among Children

Infants whose mothers smoke are 38% more likely to be hospitalized during the first year of life for pneumonia than those whose mothers do not smoke. The number of hospitalizations increases with the number of cigarettes the mother smokes each day.[4,5]

Infants with two smoking parents are more than twice as likely to have had pneumonia as are infants whose parents do not smoke.[6,7]

Exposure to ETS and Middle Ear Effusions in Children

Children whose parents smoke are about 60% more likely to develop middle ear effusion as measured by tympanometry. Although the overall fraction of middle ear effusions attributable to passive smoking is between 8% and 15%,[8] in one study a third of the cases of middle ear effusion among children were attributable to passive smoking.[9]

Exposure to ETS and Asthma

Children whose mothers smoke may be more likely to develop asthma, and those with asthma may have more frequent exacerbations and more severe symptoms.[10-12] If parents expose their asthmatic children to less cigarette smoke, their symptoms will be less severe.[13]

Exposure to ETS and Sudden Infant Death Syndrome

There is a growing body of evidence linking exposure to ETS to sudden infant death syndrome.[14] This association appears to be independent of birth weight and gestational age.[15]

Exposure to ETS and Cancer

A large number of studies have linked ETS exposure to lung cancer in adult nonsmokers who live with smokers.[16] Fewer studies have examined the relation between childhood exposure to ETS and cancer. In one study, adult leukemia and lymphoma were found to be significantly associated with exposure to maternal smoking before the age of 10 years.[17]

▌ Prevention of Exposure

Discussions related to ETS exposure and parental smoking are appropriate in pediatric visits. Most parents do not want to compromise the health of their children. Messages about risks to children from ETS may become an important factor in their decision to quit smoking. When a child has a medical condition exacerbated by ETS exposure (eg, asthma or recurrent otitis media), pediatric intervention and parent education are important elements of that child's medical care.

▌ The Pediatrician's Role in Advising Parents to Reduce Their Child's Exposure to ETS and to Attempt to Quit Smoking

Smoking cessation counseling by physicians is effective and has been found to increase smoking cessation rates almost twofold; approximately 10% of smokers who receive smoking cessation counseling from a physician stop smoking.[18] Although this rate may not seem significant within the context of an individual practice, it reflects a tremendous public health impact at the population level. If there were a 10% rate of cessation in patients in all physician practices in the United States, 2 million smokers would quit each year.[19,20] Over time, advice from physicians may also influence family members to stop smoking.

Smoking cessation among parents is the most effective means of ensuring that their children have less exposure to ETS. Even in families in which those who smoke do not quit, efforts to reduce their children's exposure to ETS may reduce their risk of disease and may also motivate those who smoke to quit. Pediatricians are often the only physician many parents of young children visit.[21] Pediatricians therefore have an extremely important role in efforts to reduce the exposure of children to ETS.

The Agency for Health Care Policy and Research (AHCPR) has released guidelines about smoking cessation.[18] In addition to a comprehensive review of the efficacy of various smoking cessation strategies, the guidelines recommend that all health care professionals routinely assess the smoking status of their patients at each medical visit. Health care professionals are urged to provide counseling at each visit and to assess the eligibility of their patients for nicotine replacement therapy.

❚ Strategies for Counseling Patients

The National Cancer Institute (NCI) has developed a "4 A's" smoking cessation educational program,[22] which includes the following components: (1) *Ask* about smoking at every appropriate opportunity, and assess smoking status with specific attention to the patient's motivation and barriers to change; (2) *Advise* the patient to quit smoking; (3) *Assist* the patient with change; and (4) *Arrange* follow-up. Although these steps are fairly brief, concern is frequently expressed about the limited time available for smoking cessation counseling during a health care visit. Even brief advice from pediatricians in the context of well child care has a positive impact on reducing maternal smoking and relapse rates.

Ask

- *Obtain a smoking history from the parents of all patients.*[23]
- *Current smoking and smoking prior to and during pregnancy should be assessed.* Pediatricians can play an important role in relapse prevention. Including a simple assessment of current and past smoking on the medical record or patient intake form is an easy way to gather this information.

Advise

- *Provide information about smoking cessation and reducing children's ETS exposure to all parents who smoke:* Recommendations include eliminating smoking in the home, in motor vehicles, and whenever children are present.
- *Look for an educational opportunity:* Parents may be more or less receptive to messages about smoking depending on the reason for their visit. Effective educational opportunities may occur in the context of office visits for recurrent otitis media, wheezing, or management of asthma.[24]
- *Engage parents in a discussion about his or her smoking:* Three main messages can be discussed: (1) the effect of ETS on the child and other family members, (2) the effect smoking has on the health of the parent, and (3) the importance of providing appropriate role modeling. Most parents are receptive to discussions of these issues, but the discussion of role modeling in particular may have a motivational impact. "Most smokers say they do not want their child to become a smoker. How do you feel about this?" can be used to

start a discussion about the increased chances of a child smoking if the parent smokes. Discuss whether the parents are ready to consider quitting or have attempted to quit in the past. Review barriers. Let the parents know that you and your staff are willing to support and assist them when they are ready to quit.

- *Personalize the child's health risk:* Many parents underestimate the impact of smoking on their child's health. Relate chronic medical conditions, such as recurrent otitis media, cough, or wheezing to ETS exposure.

Assist

- *Help parents to set goals regarding smoking cessation and reducing the child's ETS exposure:* Smoking intervention is more likely to be successful if the parents make a specific behavioral commitment, such as setting a date to quit. Just before that date, the smokers should discard all cigarettes and ashtrays. Reinforce the patient's commitment by providing a prescription with the quit date written on it. Nicotine replacement therapy and referral to outside agencies should be offered as part of an effective cessation strategy. For parents who are not ready to quit, specific goals and timelines for reducing the child's exposure to ETS should be made, such as elimination of smoking in the home and in motor vehicles.

Arrange follow-up

- *Plan to follow-up on any behavioral commitments that parents make.* Let parents see you write down commitments in the chart, and use this chart notation as a basis for discussion at the next office visit. Consider scheduling a visit or telephone follow-up call to check on progress.

∎ Strategies for Adolescents

Smoking among adolescents is a significant problem. The US Surgeon General's report has identified four categories of risk factors for adolescent use of tobacco.[25]

- *Personal:* Belief that use of tobacco will make the teenager fit better into the social scene
- *Behavioral:* Lack of strong educational goals, lack of attachment

to school and social clubs

- *Socioeconomic:*. Low socioeconomic status
- *Environmental:* Use of cigarettes by peers and/or parents, exposure to tobacco products and advertisements

Using these risk factors, pediatricians may identify certain adolescents who are at more risk for tobacco use. Table 11.1 identifies steps to help teenagers stop using tobacco.

Table 11.1. Steps to Help Teenagers Stop Using Tobacco*

Ask teenagers to consider that most adults who smoke started when they were teenagers, and wish that they had quit as teenagers.
Ask teenagers to make a list of reasons why someone might want to quit, then talk about any which could apply to them.
If the adolescent has not been smoking too long or is not yet smoking more than 10 cigarettes a day, point out that it is easier to quit before the body is more addicted.
Ask teenagers who are not willing to discontinue use to promise that they will not increase they amount they smoke.
Ask teenagers who insist that tobacco is not a problem for them: "At what point would tobacco become a problem for you?"
Ask patients who insist that they are not addicted to enter into a verbal contract with you to avoid tobacco for a week. Follow up by telephone.
Once the teenager has made a commitment to stop, the pediatrician's task is to encourage and educate. Suggest that adolescents who are determined to give up tobacco do the following:
Consider the logical arguments in favor of cessation, including health hazards.
Learn about ways to quit.
Think about how and why they use tobacco.
Develop a plan to cope with (or avoid) situations where the urge to use is great.
Make the commitment.
Get the help they need (eg, nicotine patch or gum, cessation clinics, quitting partners).
Decide on a cessation plan and stay with it.
Anticipate and prepare for occasional urges to smoke long after discontinuing use.

*Adapted from reference 26

What can the pediatrician do?

Office Interventions

Set an example: The pediatrician should serve as a role model and should not smoke, particularly in the presence of patients and office staff. The office should have signs stating the no-smoking policy.

Systematically assess parental smoking status and children's ETS exposure: Systematic strategies for identifying smokers such as stickers on the medical chart as reminders or a vital sign form that includes smoking status should be implemented. The goal is to prompt all health care professionals who have contact with patients or parents who smoke to provide information about smoking cessation. In the context of a pediatric visit, it is important to ask about parental smoking status as part of the child's health assessment. The issue of parental smoking should be placed on a problem list and addressed at each office visit.

Involve several staff members in providing information about smoking cessation: Educating additional office staff (eg, a nurse or health educator) in smoking cessation counseling can extend the physician's efforts and provide parental support.

The pediatrician as an "agenda setter": The pediatrician may serve as a catalyst for a parent to quit smoking. The pediatrician may initiate the process and provide referrals to specialists in smoking cessation and maintenance of a smoke-free lifestyle.

Provide patient education materials: Materials can be obtained free or at low cost from local affiliates of the American Lung Association, American Cancer Society, American Heart Association, and the National Cancer Institute's Cancer Information Service (see Resources section).

Utilize local resources: Local resources are available in most cities. Physician referrals should include a specific agency or program, telephone number, and description of what to expect. Self-help materials are also available from many agencies. The makers of nicotine gum and other nicotine replacement therapies also offer self-help smoking cessation programs as adjuncts to these products.

■ Frequently Asked Questions

Q *If I smoke, does it affect my breast milk?*

A Breast milk is the best food for infants. It is best to quit smoking or decrease the number of cigarettes smoked during breastfeeding because nicotine and other toxicants may be transferred through the breast milk to the infant. If you do continue to smoke, never breastfeed while smoking because your infant may be unintentionally burned. Also, a high concentration of ETS will be in close proximity to your infant.

Q *Is it useful to measure nicotine or any nicotine metabolites (such as cotinine) in infants to find out whether the infant has been exposed to tobacco smoke?*

A No, it is not useful to measure nicotine or any nicotine matabolites in the clinical setting. Although valuable as a marker in large epidemiologic studies, nicotine and cotinine measurements are not recommended for individual patient assessment or care.

Q *When visitors come to my home, they ask if they can smoke in another room. What should I tell them?*

A Because air exchanges spread smoke throughout the home, the child is exposed to smoke even when smokers use another room. Children's homes should be smoke-free. Ask your visitors to smoke outside.

Q I *can't stop smoking right now. How can I reduce my child's exposure to ETS?*

A Be sure that you only smoke outside because your child will be exposed to ETS if you smoke in any part of your home. Never smoke in your car or any vehicle in which an infant rides. Choose a smoke-free child care setting.

■ Resources

For materials about environmental tobacco smoke, contact the American Lung Association, the Office on Smoking and Health at the Centers for Disease Control and Prevention (770/488-5701), the US Environmental Protection Agency Indoor Air Quality Information

Clearinghouse (800/438-4318), the Agency for Health Care Policy and Research (800/358-9295), the National Cancer Institute (800/4-CANCER), the American Lung Association (800/LUNG-USA), or LUNGLINE/National Jewish Hospital (800/222-5864).

▋ References

1. Centers for Disease Control and Prevention. Cigarette smoking among adults –United States, 1995. *MMWR Morbid Mortal Wkly Rep.* 1997;46:1217-1220

2. Pirkle JL, Flegal KM, Bernert JT, Brody DJ, Etzel RA, Maurer KR. Exposure of the US population to environmental tobacco smoke: the Third National Health and Nutrition Examination Survey, 1988 to 1991. *JAMA.* 1996;275:1233-1240

3. Sandler DP, Everson RB, Wilcox AJ, Browder JP. Cancer risk in adulthood from early life exposure to parents' smoking. *Am J Public Health.* 1985;75:487-492

4. Colley JR, Holland WW, Corkhill RT. Influence of passive smoking and parental phlegm on pneumonia and bronchitis in early childhood. *Lancet.* 1974; 2:1031-1034

5. Fergusson DM, Horwood LJ, Shannon FT. Parental smoking and respiratory illness in infancy. *Arch Dis Child.* 1980;55:358-361

6. Harlap S, Davies AM. Infant admissions to the hospital and maternal smoking. *Lancet.* 1974;1:529-532

7. Rantakallio P. Relationship of maternal smoking to morbidity and mortality of the child up to the age of five. *Acta Paediatr Scand.* 1978;67:621-631

8. Etzel RA, Pattishall EN, Haley NJ, Fletcher RH, Henderson FW. Passive smoking and middle ear effusion among children in day care. *Pediatrics.* 1992;90:228-232

9. Ey JL, Holberg CJ, Aldous MB, Wright AL, Martinez FD, Taussig LM. Passive smoke exposure and otitis media in the first year of life. *Pediatrics.* 1995;95:670-677

10. Chilmonczyk BA, Salmun LM, Megathlin KN, et al. Association between exposure to environmental tobacco smoke and exacerbations of asthma in children. *N Engl J Med.* 1993;328:1665-1669

11. Martinez FD, Cline M, Burrows B. Increased incidence of asthma in children of smoking mothers. *Pediatrics.* 1992;89:21-26

12. Weitzman M, Gortmaker S, Walker DK, Sobol A. Maternal smoking and childhood asthma. *Pediatrics.* 1990;85:505-511

13. Murray AB, Morison BJ. The decrease in severity of asthma in children of parents who smoke since the parents have been exposing them to less cigarette smoke. *J Allergy Clin Immunol.* 1993;91:102-110

14. Taylor JA, Sanderson M. A reexamination of the risk factors for the sudden infant death syndrome. *J Pediatr.* 1995;126:887-891

15. Klonoff-Cohen HS, Edelstein SL, Lefkowitz ES, et al. The effect of passive smoking and tobacco exposure through breast milk on sudden infant death syndrome. *JAMA.* 1995;273:795-798

16. US Environmental Protection Agency, Office of Health and Environmental Assessment, Office of Research and Development. *Respiratory Health Effects of Passive Smoking: Lung Cancer and Other Disorders.* Washington, DC: US EPA; 1992

17. Sandler DP, Everson RB, Wilcox AJ, Browder JP. Cancer risk in adulthood from early life exposure to parents' smoking. *Am J Public Health.* 1985;75:487-492

18. Fiore MC, Bailey WC, Cohen SJ, et al. *Smoking Cessation: Information for Specialists. Clinical Practice Guideline. Quick Reference Guide for Smoking Cessation Specialists,* No. 18. Rockville, MD: USDHHS, Public Health Service, Agency for Health Care Policy and Research, Centers For Disease Control and Prevention; April 1996; Publication AHCPR 96-0694

19. Ockene JK. Physician-delivered interventions for smoking cessation: strategies for increasing effectiveness. *Prev Med.* 1987;16:723-737

20. Kottke TE, Battista RN, DeFriese GH, Brekke ML. Attributes of successful smoking cessation interventions in medical practice: a meta-analysis of 39 clinical trials. *JAMA.* 1988;259:2882-2889

21. Perry CL, Silvis GL. Smoking prevention: behavioral prescriptions for the pediatrician. *Pediatrics.* 1987;79:790-799

22. Glynn TJ, Manley MW. *How to Help Your Patients Stop Smoking: A National Cancer Institute Manual for Physicians.* Bethesda, MD: National Cancer Institute, US Dept of Health and Human Services, Public Health Service, National Institutes of Health; 1990. Publication NIH 90-3064

23. American Academy of Pediatrics, Committee on Environmental Health. Environmental tobacco smoke: a hazard to children. *Pediatrics.* 1997;99:639-642

24. American Academy of Pediatrics, Committee on Substance Abuse. Tobacco-free environment: an imperative for the health of children and adolescents. *Pediatrics.* 1994;93: 866-868

25. Centers for Disease Control and Prevention. *Preventing Tobacco Use Among Young People: A Report of the Surgeon General.* Atlanta, Ga: US Dept of Health and Human Services, Public Health Service, Centers for Disease Control and Prevention, National Center for Chronic Disease Prevention and Health Promotion, Office on Smoking and Health; 1994

26. Heyman RB. Tobacco: prevention and cessation strategies. *Adolesc Health Update.* 1997;9:1-8

12 Food Contaminants

T his chapter focuses on microbial contaminants in foods, pesticides, certain food additives, and mycotoxins. Other contaminants (such as lead and mercury) are described in detail in Chapters 14 and 15.

■ Pathogenic Hazards

Although the US food supply is among the safest in the world, there are still millions of people stricken by food-borne illness every year in the United States and an estimated 9000 deaths per year, mostly among the elderly and the very young.[1] The *1997 Red Book* describes the diagnosis and treatment of illnesses caused by food-borne pathogens.[2]

Pathogens in food include:

- viruses such as hepatitis A and caliciviruses including Norwalk virus;

- bacteria such as *Salmonella, Shigella, Campylobacter, Escherichia coli, Vibrio cholerae, Yersinia enterocolitica,* and *Listeria*;

- toxins from bacteria including *Staphylococcus aureus, Bacillus cereus, Clostridium perfringens, Clostridium botulinum, Escherichia coli* O157:H7;

- parasites such as *Toxoplasma gondii, Cryptosporidium parvum, Cyclospora, Giardia lamblia, Taenia,* and *Trichinosis*;

- aquatic microorganisms such as *Pfiesteria piscicida* that elaborate toxins; and
- products accumulated in the food chain of fish and shellfish, such as scombroid, saxitoxin, ciguatera toxin, and domoic acid.

Infectious organisms are ubiquitous in the environment and can enter the food supply in a multitude of ways. Chickens infected with *Salmonella* species can excrete these organisms into the eggs before the shells are formed or excrete the organisms in feces that can contaminate the shells. Shellfish and other seafood can become contaminated by pathogens, such as the hepatitis A virus in manure runoff and sewage overflows. Nitrogen pollution can stimulate the overgrowth of toxin-producing organisms such as *Pfiesteria*. When these microorganisms are present at high levels, fish can become contaminated and potentially serious neurologic illnesses may occur. Animal feces can contaminate foods via polluted irrigation water, unsafe handling of manure, and unsanitary production and processing activities. Food can become contaminated in retail facilities, institutional settings, and homes because of inappropriate food-handling.

Many pathogens are particularly virulent for children. *Salmonella, Listeria, Cyclospora, Cryptosporidium, E coli* O157:H7, *Shigella,* and *Campylobacter* are among many food-borne pathogens that pose risks to young children. The food production system is becoming more centralized and global, adding to the complexity of food-borne pathogen exposures. For example, there have been large outbreaks in the United States of infection due to *Cyclospora* associated with raspberry consumption. Extensive investigation identified the source as *Cyclospora*-contaminated irrigation water in Guatemalan raspberry fields. Severe outbreaks of hemolytic uremic syndrome and death due to *E coli* O157:H7–contaminated hamburger meat have involved the transport and blending of meats from various parts of the country, often with distribution to regions quite remote from the source of the contamination.

Standards for pathogens are established for meat, poultry, and egg products by the Food Safety and Inspection Service (FSIS) and for all other foods by the Food and Drug Administration (FDA). State public health agencies monitor the incidence of food-borne illness, along with local public health officers, and the US Environmental Protection Agency (EPA) regulates the discharge of pollutants into waters that may later contaminate food.

∎ Toxic Hazards

Toxic chemicals in food can be grouped into three broad categories:

- residues of pesticides deliberately applied to food crops or to stored or processed foods;

- colorings, flavorings, and other chemicals deliberately added to food during processing; and

- chemicals that inadvertently enter the food supply, such as afla-toxins, nitrites, polychlorinated biphenyls, heavy metals including mercury, and persistent pesticide residues such as dichlorodiphe-nyltrichloroethane (DDT).

Pesticides

Diet is a major route of exposure of children to pesticides; exposure by other routes is described in the chapter on pesticides (see Chapter 20).

Pesticides are applied extensively to food crops around the world. More than 400 different pesticidal active ingredients, formulated into thousands of products, are registered for use on agricultural products in the United States. Pesticides are used at all stages of food production to protect against pests in the field and in shipping and storage. In 1992, approximately 500 million pounds of pesticides were used on foods in the United States.[3] The EPA sets standards called tolerances for allowable levels of pesticides on food. The FDA and FSIS monitor the food supply for pesticide residues.

In 1993, the National Research Council (NRC) published a report entitled "Pesticides in the Diets of Infants and Children,"[3] which assessed health implications of pesticides on food and made numer-ous recommendations for improving assessment and regulation of pesticides. The report concluded that the government has provided inadequate attention to prenatal and postnatal developmental toxic effects and the unique food consumption patterns of children, and thus is not providing an adequate level of protection to children in establishing standards for pesticides on food. As a result, many changes are underway in the pesticide food safety area, and legisla-tion enacted in 1996 incorporates a number of the recommendations of the NRC (see Table 12.1). The 1996 Food Quality Protection Act requires that when the risks for children are uncertain, the EPA will provide an additional margin of safety, referred to as an uncertainty factor, to assure that children are safe. Consumption studies can fail to capture the dietary patterns of small children. Current food consumption data used by the EPA group all children between the ages of 2 and 6 years. More intensive studies of the foods eaten by children are underway, but results will not be available for risk assessment for a number of years.

Table 12.1. Food Quality Protection Act of 1996: Provisions Related to Protection of Infants and Children

Health-based standard: A new standard of a "reasonable certainty of no harm" that prohibits economic considerations when children are at risk.

Additional margin of safety: Requires that the EPA use an additional 10-fold margin of safety when setting standards for pesticides on food to protect children. Less than a 10-fold margin of safety may be used when there are adequate data to assess prenatal and postnatal developmental risks.

Account for children's diets: Requires the use of age-appropriate estimates of dietary consumption in establishing allowable levels of pesticides on food to account for children's unique dietary patterns.

Account for all exposures: In establishing acceptable levels of a pesticide on food, the EPA must now account for exposures that may occur via other routes, such as drinking water and residential application of the pesticide.

Cumulative effects: The EPA must now consider the cumulative effects of all pesticides that share a common mechanism of action.

Tolerance reassessments: All existing pesticide food standards must be reassessed over a 10-year period to assure that they meet the new standard to protect children.

Endocrine disruptor testing: The EPA must screen and test all pesticides and pesticide ingredients for estrogen effects and other endocrine disruptor activity.

Registration renewal: Establishes a 15-year renewal process for all pesticides to assure that they have up-to-date science evaluations over time.

Pesticide residues on individual commodities may be extremely variable. In the past, the EPA established residue levels to assure that average levels were safe. However, in 1992, the EPA discovered that it is possible for individual food items (eg, potatoes and bananas) to have high enough levels to make a child acutely ill, even when the average level for the crop is within EPA standards. Such illnesses would be expected to be sporadic, and thus not detectable by disease surveillance efforts.[4] The EPA is beginning the process of reassessing all pesticide tolerances to assure safety for children.[5]

Food Additives

Some food additives may cause adverse reactions in children. Tartrazine (also known as FD&C—food dye and coloring—yellow No. 5) is a dye used in some foods and beverages. Cake mixes, candies, canned vegetables, cheese, chewing gum, hot dogs, ice cream, orange drinks, salad dressings, seasoning salts, soft drinks, and catsup may contain tartrazine. In those who are sensitive to it, tartrazine may cause hives, urticaria, and asthma exacerbations.

Monosodium glutamate (MSG) is associated with the so-called "Chinese Restaurant Syndrome" of headache, nausea, diarrhea, sweating, chest tightness, and a burning sensation along the back of the neck. It appears to be linked to the consumption of large amounts of MSG, not only in Chinese food, but in any food in which a large concentration of MSG is used as a flavor enhancer.

Sulfites are used to preserve foods and sanitize containers for fermented beverages. They may be found in soup mixes, frozen and dehydrated potatoes, dried fruits, fruit juices, canned and dehydrated vegetables, processed seafood products, jams and jellies, relishes, and some bakery products. Some beverages, such as hard cider and beer, also contain sulfites. Because sulfites can cause asthma exacerbations in sulfite-sensitive patients, the FDA has ruled that packaged foods be labeled if they contain more than 10 parts per million of sulfites.

Mycotoxins

Mycotoxins, toxins produced by certain molds, are present in many agricultural products, such as peanuts and corn.[6] The best known mycotoxin, aflatoxin, is produced by the *Aspergillus* fungus, but others include patulin, citrinin, zearalenone, vomitoxin, and the trichothecenes. The principal human exposure to aflatoxins is from food. The International Agency for Research on Cancer has concluded that aflatoxin is a carcinogen.[7] Aflatoxin B_1 is an important risk factor for hepatocellular carcinoma in humans, based on studies conducted in areas with a high incidence of hepatocellular carcinoma, such as Asia, where the incidence of chronic hepatitis B viral infections also is high.[8-10]

▌Prevention of Food Contamination

Care must be taken during food production and preparation to prevent the introduction of pathogens into the food supply. When used in the manufacturing process, these methods are referred to as Hazard Analysis and Critical Control Point (HACCP) systems. These HACCP systems require that food manufacturers identify points at which contamination is likely to occur and implement control processes to prevent it. Also important are efforts to prevent antibiotic resistance, consumer education on proper preparation and storage of foods, pasteurization, irradiation of food, protection of animal health, prevention of discharge of pathogens and nitrogen into water bodies, and numerous other efforts to assure that pathogens are not introduced into the food supply.

Food contamination is best prevented by application of appropriate agricultural and manufacturing practices. Integrated pest management, which uses information about pest biology to control pests, is a means to reduce the risks and use of pesticides.

Enforcement of food safety laws is important in prevention at all levels. Regulation and enforcement involve a complex network of federal, state, and local laws and regulations. Some enforcement efforts involve routine monitoring and surveillance of the food supply; other efforts are in response to reports of problems and incidents. Child health care professionals have an important role in reporting food-borne illnesses to local and state public health agencies. For example, physician reports of outbreaks of hemolytic uremic syndrome caused by E coli O157:H7 led to stronger enforcement efforts to ensure that foods such as hamburger meat and apple juice are safe for consumption.

A number of steps can reduce the likelihood of food-borne illness resulting from pathogens in food:

- Thorough washing of fruits and vegetables with water removes some pathogens as well as removing many pesticide residues. Wash before you peel. Don't peel anything you wouldn't normally peel. It is unnecessary to use soap or chemicals when washing food.
- Raw eggs, fish, and meat should not be eaten, and unpasteurized milk products should not be consumed.
- Thoroughly cook meat, poultry, and eggs to ensure that pathogens are killed. For hamburgers, a thermometer inserted into the center should read 160°F.
- After poultry is prepared, cutting boards and any implements that were used on the raw poultry should be washed with soap and hot water, including hands. Cook stuffings for poultry separately rather than inside the birds.
- Store food appropriately. Refrigeration of prepared food prevents growth of many microorganisms responsible for food poisoning.
- Use of disinfectants and sterilants in the home is not necessary to prevent transmission of pathogens from food. At this time, incorporation of chemical agents into high-chair trays and cutting boards, use of disinfectants on kitchen floors and sinks, and similar practices do not have a role in preventing food-borne infections. It also is unnecessary to use chemical disinfectants for washing hands in the home; soap and water are quite effective.

∎ Frequently Asked Questions

Q *Are pesticides found on fresh vegetables in the store?*
A Pesticides are found commonly on fruits and vegetables in the store. Because no labeling is required, parents cannot tell which fruits and vegetables contain pesticides. Even organically grown fruits and vegetables are not necessarily pesticide-free.

Parents should be advised to scrub all fruits and vegetables under running water to remove superficial particle residues. Fruits and vegetables are good for children because they provide vitamins, minerals, and roughage. Because of these health benefits, children should continue to consume a wide variety of fruits and vegetables, particularly those in season.

Q *Is store-bought baby food safe?*

A Yes. Processed foods generally contain lower residues of pesticides than do fresh fruits and vegetables, in part because federal standards are stricter for processed foods. Some makers of baby foods voluntarily make their products free of all pesticide residues, although they do not advertise this action.

Q *Could cancer develop in my child because of exposure to pesticides?*

A Many factors contribute to cancer, including genetics, contact with viruses, and diet. More research is needed to determine how and why cancers develop during childhood. No causal relationship between exposure to chemicals in foods and cancer has been proven. A number of pesticides can cause tumors in laboratory animals and are associated with cancer in some farm workers exposed to very high doses.

Q *I heard that hot dogs can cause brain cancer in children. Should my children avoid hot dogs?*

A Sodium nitrite prevents the growth of *Clostridium botulinum* in meat products. In the early 1990s, consumption of nitrite-cured hot dogs was reported to be associated with brain cancer in a group of children in California. Although more research needs to be done to confirm this association, manufacturers have been working to reduce the amount of nitrite in their cured meat products. Children should eat a balanced diet, and an occasional hot dog may be a part of that diet.

■ **Resources**

The USDA Meat and Poultry Hotline number is 800/535-4555. Internet address: www.fightbac.org

Major resources for information on pesticides are the 10 regional offices of the US Environmental Protection Agency located in Boston, Mass; New York, NY; Philadelphia, Pa; Atlanta, Ga; Chicago, Ill; Dallas, Tex; Kansas City, Kan; Denver, Colo; San Francisco, Calif; and Seattle, Wash.

▮ References

1. Bean NH, Goulding JS, Lao C, Angulo FJ. Surveillance for foodborne-disease outbreaks: United States, 1988-1992. *MMWR Morb Mortal Wkly Rep.* 1996;45(SS-5):1-66

2. American Academy of Pediatrics. Peter G, ed. *1997 Red Book: Report of the Committee on Infectious Diseases.* 24th ed. Elk Grove Village, Ill: American Academy of Pediatrics; 1997

3. National Research Council. *Pesticides in the Diets of Infants and Children.* Washington, DC: National Academy Press; 1993

4. Goldman LR. Children—unique and vulnerable: environmental risks facing children and recommendations for response. *Environ Health Perspect.* 1995;103 (suppl 6):13-18

5. US Environmental Protection Agency. *Environmental Health Threats to Children.* Washington, DC: Environmental Protection Agency; 1996

6. Morgan MRA, Fenwick GR. Natural foodborne toxicants. *Lancet.* 1990; 336:1492-1495

7. *Aflatoxins: Naturally Occurring Aflatoxins (Group 1). Aflatoxin M1 (Group 2B).* IARC Monographs. Leon, France: International Agency for Research in Cancer; 1993;56

8. Alpert M, Hutt M, Wogan G, et al. The association between aflatoxin content of food and hepatoma frequency in Uganda. *Cancer.* 1971;28:253-260

9. Yeh FS. Aflatoxin consumption and primary liver cancer: a case control study in the USA. *J Cancer.* 1989;42:325-328

10. Yeh FS. Hepatitis B virus, aflatoxins, and hepatocellular carcinoma in Southern Guangxi, China. *Cancer Res.* 1989;49:2506-2509

13 | Indoor Air Pollutants

Indoor air quality has become a health concern in recent years because energy costs have led to building designs that reduce air exchanges and because new synthetic materials have become more widely used in home furnishings. Research has shown that exposure to indoor air contaminants may have adverse effects on health. Indoor environments have a range of airborne pollutants, including particulate matter, gases, vapors, biological materials, and fibers.[1,2] In the home, common sources of air pollutants include tobacco smoke, gas and wood stoves, and furnishings and construction materials that release organic gases and vapors. Allergens and biologic agents include animal dander, fecal material from house dust mites and other insects, mold spores, and bacteria. Pollutants such as particulate matter may be brought into the indoor environment from the outdoor air by natural and mechanical ventilation. This chapter focuses on indoor air pollutants other than tobacco smoke, ie, combustion products, volatile organic compounds (VOCs), and molds.

■ Combustion Products

Combustion pollutants in the home arise primarily from gas ranges, particularly when they malfunction or are used as space heaters, and from improperly vented wood stoves and fireplaces. Combustion of natural gas results in the emission of nitrogen dioxide (NO_2) and carbon monoxide (CO). Levels of NO_2 in the home are generally increased during the winter when ventilation is reduced to conserve energy. During the winter, average indoor concentrations of NO_2 in homes with gas cooking stoves are as much as twice as high as outdoor levels. Some of the highest indoor NO_2 levels have been measured in homes where ovens were used as space heaters.[3] Residential levels of CO are generally low. Cooking or heating with wood results in the emission of liquids (suspended droplets), solids (suspended particles), and gases such as NO_2 and sulfur dioxide (SO_2).[3] The aerosol mixture of very fine solid and liquid particles or "smoke" contains particles in the inhalable range, less than 10 μm in diameter. Few measurements of wood smoke in indoor environments in the United States have been done. In several studies, concentrations of inhalable particles were higher in homes with wood-burning stoves, compared to homes without wood stoves. Depending on the frequency and duration of cooking or heating with wood and the adequacy of ventilation, the concentration of inhalable particles may exceed outdoor air standards. With adequate ventilation, however, operating a wood stove or fireplace may not adversely affect indoor air quality.

■ Volatile Organic Compounds

Many household furnishings and products contain VOCs as residues or carriers.[1,2] These include chemicals such as aliphatic and aromatic hydrocarbons (including chlorinated hydrocarbons), alcohols, and ketones in products such as finishes, rug and oven cleaners, paints and lacquers, and paint strippers. Formaldehyde is found primarily in building materials and home furnishings.[1,2,4,5] Since product labels may not always specify the presence of organic compounds, the specific chemical(s) to which a product user may be exposed may be difficult to discern. Over the normal range of room temperatures, VOCs are released as gases or vapors from furnishings or consumer products. Volatile organic compound measurements in residential and nonresidential buildings show that exposure to VOCs is widespread and highly variable.[6,7] In general, VOCs are likely to be higher in recently constructed or renovated buildings compared to older buildings. Once building-related emissions decrease, consumer products are likely to remain the predominant source of exposure to VOCs. Studies have shown that indoor concentrations of VOCs (measured using a personal monitor) are greater than outdoor concentrations, breath levels correlate better with air exposures in a person's breathing zone than with outdoor air levels, and inhalation accounts for more than 99% of exposure for many VOCs.[8]

Formaldehyde is one of the most ubiquitous indoor air contaminants. It is used in hundreds of products such as urea-formaldehyde and phenol-formaldehyde resin, used to bond laminated wood products and to bind wood chips in particle board; as a carrier solvent in dyeing textiles and paper products; and as stiffeners, wrinkle resistants, and water repellents in floor coverings (eg, rugs and linoleums).[1-3] Urea-formaldehyde foam insulation, one source of formaldehyde used in home construction until the early 1980s, is no longer used. The addition of new furniture to a home increases formaldehyde concentrations. Mobile homes, which have small enclosed spaces, low air exchange rates, and many particle board furnishings, may have much higher concentrations of formaldehyde than other types of homes.[1] Table 13.1 lists common VOCs and their uses.

∎ Molds

Molds are ubiquitous in the outdoor environment, and can enter the home through doorways, windows, heating, ventilation systems, and air conditioning systems. Molds proliferate in environments that contain excessive moisture, such as from leaks in roofs, walls, plant pots, or pet urine. The most common indoor molds are *Cladosporium, Penicillium, Aspergillus,* and *Alternaria.*[9]

∎ Routes of Exposure

Exposure to combustion products occurs by way of inhalation. Exposure to VOCs and to molds occurs via both inhalation of contaminated air and dermal contact with surfaces where they are deposited. Exposure to molds occurs via both routes, inhalation and dermal.

∎ Systems Affected

The mucous membranes of the eyes, nose, throat, and respiratory tract are affected by exposure to combustion products, VOCs, and molds.

Table 13.1. Commonly Used Volatile Organic Compounds

1,1,1-Trichloroethane	Used as a dry-cleaning agent, a vapor degreasing agent, and a propellant
1,4-Dichlorobenzene	Used as an air deodorant and an insecticide
2-Butanone	Used as a solvent, and in the surface coating industry, in manufacturing synthetic resins
Acetone	Used as a solvent, in the production of lubricating oils and as an intermediate in pharmaceuticals and pesticides
Benzene	Constituent in motor fuels, solvent for fats, inks, oils, paints, plastics, and rubber. Also used in the manufacturing of detergents, pharmaceuticals, explosives, and dyestuffs
Chlorobenzene	Used in the manufacture of dyestuffs and pesticides
Chloroform	Used as a solvent; widely distributed in atmosphere and water
Ethylbenzene	Used as a solvent and in the manufacture of styrene-related products; emitted vapors at filling stations and from motor vehicles
Formaldehyde	Used in particleboard, insulation (UFFI), mobile homes
m-/p-Xylene and o-Xylene	Used as solvents, as constituents of paint, lacquers, varnishes, inks, dyes, adhesives, cement, and aviation fluids. Also used in the manufacture of perfumes, insect repellants, pharmaceuticals, and the leather industry
Perchloroethylene	Used in dry cleaning
Styrene	At high temperature becomes a plastic; used in the manufacture of resins, polyesters, insulators, and in drug manufacturing
Tetrachloroethylene	Used as a solvent and in degreasing and dry cleaning
Toluene	Used in the manufacture of benzene, as a solvent for paints and coatings, or as a component of car and aviation fuels
Trichloroethylene	Used as a solvent in vapor degreasing. Used for extracting caffeine from coffee, as a dry-cleaning agent, and as an intermediate in production of pesticides, waxes, gums, resins, tars, and paints

∎ Clinical Effects

Combustion Products

The effects of exposure to CO are discussed in Chapter 7.

Exposure to high levels of NO_2 and SO_2 may result in acute muco-cutaneous irritation and respiratory effects. The relatively low water solubility of NO_2 results in minimal mucous membrane irritation of the upper airway; the principal site of toxicity is the lower respiratory tract.[10] In contrast, the high water solubility of SO_2 makes it extremely irritating to the eyes and upper respiratory tract. Whether exposure to the relatively low levels of these gases attained in houses is associated with any health effects remains to be determined.

Exposure to inhalable particles in wood smoke may result in irritation and inflammation of the upper and lower respiratory tract resulting in rhinitis, cough, wheezing, and worsening of asthma.[11-13]

Volatile Organic Compounds

Exposure to VOCs may result in dermal, mucocutaneous, and non-specific effects.[14]

Depending on the dominant compounds and route and level of exposure, signs and symptoms may include upper respiratory tract and eye irritation, rhinitis, nasal congestion, rash, pruritus, headache, nausea, and vomiting.[15-17]

Volatile organic compounds have only recently attracted study, and studies are ongoing to determine which VOCs are associated with specific health effects.[18]

The effects of exposure to formaldehyde have received more attention. Exposure to airborne formaldehyde may result in conjunctival and upper respiratory tract irritation (ie, burning or tingling sensations in eyes, nose, and throat); these symptoms are temporary and resolve with cessation of exposure.[19,20] Formaldehyde may exacerbate asthma in some infants and children,[21,22] and has been linked to nasopharyngeal cancer in occupationally exposed adults.[23]

Molds

The clinical effects of exposure to molds may be allergic or toxic. Some children who are exposed to molds have persistent upper respiratory tract symptoms such as rhinitis, sneezing, eye irritation, as well as lower respiratory tract symptoms such as coughing and wheezing.[24-26]

Toxic effects of molds may be due to inhalation of mycotoxins, lipid-soluble toxins readily absorbed by the airways.[27] Species of mycotoxin-producing molds include *Fusarium, Trichoderma,* and *Stachybotrys.* Exposure to *Stachybotrys* and other molds has been associated with acute pulmonary hemorrhage among young infants in Cleveland.[28-31]

■ Diagnostic Methods

If CO poisoning is suspected, a carboxyhemoglobin level should be promptly measured (see Chapter 7).

For an indoor air pollution-related respiratory illness, a specific etiology may be difficult to establish because most respiratory signs and symptoms are nonspecific and may occur only in association with significant exposures. Effects of lower exposures may be milder and more vague. Furthermore, signs and symptoms in infants and children may be atypical. Multiple pollutants may be involved in a given situation. Establishing the environmental cause of a given respiratory illness is further complicated by the similarity of effects to those associated with allergies and respiratory infections. Clinicians should be aware of whether their patients live in mobile homes or new houses, or burn wood.

Combustion Products
Use of space heaters, kerosene lamps or heaters, and gas ovens or ranges as home heating devices should raise concerns about exposure to combustion products, particularly if there is any indication that appliances may not be properly vented to the outside, or that heating equipment may be in disrepair. Burning wood indoors in a wood stove or fireplace may suggest the source of a respiratory problem.

Volatile Organic Compounds
Several questions may help to identify potential exposure. These include: Does the family live in a new home with large amounts of pressed wood products? Is there new pressed wood furniture? Have household members recently worked on craft or graphic materials? Are chemical cleaners used extensively? Has remodeling recently been done? Has anyone recently used paints, solvents, or sprays in the home? Do the child's symptoms clear when he is removed from

the home and reappear when he returns?

Molds and Mycotoxins

Several questions may help to identify exposure to molds. They include: Has the home been flooded? Is there any water-damaged wood or cardboard in the house? Has there been a roof or plumbing leak? Have occupants seen any mold or noticed a musty smell? Testing the environment for specific molds is usually not necessary. There is currently no diagnostic test for mycotoxins in human tissue.

∎ Treatment

Clinical symptoms due to exposure to indoor air pollutants are usually acute, short-lived, and cease with elimination of exposure. Treatment of most indoor air pollution related illnesses includes relief of symptoms and elimination of the pollution source. Children with persistent respiratory symptoms may require evaluation for possible infection, allergy, and asthma.

∎ Prevention of Exposure

Combustion Products

Measures that may help to minimize exposure include periodic professional inspection and maintenance of furnaces, gas water heaters, and clothes dryers, venting such equipment directly to the outdoors, and regular cleaning and inspection of fireplaces and wood stoves. Charcoal (in a hibachi or grill) should never be burned indoors.

Volatile Organic Compounds

Prevention strategies include increasing ventilation and avoiding storage of opened containers of unused paints and similar materials within the home. If formaldehyde is thought to be the cause of the problem, the source should be identified, and, if possible, removed. Measuring levels of formaldehyde in the air is usually not necessary. If it is not possible to remove the source, the exposure can be reduced by coating cabinets, paneling, and other furnishings with polyurethane or other nontoxic sealants, and by increasing the amount of ventilation in the home. Formaldehyde concentrations decrease rapidly over the first year after a product is manufactured.

Molds

Prevention strategies include cleaning up water and removing all water-damaged items (including carpets) within 24 hours of a flood or leak. If this is done, toxic mold will not have the opportunity to grow. If some mold is already present, the affected area needs to be washed with soap and water, followed with a solution of 1 part bleach to 4 parts water. Protective gloves should be worn during clean up.

▌ Frequently Asked Questions

Q *What are the most important things I can do to protect my child from indoor air pollution?*

A Do not smoke. Preventing children from being exposed to environmental tobacco smoke is important. Keep your home dry. Wood stoves and fireplaces need to be checked yearly by a professional to make sure they are clean and running efficiently. Gas ovens should not be used to provide supplemental heat. Children should not come into contact with mothballs because they contain dangerous chemicals.

Q *My child has had a persistent runny nose. Could this be due to the new carpet we installed last month?*

A The symptom could be due to viruses, bacteria, or allergies. It is also possible that the symptoms relate to something in the child's environment such as environmental tobacco smoke or the chemical compounds released from a new carpet. Sometimes an exact diagnosis is difficult to determine. Symptoms from colds are temporary, and symptoms from environmental irritants tend to improve once exposure to the irritant is eliminated. If possible, have the child play and sleep in another room to see if symptoms improve. It may take some time to determine the cause of the child's symptoms.

Q *Are air fresheners dangerous?*

A Currently no information indicates that air fresheners are dangerous. However, the long-term effects have not been studied.

Q *My child's asthma inhaler contains chlorofluorocarbons (CFCs). Does this harm him?*
A Using an inhaler that contains CFCs does not harm the child's health. However, CFCs harm the environment by contributing to the depletion of the stratospheric ozone layer. The EPA has mandated that CFCs be phased out over the next several years as replacement products become available.

Q *What are the effects of exposure to mothballs?*
A Two products, p-dichlorobenzene (PDCB) and naphthalene, are used as moth repellents. Reports of occupational exposure to the active ingredients of mothballs are available. Studies documenting health effects from residential exposure are limited. The active ingredient in mothballs is usually PDCB. Exposure to PDCB may cause irritation of the eyes, nose, and throat, periorbital swelling, headache, and rhinitis, which usually subside 24 hours after cessation of exposure. Prolonged occupational exposure to PDCB may result in anorexia, nausea, vomiting, weight loss, and liver damage. A case of allergic purpura induced by PDCB has been reported.

Naphthalene may also be used as a moth repellent. Exposure to large amounts of naphthalene may result in hemolytic anemia, resulting in jaundice and hemoglobinuria in children with glucose-6-phosphate dehydrogenase deficiency. Nausea, vomiting, and diarrhea may also occur.

Q *What can be done to reduce the levels of particulates from wood stoves and fireplaces?*
A Measures to reduce the levels of particulate matter from a wood stove include ensuring that the stove is placed in a room with adequate ventilation and properly vented directly to the outdoors. Newer stoves are designed to emit less particulate matter into the air.

Q *What are ionizers and other ozone-generating air cleaners? Should they be used?*
A Ion generators act by charging the particles in a room so that they are attracted to walls, floors, tabletops, draperies, or occupants. Abrasion can result in resuspension of these particles into the air. In some cases these devices contain a collector to attract

the charged particles back to the unit. While ion generators may remove small particles (eg, those in tobacco smoke), they do not remove gases or odors and may be relatively ineffective in removing large particles such as pollen and house dust allergens. Ozone generators are specifically designed to release ozone in order to purify the air.

Ozone is produced indirectly by ion generators and some electronic air cleaners and produced directly by ozone generators. While indirect ozone production is of concern, there is even greater concern with the direct and purposeful introduction of ozone into indoor air. No difference exists, despite the claims of some marketers, between ozone in smog outdoors and ozone produced by ozone generators. Under certain conditions, these devices can produce levels of ozone high enough to be harmful to a child. They are not recommended for use in homes or schools.

Q *Can other air cleaners help?*

A Other air cleaners include mechanical filter, electronic (eg, electrostatic precipitators), and hybrid air cleaners utilizing two or more techniques. The value of any air cleaner depends on its efficiency, proper selection for the pollutant to be removed, proper installation, and appropriate maintenance. Drawbacks include inadequate pollutant removal, redispersement of pollutants, deceptive masking of the pollutant rather than its removal, generation of ozone, and unacceptable noise levels. The EPA and CPSC have not taken a position either for or against the use of these devices.

Effective control at the source of a pollutant is key. Air cleaners are not a solution but are adjunct to source control and adequate ventilation. The National Heart, Lung and Blood Institute recommends that a good filter be installed in furnaces.

Q *When I bring clothes home from the dry cleaners, are the chemicals that are released from the clothes dangerous to my child?*

A A very small amount of the chemicals used in the dry cleaning process will be released from clothes. The quantity is probably not significant enough to cause health problems in a child. Of more concern is whether the home is located directly above or adjacent to a dry cleaning establishment. If so, the amount of daily exposure may be enough to cause health concerns.

Q *Can carpet exposure make people sick?*

A New carpet may emit VOCs, as do products that accompany carpet installation such as adhesives and padding. Some people report symptoms such as eye, nose, and throat irritation; headaches; skin irritation; shortness of breath or cough; and fatigue, which they may associate with new carpet installation. Carpet can also act as a "sink" for chemical and biological pollutants including pesticides, dust mites, and molds.

Anyone involved in purchasing new carpet should ask retailers for information to help them select lower emitting carpet, padding, and adhesives. Before new carpet is installed, the retailer should unroll and air out the carpet in a clean, well-ventilated area. Opening doors and windows reduces the level of chemicals released. Ventilation systems should be in proper working order and operated during installation, and for 48 to 72 hours after the new carpet is installed.

Q *Can plants control indoor air pollution?*

A Reports in the media and promotions by representatives of the decorative houseplant industry characterize plants as "nature's clean air machine," claiming that National Aeronautics and Space Administration research shows plants remove indoor air pollutants. While it is true that plants remove carbon dioxide from the air, and the ability of plants to remove certain other pollutants from water is the basis for some pollution control methods, the ability of plants to control indoor air pollution is less well established. The only available study of the use of plants to control indoor air pollutants in an actual building could not determine any benefit from the use of plants. As a practical means of pollution control, the plant removal mechanisms appear to be inconsequential when compared with common ventilation and air exchange rates. Overdamp planter soil conditions may promote growth of molds.

Q *How do I keep my fireplace safe?*

A The box lists measures to increase fireplace safety.

Fireplace Safety
1. If possible, keep a window cracked open while the fire is burning.
2. Be certain the damper or flue is open before starting a fire. Keeping the damper or flue open until the fire is out will draw smoke out of the house. The damper can be checked by looking up into the chimney with a flashlight.
3. Use dry and well-aged wood. Wet or green wood causes more smoke and contributes to soot buildup in the chimney.
4. Smaller pieces of wood placed on a grate burn faster and produce less smoke.
5. Levels of ash at the base of the fireplace should be kept to 1 inch or less because a thicker layer restricts the air supply to logs, resulting in more smoke.
6. The chimney should be checked annually by a professional. Even if the chimney is not due for cleaning, it is important to check for animal nests or other blockages that could prevent smoke from escaping.

▌Resources

For information on how to deal with known or suspected adverse effects from indoor air pollution, contact the US EPA Indoor Air Quality Information Clearinghouse (800/438-4318) or the American Lung Association (800-LUNG-USA). Additional resources include EPA regional offices, and state and local departments of health and environmental quality. For information on particular product hazards, contact the US Consumer Product Safety Commission (800/638-CPSC); and on regulation of specific pollutants, contact the EPA Toxic Substances Control Act (TSCA) Assistance Information Service (202/554-1404).

∎ References

1. Spengler JD. Sources and concentrations of indoor air pollution. In: *Indoor Air Pollution. A Health Perspective.* Samet JM, Spengler JD; eds. Baltimore, MD: The John Hopkins University Press; 1991

2. US Environmental Protection Agency. Indoor air pollution: an introduction for health professionals. US EPA Office of Air and Radiation. EPA 523-217/81322. Washington, DC: US Government Printing Office; 1994

3. Lambert WE, Samet JM. Indoor air pollution. In: *Occupational and Environmental Respiratory Disease.* Harber P, Schenker MB, Balmes JR, eds. St Louis, Mo: Mosby 1996;784-807

4. Wallace LA. Volatile organic compounds. In: *Indoor Air Pollution: A Health Perspective.* Samet JM, Spengler JD, eds. Baltimore, MD: John Hopkins University Press; 1991; 252-272

5. Molhave L. Indoor air pollution due to organic gases and vapours of solvents in building materials. *Environ Int.* 1982;8:117-127

6. Wallace LA. Human exposure to environmental pollutants: a decade of experience. *Clin Exp Allergy.* 1995;25:4-9

7. Ott WR, Roberts JW. Everyday exposure to toxic pollutants. *Sci Am.* 1998;278:86-91

8. Wallace LA. Comparison of risks from outdoor and indoor exposure to toxic chemicals. *Environ Health Perspect.* 1991;95:7-13

9. American Academy of Pediatrics, Committee on Environmental Health. Toxic effects of indoor molds. *Pediatrics.* 1998;101:712-714

10. Samet JM, Lambert WE, Skipper BJ, et al. Nitrogen dioxide and respiratory illnesses in infants. *Am Rev Respir Dis.* 1993;148:1258-1265

11. Robin LF, Lees PS, Winget M, et al. Wood-burning stoves and lower respiratory illnesses in Navajo children. *Pediatr Infect Dis J.* 1996;15:859-865

12. Honicky RE, Osborne JS. Respiratory effects of wood heat: clinical observations and epidemiologic assessment. *Environ Health Perspect.* 1991;95:105-109

13. Morris K, Morgenlander M, Coulehan JL, Gahagen S, Arena VC. Wood-burning stoves and lower respiratory tract infection in American Indian Children. *Am J Dis Child.* 1990;144:105-108

14. Norback D, Torgen M, Edling C. Volatile organic compounds, respirable dust, and personal factors related to prevalence and incidence of sick building syndrome in primary schools. *Br J Ind Med.* 1990;47:733-741

15. Gold DR. Indoor air pollution. *Clin Chest Med.* 1992;13:215-229

16. Wieslander G, Norback D, Bjornsson E, Janson C, Boman G. Asthma and the indoor environment: the significance of emission of formaldehyde and volatile organic compounds from newly painted indoor surfaces. *Int Arch Occup Environ Health.* 1997;69:115-124

17. Norback D, Bjornsson E, Janson C, Widstrom J, Boman G. Asthmatic symptoms and volatile organic compounds, formaldehyde, and carbon dioxide in dwellings. *Occup Environ Med.* 1995;52:388-395

18. Jo WK, Weisel CP, Lioy PJ. Chloroform exposure and the health risk associated with multiple uses of chlorinated tap water. *Risk Anal.* 1990;10:581-585

19. Wantke F, Demmer CM, Tappler P, Gotz M, Jarisch R. Exposure to gaseous formaldehyde induces IgE-mediated sensitization to formaldehyde in school children. *Clin Exp Allergy.* 1996;26:276-280

20. Liu KS, Huang FY, Hayward SB, Wesolowski J, Sexton K. Irritant effects of formaldehyde exposure in mobile homes. *Environ Health Perspect.* 1991;94:91-94

21. Krzyzanowski M, Quackenboss JJ, Lebowitz MD. Chronic respiratory effects of indoor formaldehyde exposure. *Environ Res.* 1990;52:117-125

22. Smedje G, Norback D, Edling C. Asthma among secondary school children in relation to the school environment. *Clin Exp Allergy.* 1997;27:1270-1278

23. West S, Hildesheim A, Dosemeci M. Non-viral risk factors for nasopharyngeal carcinoma in the Philippines: results from a case-control study. *Int J Cancer.* 1994;58:722-727

24. Dales RE, Zwanenburg H, Burnett R, Franklin CA. Respiratory health effects of home dampness and molds among Canadian children. *Am J Epidemiol.* 1991;134:196-203

25. Jaakkola JJK, Jaakkola N, Ruotsalainen R. Home dampness and molds as determinants of respiratory symptoms and asthma in pre-school children. *J Expo Anal Environ Epidemiol.* 1993;3(suppl):129-142

26. Verhoeff AP, ven Strien RT, van Wijnen JH, Brunekreef B. Damp housing and childhood respiratory symptoms: the role of sensitization to dust mites and molds. *Am J Epidemiol.* 1995;141:103-110

27. Croft WA, Jarvis BB, Yatawara CS. Airborne outbreak of trichothecene toxicosis. *Atmos Environ.* 1986;20:549-552

28. Centers for Disease Control and Prevention. Update: pulmonary hemorrhage/hemosiderosis among infants—Cleveland, Ohio, 1993—1996. *MMWR Morb Mortal Wkly Rep.* 1997;46:33-35

29. Montaña E, Etzel RA, Allan T, Horgan TE, Dearborn DG. Environmental risk factors associated with pediatric idiopathic pulmonary hemorrhage and hemosiderosis in a Cleveland community. *Pediatrics.* 1997;99:E5. Available at: http://www.pediatrics.org/cgi/content/full/99/1/e5

30. Etzel RA, Montaña E, Sorenson WG, et al. Acute pulmonary hemorrhage in infants associated with exposure to *Stachybotrys atra* and other fungi. *Arch Pediatr Adolesc Med.* 1998;152:757-762

31. Jarvis BB, Sorenson WG, Hintikka EL, et al. Study of toxin production by isolates of *Stachybotrys chartarum* and *Memnoniella echinata* isolated during a study of pulmonary hemosiderosis in infants. *Appl Environ Microbiol.* 1998;64: 3620-3625

14 Lead

C hildhood lead toxicity has been recognized for at least 100 years. With the accumulation of better epidemiologic and toxicologic data, understanding of the nature of the condition has steadily changed. As recently as the 1940s, it was believed that children who had experienced lead poisoning and did not die during the acute toxic episode had no residual effects from the event. After pediatricians recognized the high prevalence of learning and behavior disorders in children who recovered from acute toxicity, it was believed that only children with frank symptoms suffered neurobehavioral deficits. In the 1970s and 1980s, studies worldwide demonstrated that some asymptomatic children with elevated levels of lead had lower IQ scores, more language difficulties, attention problems, and behavior disorders.[1]

With better epidemiologic studies, the definition of a harmful level of lead has changed dramatically. As recently as 1970, children with blood lead levels less than 60 µg/dL were considered healthy. The US Environmental Protection Agency (EPA)[2] and the Agency for Toxic Substances and Disease Registry (ATSDR)[3] have asserted that toxicity in children may begin at less than 10 µg/dL. The definition of the lead level of concern continues to change as new data emerge.

The past 20 years have witnessed a remarkable decline in childhood exposure to lead in the United States.[4,5] On the basis of data from the National Health and Nutrition Examination Survey (NHANES III), blood lead levels have fallen by more than 80% as a result of public health efforts to reduce lead in air, water, and food. In 1991–1994 the average blood lead level in American children was 2 to 4 µg/dL.[6,7] The prevalence of blood lead levels 10 µg/dL or greater in 1991–1994 was approximately 4.4%, meaning that an estimated 890,000 children in the United States had blood lead levels 10 µg/dL or greater.

Human activity has concentrated lead in the biosphere. Natural concentrations of lead in soil, air, and water are extremely low. With the removal of lead from gasoline beginning in the mid-1970s, airborne lead concentrations dropped, and a reduction in the average blood lead levels followed. In the United States, airborne lead is now a hazard only to those who live close to smelters that use or produce lead-containing materials. Lead in paint is currently the most important threat for children. Use of high concentrations of lead in paint decreased markedly after 1946. Although use of lead in paint intended for household use has been almost eliminated since 1977, many houses continue to have surfaces that contain lead. Approximately 70% of the houses built before 1980 contain some lead-based paint. There are about 2 to 3 million housing units in the United States built before 1950 in which children live with deteriorated lead paint.[8,9] These children are at the highest risk for lead poisoning.

■ Routes of Exposure

Children are most often exposed to lead through the unintentional ingestion of lead-containing particles such as dust, paint, water, soil, or foreign bodies. However, lead can be absorbed from the pulmonary tract if inhaled as fumes or respirable particles. Table 14.1 lists risk factors for lead exposure and prevention strategies.

■ Systems Affected

The mechanisms by which lead interferes with function are manifold. Lead binds tightly to sulfhydryl groups, altering the structure and function of many proteins. As a result, the activity of many enzymes is altered. Many of these changes occur at extremely low concentrations of lead. Porphobilinogen synthetase, an enzyme important in heme synthesis, is extremely sensitive to lead.[10] Other enzymes affected are guanine hydroxylase, ferrochelatase, and 5¹ pyrimidine nucleotidase.[11]

In addition to its actions in the central nervous system, lead is concentrated in the kidney and at high concentrations may produce Fanconi syndrome.[12] Chronic lead poisoning is associated with gouty nephropathy and renal failure in adults, although there are no cases reported in children. Effects of lead on myocardial excitability[13] and thyroid function have been reported.[14]

Table 14.1. Risk Factors for Lead Exposure and Prevention Strategies

Risk Factor	Prevention Strategy
Environmental	
Paint	Identify and abate
Dust	Wet mop, frequent hand washing
Soil	Restrict play in area, ground cover, frequent hand washing
Drinking water	2-min flush of water faucet in the morning; use of cold water for cooking and drinking
Folk remedies	Avoid use
Old ceramic or pewter cookware, old urns/kettles	Avoid use
Some imported cosmetics, toys, crayons	Avoid use
Parental occupations	Remove work clothing at work
Hobbies	Proper use, storage, and ventilation
Home renovation	Proper containment, ventilation
Buying or renting a new home	Inquire about lead hazards
Host	
Hand-to-mouth activity (or pica)	Frequent hand washing
Inadequate nutrition	High iron and calcium, low-fat diet
Developmental disabilities	Frequent screening

■ Clinical Effects

Children with extremely high concentrations of lead in their blood (generally >60 µg/dL) may complain of headaches, abdominal pain, loss of appetite, constipation, and display clumsiness, agitation, or decreased activity and somnolence. These are premonitory symptoms of central nervous system involvement and may rapidly proceed to vomiting, stupor, and convulsions. Symptomatic lead toxicity should be treated as an emergency. Fortunately, this is a rare event. Because symptoms may be nonspecific (malaise or irritability) or nonexistent at lesser concentrations of blood lead, the diagnosis of lead intoxication in these children depends on the measurement of blood lead.

■ Subclinical Effects

Many studies in the 1970s and 1980s of children in the United States, Europe, and Scandinavia demonstrated that having elevated amounts of lead in the blood or deciduous teeth, in the absence of any symptoms, was associated with lower IQ scores and behavioral changes.[1] Lead also affects behavior in school. Teachers reported that students with elevated tooth lead levels were more inattentive, hyperactive, disorganized, and less able to follow directions than those without elevated levels of lead.[15-17] In epidemiologic studies of large populations, elevated lead levels have been found to be associated with decreased growth,[18] decreased hearing acuity,[19] and elevated blood pressure.[20] Most recently, elevated bone lead concentrations were reported to be associated with increased attentional dysfunction, aggression, and delinquency.[21]

■ Diagnostic Measures

Lead poisoning can be confirmed only through direct measurement of lead by capillary (fingerstick) sampling or venipuncture. Venipuncture is the preferred method, although capillary sampling, when properly performed, may approach the same level of accuracy as venipuncture.[22] Bone lead measurements are currently not available for clinical assessment.

∎ Management of Clinical and Low Level Lead Toxicity

Currently, a blood lead concentration of 20 µg/dL requires a medical evaluation[5] (See Table 14.2). Proper management includes finding and eliminating the source of the lead, instruction in proper hygienic measures (both personal and household), optimizing the child's diet, and close follow-up by the pediatrician.

Table 14.2. Clinical Evaluation

Medical history

Ask about:

• Symptoms

• Developmental history

• Mouthing activities

• Pica

• Previous blood lead levels measurements

• Family history of lead poisoning

Environmental history

Ask about:

• Age, condition, and ongoing remodeling of repainting of primary residence and other places that the child spends time (including secondary homes and child care settings).

• Determine whether the child may be exposed to lead-based paint hazards at any or all of these places.

• Occupational and hobby histories of adults with whom the child spends time. Determine whether the child is being exposed to lead from an adult's workplace or hobby.

• Other local sources of potential lead exposure.

Nutritional history

• Take a dietary history.

• Evaluate the child's iron status using appropriate laboratory tests.

• Ask about history of food stamps or WIC participation.

Physical examination

• Pay particular attention to the neurologic examination and to the child's psychosocial and language development.

Successful therapy depends on eliminating the child's exposure to lead. Any treatment regimen that does not eliminate exposure is considered inadequate. A thorough investigation of the child's environment and lifestyle for sources of lead should be conducted. In addition to paint, diet, water supply, tableware, and foods from cans with soldered seams should be evaluated. Other rare sources include cosmetics such as surma and kohl, used by many of Asian or Arabic origin. Some dietary supplements of calcium such as bone meal and ground oyster shell may have high amounts of lead. Lead exposure of parents in the workplace has caused elevated blood lead levels in their children, as have certain activities such as reloading ammunition in the home, casting toy soldiers, or construction of stained glass windows. Children who live near a smelter that uses or produces lead-containing materials may be exposed to lead in the air and the soil. In this environment, children who bite their nails or suck their thumbs may absorb a considerable amount of lead. Specific attention should be paid to treating iron deficiency and to assuring adequate calcium and zinc intake.[23]

If the blood lead level is greater than 45 µg/dL and the chain of exposure has been interrupted, treatment with a chelating agent such as succimer should begin. A pediatrician experienced in managing children with lead poisoning should be consulted. Successful therapy depends on providing a lead-free environment and maintaining the child's medication regimen.[24] A brief hospital stay for 2 to 3 days may be worthwhile to obtain baseline data and ensure regimen compliance. At this time, baseline hepatocellular enzymes, a complete blood count, and differential should be obtained; the first dose of succimer should be given while the parent observes the procedure; and the parent should administer the subsequent three doses of succimer under physician supervision. The initial dose is 30 mg/kg every 24 hours, divided into 3 doses. The dose is calculated to the nearest 100 mg, and the 100-mg capsules are emptied into palatable foods such as jello, peanut butter, or applesauce (the capsules dissolve in warm water). This regimen is continued for 5 days. The dose is then reduced to 20 mg/kg every 24 hours for an additional 14 days. Hepatocellular enzymes and a complete blood count should be obtained on the fourth day after the initial dose and at the conclusion of the course of therapy.

The most common side effects of succimer are abdominal distress, a transient rash, elevated hepatocellular enzyme levels, and neutropenia. If side effects occur, the drug treatment should be stopped and then cautiously resumed after the side effects abate. If the side effects do not recur, treatment may be completed.

Calcium disodium EDTA is an alternative therapy for a child whose blood lead level is greater than 45 µg/dL. It should be given intravenously at a dose of 35 to 50 mg/kg per day in a dextrose and saline solution at a concentration not greater than 0.5%. The drug is administered for 3 to 5 days.

If a child is symptomatic or the blood lead level is greater than 70 µg/dL, treatment should be urgently started with EDTA and dimercaprol (BAL). Dimercaprol is given intramuscularly at a dose of 15 to 25 mg/kg per day in four doses. Iron therapy should be withheld while BAL is administered.

Management of lead encephalopathy should only be undertaken in consultation with experienced pediatric intensivists. The patient's fluid intake should be restricted to reduce intracranial pressure while maintaining adequate perfusion of the kidneys for lead excretion.

∎ Persistence of Lead Effects

The early effects of untreated lead exposure during childhood may be permanent. An 11-year follow-up of children from Massachusetts demonstrated that having high levels of lead in deciduous teeth was associated with a much higher rate of failure to graduate from high school, reading disabilities, greater absenteeism in the final year of high school, and other behavioral deficits when compared with those without high levels of lead.[25] These data indicate that lead exposure may interfere with a child's chances for success in life.

∎ Screening for Elevated Blood Lead Levels

The Centers for Disease Control and Prevention (CDC) has proposed a basis for state and local public health authorities to decide on appropriate lead screening policies using local blood lead level data and/or housing data collected by the US Bureau of the Census.[26, 27] Universal screening is encouraged for communities with 27% or more of the housing built before 1950 and in populations in which the percentage of 1- and 2-year-olds with elevated blood lead levels is 12% or more. In areas that have a lower prevalence of elevated blood lead levels or homes built before 1950, targeted (selective) screening is appropriate. In areas in which targeted screening is recommended, the pediatrician's focus should be on children who are at risk: (1) children in the first and second year of life who live in housing built prior to 1950; (2) children living in poverty; (3) children who may be exposed to lead-containing folk remedies; (4) children with developmental delay whose oral behaviors place them at risk; (5) victims of abuse or neglect; (6) children whose parents are exposed to lead; and (7) immigrant children, including adoptees. The determination of which children should be screened can also be based on the parent's response to a personal-risk questionnaire (see Table 14.3).

Follow-up should be dictated by the measurement result (see Table 14.4).

Table 14.3. A Basic Personal-Risk Questionnaire*

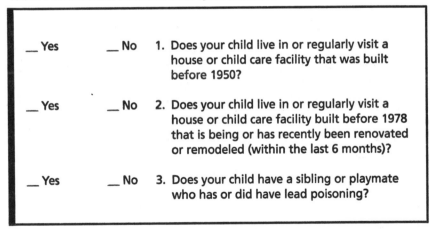

__ Yes	__ No	1. Does your child live in or regularly visit a house or child care facility that was built before 1950?
__ Yes	__ No	2. Does your child live in or regularly visit a house or child care facility built before 1978 that is being or has recently been renovated or remodeled (within the last 6 months)?
__ Yes	__ No	3. Does your child have a sibling or playmate who has or did have lead poisoning?

*Adapted from reference 26.

If the answers to the questions are "no," then a screening test is not required, although the pediatrician should explain why the questions were asked to reinforce anticipatory guidance. If the answer to one or more questions is "yes" or "not sure," a screening test should be considered.

The state or local health department may recommend alternative or additional questions based on local conditions.

Table14.4. Recommended Follow-up Actions, According to Diagnostic Blood Lead Level*

Blood Lead Level (µg/dL)	Actions
<10	No action required
10-14	Obtain a confirmatory venous BLL within 1 month; if still within this range, • Provide education to decrease lead exposure • Repeat BLL test within 3 months
15-19	Obtain a confirmatory venous BLL within 1 month; if still within this range, • Take a careful environmental history • Provide education to decrease lead exposure and to decrease lead absorption • Repeat BLL test within 2 months
20-44	Obtain a confirmatory venous BLL within 1 week; if still within this range, • Conduct a complete medical history (includng an environmental evaluation and nutritional assessment) and physical examination • Provide education to decrease lead exposure and to decrease lead absorption • Either refer the patient to the local health department or provide case management that should include a detailed environmental investigation with lead hazard reduction and appropriate referrals for support services • If BLL >25 µg/dL, consider chelation (not currently recommended for BLLs <45 µg/dL), after consultation with clinicians experienced in lead toxicity treatment
45-69	Obtain a confirmatory venous BLL within 2 days; if still within this range, • Conduct a complete medical history (including an environmental evaluation and nutritional assessment) and a physical examination • Provide education to decrease lead exposure and to decrease lead absorption • Either refer the patient to the local health department or provide case management that should include a detailed environmental investigation with lead hazard reduction and appropriate referrals for support services • Begin chelation therapy in consultation with clinicians experienced in lead toxicity therapy
>70	Hospitalize the patient and begin medical treatment immediately in consultation with clinicians experienced In lead toxicity therapy. • Obtain a confirmatory BLL immediately • The rest of the management should be as noted for management of children with BLLs between 45 and 69 µg/dL

■ Frequently Asked Questions

Q *How do I know if my child needs to have a blood lead screening test?*

A The need for your child to be screened is based on criteria provided by the health department (either state or local). These criteria include:

- Residence in a high-risk neighborhood
- Membership in a subpopulation that is at an increased risk of lead exposure
- Answers to a personal-risk questionnaire. Such a questionnaire would be developed by the health department and be based on local risks of lead exposure.

Q *Do all young children living in housing constructed before 1950 need to have a blood lead screening test?*

A It depends on how the home is maintained. Poorly maintained older housing may be the best predictor of elevated blood lead levels in young children. Most dangerous are the homes constructed before 1950 with decaying or deteriorating lead paint However, if older housing is well maintained, the risk of exposure to lead is not as great.

Q *We have imported ceramic dishes. Is it safe to use them?*

A Some imported ceramic dishes contain lead. Such dishes should not be used to serve acidic substances, since the acids can leach large amounts of lead from the dishes into the food.

Q *We have vinyl miniblinds. Should I get rid of them?*

A In the mid-1990s, some imported, non-glossy vinyl miniblinds were found to contain lead. Sunlight and heat can break down the blinds and may release lead-contaminated dust. Children who touch these miniblinds and put their fingers in their mouths may ingest small amounts of lead. If you purchase new miniblinds, look for products with labels that say "New Formulation" or "non-leaded formula."

Q *Can food be a source of lead?*

A Occasionally lead may contaminate food. Soil lead is taken up by root vegetables and atmospheric lead may fall onto leafy vegetables. Cans with soldered seams can also add lead to foods. In the United States, soldered cans have largely been replaced by seamless aluminum containers, but some imported canned products and large commercial-sized cans still have lead-soldered seams.

Q *What about testing for lead in water?*

A If you have an infant and are using tap water to reconstitute infant formula, you may want to know whether your water contains lead. To help determine whether your water might contain lead, call either the EPA Safe Drinking Water Hotline at 1-800-426-4791 or your local health department to find out about testing your water.

∎ Resources

Three important resources for more information on the effects of lead exposure are as follows: the Child and Maternal Health Clearinghouse at 202/625-8410; the National Center for Environmental Health, Centers for Disease Control and Prevention at 770/488-7330; and the National Lead Information Center at 800/532-3394.

∎ References

1. National Research Council. Committe on Measuring Lead in Critical Populations. *Measuring Lead Exposure in Infants, Children, and Other Sensitive Populations.* Washington, DC: National Academy Press; 1993

2. US Environmental Protection Agency. *Air Quality Criteria for Lead.* EPA-600/8-83/028dF; 1986

3. Agency for Toxic Substances and Disease Registry. *The Nature and Extent of Lead Poisoning in Children in the United States: A Report to Congress.* Atlanta, Ga: Dept of Health and Human Services; 1988

4. Brody DJ, Pirkle JI, Kramer RA, et al. Blood lead levels in the US population: phase I of the third National Health and Nutrition Examination Survey (NHANES III, 1988 TO 1991). *JAMA.* 1994;272:277-283

5. American Academy of Pediatrics, Committee on Environmental Health. Screening for elevated blood lead levels. *Pediatrics.* 1998;101:1072-1078

6. Centers for Disease Control and Prevention. Update: blood lead levels–United States, 1991-1994. *MMWR Morb Mortal Wkly Rep.* 1997; 46:141-146

7. Centers for Disease Control and Prevention. Erratum: vol 46, no. 7. *MMWR Morb Mortal Wkly Rep.* 1997; 46:607

8. Centers for Disease Control and Prevention. *Preventing Lead Poisoning in Young Children.* October 1991

9. American Academy of Pediatrics, Committee on Environmental Health. Lead poisoning: from screening to primary prevention. *Pediatrics.* 1993;92:176-183

10. Hernberg S, Nikkanen J, Mellin G, Lilius H. Delta-aminolevulinic acid dehydrase as a measure of lead exposure. *Arch Environ Health.* 1970;21:140-145

11. Paglia DE, Valentine WN, Fink W. Lead poisoning: further observations on erythrocyte pyrimidine nucleotidase deficiency and intracellular accumulation of pyrimidine nucleotides. *J Clin Invest.* 1977;60:1362-1366

12. Chisolm JJ. Aminoaciduria as a manifestation of renal tubular injury in lead intoxication and a comparison with patterns of aminoaciduria seen in other diseases. *J Pediatr.* 1962;60:1-17

13. Silver W, Rodriguez-Torres R. Electrocardiographic studies in children with lead poisoning. *Pediatrics.* 1968;41:1124-1127

14. Huseman CA, Moriarty CM, Angle CR. Childhood lead toxicity and impaired release of thyrotropin stimulating hormone. *Environ Res.* 1987;42:524-533

15. Needleman HL, Gunnoe C, Leviton A, Peresie H, Maher C, Barret P. Deficits in psychological and classroom performance of children with elevated dentine lead levels. *N Engl J Med.* 1979;300:689-695

16. Sciarillo WG. Lead exposure and child behavior. *Am J Public Health.* 1992; 82:1356-1360

17. Lansdown R, Yule W, Urbanowicz M, Millar IB. Blood lead, intelligence, attainment and behaviour in school children: overview of a pilot study. In: Rutter M, Jones RR, eds. *Lead Versus Health.* New York, NY: John Wiley and Sons; 1983

18. Schwartz J, Angle C, Pitcher H. Relationship between childhood blood lead levels and stature. *Pediatrics.* 1986;77:281-288

19. Schwartz J, Otto D. Blood lead, hearing thresholds and neurobehavioral development in children and youth. *Arch Environ Health.* 1987;42:153-160

20. Schwartz J. The relationship between blood lead and blood pressure in the NHANES II survey. *Environ Health Persp.* 1988;78:15-22

21. Needleman HL, Riess JA, Tobin MJ, Biesecker GE, Greenhouse JB. Bone lead levels and delinquent behavior. *JAMA.* 1996;275:363-369

22. Schlenker TL, Fritz CJ, Mark D, et al. Screening for pediatric lead poisoning: comparability of simultaneously drawn capillary and venous blood samples. *JAMA.* 1994;271:1346-1348

23. Mahaffey KR. Environmental lead toxicity: nutrition as a component of intervention. *Environ Health Perspect.* 1990;89:75-78

24. American Academy of Pediatrics, Committee on Drugs. Treatment guidelines for lead exposure in children. *Pediatrics.* 1995;96:155-160

25. Needleman HL, Schell A, Bellinger D, Leviton A, Allred EN. The long-term effects of exposure to low doses of lead in childhood: an 11-year follow-up report. *N Engl J Med.* 1990;322:83-88

26. Centers for Disease Control and Prevention. *Screening Young Children for Lead Poisoning: Guidance for State and Local Public Health Officials.* November 1997

27. Harvey B. New lead screening guidelines from the Centers for Disease Control and Prevention: how will they affect pediatricians? *Pediatrics.* 1997; 100:384-388

15 Mercury

M ercury (Hg) occurs in three forms: the metallic element (Hg^0, quicksilver or elemental mercury); inorganic salts (Hg^{1+}, or mercurous salts, and Hg^{2+}, or mercuric salts); and organic compounds (methyl mercury, ethyl mercury, and phenyl mercury). Solubility, reactivity, biological effects, and toxicity vary among these forms. Mercury has been used for over 3000 years in medicine and industry.

Naturally occurring mercury sources include cinnabar (ore) and fossil fuels, such as coal and petroleum. Environmental contamination has resulted from mining, smelting, and industrial discharges. Mercury in lakes and stream sediments can be converted by bacteria into organic mercury compounds (eg, methyl mercury) that accumulate in the food chain. Consumption of fish with high levels of methyl mercury by pregnant women in Minamata Bay, Japan, in the 1950s resulted in at least 30 cases of infantile cerebral palsy.[1] To prevent this from occurring, several states have issued advisories about consumption of fish from contaminated waters (see Chapter 24). Large ocean fish, such as tuna, swordfish, and shark, may have increased methyl mercury content owing to exposure from naturally occurring sources of mercury pollution.

Elemental mercury is used in sphygmomanometers, thermometers, and thermostat switches. Dental amalgams contain mercury as well as silver and other metals. Fluorescent light bulbs (usually 2-4 foot tubes) and disc ("button") batteries also contain mercury. Indiscriminate disposal of these items is a major source of environmental mercury contamination when they are buried in landfills or burned in waste incinerators rather than recycled. Elemental mercury is also used in some folk remedies, such as those of Santeria, practiced by some groups of Hispanic Americans.

Methyl mercury has been used as a fungicide on seed grains and is an industrial waste product. When grain in Iraq treated with a mercury fungicide was accidentally eaten by people in Iraq between 1959 and 1972, mercury poisoning occurred in thousands of people.[2]

■ Routes of Exposure

Elemental Mercury

Elemental mercury is a liquid at room temperature and readily volatilizes to a colorless and odorless vapor. When inhaled, elemental mercury vapor easily passes through pulmonary alveolar membranes and enters the blood, where it distributes primarily into red blood cells and the central nervous system. In contrast, less than 0.1% of elemental mercury is absorbed from the gastrointestinal tract after ingestion, and only minimal absorption occurs with dermal exposure.[3]

Inorganic Mercury

Inorganic mercury salts are poorly absorbed after ingestion, although mercuric salts tend to be extremely caustic. Dermal exposure has resulted in toxic effects in animals. Merthiolate used to irrigate the external auditory canals in a child with tympanostomy tubes caused fatal mercury poisoning.

Organic Mercury

In general, organic mercury compounds are lipid soluble and are well absorbed from the gastrointestinal tract. Methyl mercury is essentially 100% absorbed after ingestion, contributing to concern about consumption of methyl mercury-contaminated fish.[3] Methyl mercury passes through the placenta and is excreted into breast milk. This form of mercury also is well absorbed after inhalation. Phenyl mercury is well absorbed after ingestion and dermal contact. In contrast to other organic mercury compounds, the carbon-mercury chemical bond of phenyl mercury is relatively unstable, resulting in the release of elemental mercury that can be inhaled and absorbed across pulmonary membranes.

▌ Systems Affected and Clinical Effects

Elemental Mercury

At high concentrations, mercury vapor inhalation produces an acute necrotizing bronchitis and pneumonitis, which can lead to death due to respiratory failure.[4] Fatalities have resulted from heating elemental mercury in inadequately ventilated areas.[5]

Long-term exposure to mercury vapor primarily affects the central nervous system. Early nonspecific signs include insomnia, forgetfulness, loss of appetite, and mild tremor and may be misdiagnosed as psychiatric illness. Continued exposure leads to progressive tremor and erethism, characterized by red palms, emotional lability, and memory impairment.[6-8] Salivation, excessive sweating, and hemoconcentration are accompanying autonomic signs. Mercury also accumulates in kidney tissues. Renal toxicity includes proteinuria or nephrotic syndrome, alone or in addition to other signs of mercury exposure.[9-10] Isolated renal effects may be immunologic in origin.

Mercury exposure from dental amalgams has provoked concerns about subclinical or unusual neurologic effects, ranging from such subjective complaints as chronic fatigue to demyelinating neuropathies including multiple sclerosis.[11] Although dental amalgams are a source of mercury exposure and are associated with slightly higher urinary mercury excretion, there is no scientific evidence for any measurable clinical toxic effects other than rare hypersensitivity reactions.[12-14] The United States Public Health Service concluded that dental amalgams do not pose a health risk and should not be replaced merely to reduce mercury exposure.[13]

Inorganic Salts

Mercuric bichloride (Hg^{2+}) is well described by its common name, corrosive sublimate. Ingestions are usually inadvertent or with suicidal intent, and gastrointestinal ulceration or perforation and hemorrhage are rapidly produced, followed by circulatory collapse. Breakdown of intestinal mucosal barriers leads to extensive mercury absorption and distribution to the kidneys. Acute renal toxic effects consist of proximal tubular necrosis and anuria.

Acrodynia, or childhood mercury poisoning, was frequently reported in the 1940s among infants exposed to calomel teething powders containing mercurous chloride.[15,16] Cases also have been reported in infants exposed to phenyl mercury used as a fungicidal diaper rinse[17] and in children exposed to phenyl mercuric acetate from interior latex paint.[18] Children's individual susceptibility to develop acrodynia is poorly understood, but a maculopapular rash, swollen and painful extremities, peripheral neuropathy, hypertension, and renal tubular dysfunction develop in affected children.

Organic Mercury

Organic mercury toxicity occurs with long-term exposure and affects the central nervous system. Signs progress from paresthesias to ataxia, followed by generalized weakness, visual and hearing impairment, tremor and muscle spasticity, and then coma and death. Organic mercury also is a potent teratogen, causing disruption of the normal patterns of neuronal migration and nerve cell histology in the developing brain. In the Minamata Bay disaster, with contaminated fish, and the Iraq epidemic, with contaminated seed grain, mothers who were asymptomatic or showed mild toxic effects gave birth to severely affected infants. Typically, the infants appeared normal at birth, but psychomotor retardation, blindness, deafness, and seizures developed over time.[19]

Because the fetus and infant are more susceptible to the neurotoxic effects of methyl mercury, investigators have looked for subclinical effects among children whose mothers' diets include large amounts of fish or marine mammals containing methyl mercury and whose blood mercury levels are higher than those commonly seen in the United States. There are two such longitudinal studies—one in the Seychelles (islands in the Indian Ocean about 1000 miles off the east coast of Africa), the other in the Faroes (islands off the coast of Iceland). Among 917 Faroese children evaluated at 7 years of age, higher maternal hair mercury levels were associated with deficits in language, attention, and memory.[20] However, despite similar exposures, these deficits were not seen among 711 children examined at 66 months of age in the Seychelles.[21] Further research is necessary before the clinical and public health implication of these findings are clear.

▌ Diagnostic Methods

Diagnosis of mercury poisoning is usually made by history and physical examination. In addition, laboratory tests may demonstrate elevated mercury levels. Normal blood mercury levels, however, do not exclude mercury poisoning.

Metallic Mercury

Increased mercury vapor concentrations can be measured in exhaled air from persons with dental amalgams, but the biological significance is uncertain. Also unclear is the significance of the slight increase in urinary mercury excretion detected after dental amalgams are placed.

Inorganic Mercury

Inorganic mercury exposure can be measured by urinary mercury determination, preferably using a 24-hour urine collection. Results greater than 10 to 20 µg/L are evidence of excessive exposure, and neurologic signs may be present at values greater than 100 µg/L. However, the urinary mercury concentration does not necessarily correlate with chronicity or severity of toxic effects, especially if the mercury exposure has been intermittent or variable in intensity. Whole blood mercury can be measured, but values tend to return to normal (<0.5 to 1.0 µg/dL) within 1 to 2 days after the exposure to metallic mercury vapor ends.

Organic Mercury

Organic mercury compounds concentrate in red blood cells, so whole blood may be used to diagnose excessive exposure. Blood mercury levels rarely exceed more than 1.5 µg/dL in the unexposed population, and a blood concentration of 5 µg/dL or greater is considered the threshold for symptoms of toxicity. Methyl mercury also distributes into growing hair, thus providing a noninvasive means to estimate body burden and blood concentration over time. In the general population, the mercury level in hair is usually 1 ppm or less.[22-25]

∎ Treatment

The most important and most effective treatment is to identify the mercury source and end the exposure.

Inorganic Mercury

Mercury accumulates in blood and central nervous system and renal tissues and is very slowly eliminated. Chelating agents have been used to enhance mercury elimination, but whether chelation reduces toxic effects or speeds recovery in persons who have been poisoned is unclear. Dimercaprol (BAL in oil) has been used for severe cases of inorganic mercury poisoning and can be administered to patients in renal failure because it is eliminated by hepatic excretion. d-Penicillamine is an oral chelator that enhances urinary excretion of inorganic mercury but has a 10% to 30% rate of adverse drug reactions. Newer derivatives of BAL, such as dimercaptosuccinic acid (DMSA, succimer) and 2,3-dimercaptopropane-1-sulfonate (DMPS, dimaval) have been more effective than BAL in experimental studies. Succimer, an oral chelating agent for the treatment of childhood lead poisoning, increases urinary mercury excretion, but its efficacy is uncertain and it must be considered experimental therapy for mercury poisoning. The dimaval-mercury challenge test holds great promise as a diagnostic test for mercury exposure.[26-28] Mercury poisoning should be treated in consultation with a physician experienced in managing children with mercury poisoning.

Organic Mercury

There is no chelating agent approved by the US Food and Drug Administration that is effective for methyl mercury poisoning. Dimercaprol may increase the mercury concentration in the brain and should not be used in cases of methyl mercury poisoning.[29]

Children who have had mercury poisoning should undergo periodic follow-up neurologic examinations by a pediatrician.

❚ Prevention

Many mercury compounds are no longer sold in the United States. Organic mercury fungicides, including phenyl mercury (once used in latex paints), are no longer licensed for commercial use. Electronic equipment has replaced many mercury-containing oral thermometers and sphygmomanometers in medical settings. Newer enclosed methods for preparing mercury amalgams have reduced the likelihood of mercury spillage and exposure during dental amalgam preparation. Inorganic salts have limited use as antiseptics, although merthiolate and thimerosal are still available.

The amount of mercury in thermometers is small and usually insufficient to produce clinically significant exposure. If a mercury thermometer breaks, the bead of elemental mercury should be carefully rolled onto a sheet of paper and then put in a jar or an airtight container for appropriate disposal. Use of a vacuum cleaner should be avoided because it causes elemental mercury to vaporize in the air, creating greater health risks.[30] In the event of a larger elemental mercury spill, consultation with a certified environmental cleaning company is advised. They are often listed in the telephone directory yellow pages under "environmental or ecological services."

Most regulatory standards or advisories pertain to the workplace. Nonoccupational standards have been established by the Environmental Protection Agency for drinking water (2 µg/L) and by the Food and Drug Administration for fish (1 ppm) and bottled drinking water (2 µg/L). Although the levels of mercury in commercial fish are regulated by the FDA, the federal government does not regulate the levels of mercury in fish caught for sport. Because of the potential for mercury contamination, 41 states have issued advisories recommending that the public limit or avoid consumption of certain fish caught for sport from specific bodies of water.

Although there are no regulatory standards for home air, the Agency for Toxic Substances and Disease Registry suggests that acceptable residential air mercury levels should not exceed 0.5 µg/m³.[31]

∎ Frequently Asked Questions

Q *Will toxic effects result after ingesting mercury from an oral thermometer?*

A Elemental mercury in these thermometers is poorly absorbed from the gastrointestinal tract. No treatment is needed. (The fragments of broken glass are of greater concern.)

Q *Should pregnant women or women planning pregnancy avoid eating fish?*

A There is no known risk that outweighs the benefit of eating commercially caught fish. However, the consumption of tuna, shark and swordfish should be limited. For fish that are caught from local waters, check with your state health department to find out whether pregnant women should limit their fish intake (see Chapter 24).

Q *Should my child have nonmercury fillings, or should the mercury fillings be replaced?*

A Mercury amalgams (fillings) are a durable material for filling dental caries. There is no scientific evidence that this commonly used dental material is a health hazard, although mercury exposure may occur from the presence of dental amalgams. It is not necessary to replace amalgams just because of the mercury content; furthermore, the removal process may weaken the tooth.

Q *Is it true that latex paint containing mercury can be hazardous to a child's health?*

A Before 1991, it was permissible to add phenylmercuric acetate to interior latex paint as a preservative. This is no longer permitted. Therefore, paints produced in the United States since 1991 for indoor use should not contain mercury compounds.

Since mercury is emitted from the wall in the first year after the paint is applied, there is no need to remove paint that contained mercury compounds.

Q *Someone spilled some mercury at my child's school. How should it be cleaned up?*

A It is necessary to enlist a specialist's help to clean up even small mercury spills in schools. The janitor should not vacuum it up, as this may spread the mercury aerosol. The local health department can provide the names of local environmental companies with expertise in mercury clean-up. School children should not play with the spilled mercury or take it home from the school.

Q *Do vaccines contain mercury?*

A Since the 1930s, some but not all of the vaccines routinely recommended for children have contained small amounts of thimerosal, a mercury-containing preservative. Because some infants who receive thimerosal-containing vaccines during the early months of life could be exposed to more mercury than recommended by Federal guidelines, in July 1999 the US government asked manufacturers to eliminate or reduce as expediciously as possible the mercury content of their vaccines.[32]

■ Resources

Regional poison control centers may be resources for clinical and therapeutic information about mercury poisoning. State and local public health and environmental agencies may be of assistance if a mercury spill occurs, if clinically significant poisoning is suspected, or to evaluate possible environmental exposure sources.

Environmental Protection Agency website: www.epa.gov/OST.fish/

▌ References

1. Study Group of Minamata Disease. *Minamata Disease*. Kumamato, Japan: Kumamato University; 1968

2. Bakir F, Damlugi SF, Amin-Zaki L, et al. Methylmercury poisoning in Iraq. *Science*. 1973;181:230-241

3. Clarkson TW. The pharmacology of mercury compounds. *Annu Rev Pharmacol*. 1972;12:375-406

4. Jaffe KM, Shurtleff DB, Robertson WO. Survival after acute mercury vapor poisoning. *Am J Dis Child*. 1983;137:749-751

5. Kanluen S, Gottlieb CA. A clinical pathologic study of four adult cases of acute mercury inhalation toxicity. *Arch Pathol Lab Med*. 1991;115:56-60

6. Taueg C, Sanfilippo DJ, Rowens B, Szejda J, Hesse JL. Acute and chronic poisoning from residential exposures to elemental mercury—Michigan, 1989-1990. *J Toxicol Clin Toxicol*. 1992;30:63-67

7. Fawer RF, De Ribaupierre Y, Guillemin MP, Berode M, Lob M. Measurement of hand tremor induced by industrial exposure to metallic mercury. *Br J of Ind Med*. 1983;40:204-208

8. Smith PJ, Langolf GD, Goldberg J. Effects of occupational exposure to elemental mercury on short term memory. *Br J Ind Med*. 1983;40:413-419

9. Agner E, Jans H, Mercury poisoning and nephrotic syndrome in two young siblings. *Lancet*. 1978;2:951

10. Tubbs RR, Gephardt GN, McMahon JT, Pohl MC, Vidt DG, Barenberg SA, Valenzuela R. Membranous glomerulonephritis associated with industrial mercury exposure: study of pathogenic mechanisms. *Am J Clin Pathol*. 1982;77:409-413

11. Mortensen ME. Mysticism and science: the amalgam wars. *J Toxicol Clin Toxicol*. 1991;29:vii-xii

12. Clarkson TW, Friberg L, Hursh JB, Nylander M. The prediction of intake of mercury vapor from amalgams. In: Clarkson TW, Friberg L, Nordberg GF, Sager PR, eds. *Biological Monitoring of Toxic Metals*. New York, NY: Plenum Press; 1988:247-264

13. Eley BM. The future of dental amalgam: a review of the literature. Part 4: Mercury exposure hazards and risk assessment. *Br Dent J* 1997;182:373-381

14. Eley BM. The future of dental amalgam: a review of the literature. Part 6: Possible harmful effects of mercury from dental amalgam. *Br Dent J* 1997; 182:455-459

15. Cheek DB. Acrodynia. In: Kelley V, ed. *Brenneman's Practice of Pediatrics*. vol I. New York, NY: Harper and Row Publishers; 1977; 17D:1-12

16. Warkany J. Acrodynia—postmortem of a disease. *Am J Dis Child*. 1966;112:147-156

17. Gotelli CA, Astolfi, E, Cox C, Cernichiari E, Clarkson TW. Early biochemical effects of an organic mercury fungicide on infants: "dose makes the poison." *Science*. 1985;227:638-640

18. Agocs MM, Etzel RA, Parrish RG, et al. Mercury exposure from interior latex paint. *N Engl J Med.* 1990;323:1096-1101

19. Amin-Zaki L, Majeed MA, Elhassani SB, et al. Prenatal methylmercury poisoning: clinical observations over five years. *Am J Dis Child.* 1979;133:172-177

20. Grandjean P, Weihe P, White RF, et al. Cognitive deficit in 7-year-old children with prenatal exposure to methylmercury. *Neurotoxicol Teratol.* 1997;6:417-428

21. Davidson PW, Myers GJ, Cox C, et al. Effects of prenatal and postnatal methylmercury exposure from fish consumption on neurodevelopment: Outcomes at 66 months of age in the Seychelles Child Development Study. *JAMA.* 1998;280:701-707

22. Dickman MD, Lueng CK, Leong MK. Hong Kong male subfertility links to mercury in human hair and fish. *Sci Total Environ.* 1998;214:165-174

23. Batista J, Schuhmacher M, Domingo JL, Corbella J. Mercury in hair for a child population from Tarragona Province, Spain. *Sci Total Environ.* 1996;193:143-148

24. Saeki K, Fujimoto M, Kolinjim D, Tatsukawa R. Mercury concentrations in hair from populations in Wau-Bulolo area, Papua New Guinea. *Arch Environ Contam Toxicol.* 1996;30:412-417

25. Katz SA, Katz RB. Use of hair analysis for evaluating mercury intoxication of the human body: a review. *J Appl Toxicol.* 1992;12:79-84

26. Garza-Ocanas L, Torres-Alanis O, Pineyro-Lopez A. Urinary mercury in twelve cases of cutaneous mercurous chloride (calomel) exposure: effect of sodium 2,3-dimercaptopropane-1-sulfonate (DMPS) therapy. *J Toxicol Clin Toxicol.* 1997;35:653-655

27. Hohage H, Otte B, Westermann G, Witta J, Welling U, Zidek W, Heidenreich S. Elemental mercury poisoning. *South Med J.* 1997;90:1033-1036

28. Gonzalez-Ramirez D, Zuniga-Charles M., Narro-Juarez A, Molina-Recio Y, Hurlbut KM, Dart RC, Aposhian HV. DMPS (2,3-dimercaptopropane-1-sulfonate, dimaval) decreases the body burden of mercury in humans exposed to mercurous chloride. *J Pharmacol Exp Ther.* 1998;287:8-12

29. Agency for Toxic Substances and Disease Registery. Mercury toxicity. *Am Fam Physician.* 1992;46:1731-1741

30. Bonhomme C, Gladyszaczak-Kholer J, Cadou A, Ilef D, Kadi Z. Mercury poisoning by vacuum-cleaner aerosol. *Lancet.* 1996;347:1044-1045

31. Agency for Toxic Substances and Disease Registry. Mercury toxicity. In: *Case Studies in Environmental Medicine.* vol 17. Atlanta, GA: US Public Health Service, Agency for Toxic Substances and Disease Registry; March 1992

32. American Academy of Pediatrics. Committees on Infectious Diseases and Environmental Heath. Thimerosal in vaccines: an interim report to clinicians. *Pediatrics.* 1999;104:570-574

16 Human Milk

Nursing infants feed from the top of the food chain. This exposes them to bioconcentrating pollutant chemicals, especially persistent halogenated pesticides and industrial chemicals dissolved in the fat of their mothers' milk. These residues are present in the breast milk of women without occupational or other special exposure (see Table 16.1).[1] Infant formula is free of these residues because the lipid comes from coconuts or other sources low on the food chain. Dairy cows do not have much exposure; in addition, a cow makes tons of milk during her lifetime production, keeping the concentrations of pollutants in any given volume of milk low.

Breastfeeding is good for infants. The American Academy of Pediatrics (AAP) and the World Health Organization have considered the problem of environmental contaminants in human milk and continue to recommend breastfeeding. So far, despite a literature that is now almost 50 years old, there are very few instances in which morbidity has occurred in a nursling from a pollutant chemical in milk.[2] There is good evidence that no such morbidity is occurring from the commoner and well-studied chemical agents. It is likely, nonetheless, that practitioners will be asked about this issue, and new reports of toxic chemicals found in breast milk will appear in the popular press. Thus, this chapter describes the types of chemicals that have been found in breast milk, related studies, and the likelihood of human toxicity.

For the last 4 decades, the insecticide DDT or one of its deriva-

Table 16.1. Environmental Pollutants That May Be Found in Human Milk*

Chemical Agent	Potential Health Effects
DDT, DDE	Estrogenic, antiandrogenic activity
PCB/PCDF	Ectodermal defects, developmental delay
TCDD (Dioxin)	Chloracne
Chlordane	Neurotoxicity
Heptachlor	Neurotoxicity
Hexachlorobenzene	Hypotonia, seizures, rash
Volatile organic compounds	
Tetrachloroethylene, trichloroethylene	Hepatotoxicity
Halothane	Hepatotoxicity
Carbon disulfide	Neurotoxicity
Nicotine	Neurotoxicity
Metals	
Lead	Renal, central nervous system injury
Methyl mercury	Central nervous system toxicity

*From reference 1.

tives, usually the very stable metabolite DDE, has been found in the lipid of essentially all human milk tested worldwide. Hexachlorobenzene, the cyclodiene pesticides or their metabolites, such as dieldrin, heptachlor, and chlordane, and industrial chemicals, such as polychlorinated biphenyls (PCBs) and similar compounds, have all been and, in some cases, continue to be, common contaminants.

Human milk is the major dietary source of these stable pollutants for young children. The quantities transferred, 20% or more of maternal body burden in 6 months of lactation, are much larger than children would receive otherwise and leave breastfed children with a detectable higher body burden of pollutants for years.[3]

The relatively high concentration of fat in breast milk means that fat-soluble substances will, in effect, concentrate there. The persistent fat-soluble agents that are discussed here are the best-studied human milk contaminants, but volatile organic hydrocarbons, metals, and organometals can contaminate milk, although almost always at levels that are of much less toxicologic concern than the persistent fat-soluble agents. Asbestos fibers or fine particulate air pollution are not found in human milk. Alcohol, components of tobacco smoke, and many drugs may be detected, but are not included in this discussion.

▌ Specific Agents

Dichlorodiphenyltrichloroethane (DDT) and Dichlorodiphenyldichloroethane (DDE)

Dichlorodiphenyltrichloroethane, a pesticide once used widely in the United States, was banned from manufacture in 1972, after 4 decades of extensive global use. This decision was based on, among other things, its widespread appearance in human tissue and its effects on wildlife, especially reproduction in pelagic birds. The pesticide is not acutely toxic. At extremely high doses, DDT is an excitatory neurotoxin. At much lower levels, *o,p*-DDT and DDE are weak estrogens and *p,p*-DDE is a potent antiandrogen.[4] One prospective study of more than 700 children from North Carolina measured DDE in the breast milk they were being fed; the children were followed up medically and developmentally.[5] All of the breast milk had detectable levels of DDE. No illness or lasting neurologic or developmental abnormality was related to DDE exposure; however, there was a large difference in lactation performance between women at the extremes of the DDE distribution. The 75 women with DDE levels above 5 ppm in fat had median durations of lactation of 10 weeks, whereas 259 women whose levels were below 2 ppm breastfed for 26 weeks. In a similar study of approximately 230 women in Mexico, where levels of DDE in breast milk were higher, women showed a similar decrease in the length of lactation, at least among second and later children.[6] This is plausibly related to the estrogenicity of DDE, since prolactin is inhibited peripherally by the high estrogen levels during pregnancy, and lactation is initiated at very low levels of estrogen postpartum.

Polychlorinated Biphenyls and Polychlorinated Dibenzofurans (PCDFs)

In newborns, background exposure to PCBs is associated with developmental delay and possible subclinical effects on thyroid function.[7] Prenatal exposure to PCBs from the mother's body burden, rather than exposure through breast milk, seems to account for the findings.[1]

157

No episode has occurred in which persons were exposed only to PCDFs because they appear as degradation products in used PCBs.[8] They also may contaminate the municipal and industrial solid waste; background exposure probably comes mostly from fish. With good analytical methods, PCDFs can be detected in human milk (see Chapter 21).

Chlordane

In 1970, inadvertent injection of chlordane, an organochlorine insecticide, into the heating ducts of a military home resulted in air contamination when the heat was turned on. Similar incidents happened over the next few years in homes in which drench application of chlordane was done under the slab or ditch application was done around houses with heating ducts that were either in or beneath the slab, which resulted in unacceptably high levels of chlordane in the air when the heat was used. Eventually, the US Air Force performed studies in almost 500 dwellings and found that while most homes had very little chlordane in the air, occasionally values were as high as 260 µg/m³. At the higher levels of chlordane, symptoms of irritation and a strong "organic" odor were noted by people who lived in the building. The symptoms abated and the air cleared when appropriate repairs were made. Among those women who lived in homes treated with chlordane, breast milk levels of chlordane increased during the following 5 years.[9] There are no reports of morbidity due to this exposure.

Hexachlorobenzene

The fungicide hexachlorobenzene in human milk has caused disease in nurslings. After an epidemic of hexachlorobenzene poisoning in Turkey in 1957-1959, breastfed children did not get porphyria as seen in adults, but rather *pembe yara* (pink sore), characterized by weakness, convulsions, and an annular papular rash. The case fatality rate was approximately 95%, and cohorts of children died in some of the villages. The chemical was present in human milk but not quantitated at the time; 20 years later, 20 samples had an average of 0.23 ppm of hexachlorobenzene.[10] If it is assumed that analysis was per gram of milk fat, then levels were still at about 15 times background.

Volatile Organic Compounds (VOCs)

There is a single case report of a child who developed cholestatic jaundice while being breastfed.[11] His mother lunched daily with her husband, who was a dry cleaner, and perchloroethylene was found in her milk. The child's jaundice resolved with cessation of breastfeeding. In the many years since this case was reported, there have been no other reported occurrences, and so it may have been coincidence or the levels of perchloroethylene may now be low enough so that it does not occur.

Because halothane has been detected in the milk of a lactating anesthesiologist, it may be presumed to be present in lactating women who undergo anesthesia using halothane. Volatile agents similar to anesthetic gases may be excreted through expired air, and their concentration in human milk should decline rapidly once exposure ceases. Many other commonly encountered VOCs, such as benzene, freon, and methylene chloride, have been found in breast milk, but are of no known clinical significance.

Nicotine

Nicotine, its metabolites, and probably other components of cigarette smoke appear in the milk of smokers. Smokers tend to wean early, but whether this is caused by smoking is not known. There is no evidence of an effect from breastfeeding independent of an effect from passive inhalation in the child, and there are no data on the occurrence of components of smoke in the milk of passively smoking breastfeeders.

Metals

Lead was known historically to be toxic to the nurslings of women who worked with it. Earlier this century, there may have been more lead in canned formula and evaporated milk than in breast milk, but seams in cans for food no longer contain lead. Lead levels in human milk are low, and there are no modern reports of lead toxicity in a nursed child from an asymptomatic mother. Both a mother and her child have been poisoned by a lead-containing toilet powder she used. Another child has been poisoned by nursing through a lead nipple shield.[13]

Levels of cadmium, arsenic, and metallic mercury are low in human milk. Methyl mercury, although relatively nonpolar, associates with protein and appears in milk at levels lower than those in serum. In Iraq in 1972, seed wheat treated with methyl mercury used in making bread produced levels in human milk of about 200 ppb, which is 50 to 100 times background exposure. There were thousands of cases of illness (see Chapter 15), including some that may have resulted from exposure to human milk alone. The upper end of background exposure to methyl mercury has been studied among children in the Seychelles Islands, who have relatively high dietary exposure from ocean fish but have not experienced morbidity or developmental delay attributable to methyl mercury.[14]

▌ Diagnostic Methods

Many laboratories have equipment to measure some or all of the contaminant residues in human milk. However, any such analysis must be regarded as research, because there are no standard quality assurance methods, no established normal values, and some evidence that, at least for PCBs, the variability of test results between laboratories is too great to allow a single sample to be interpretable. It is difficult to imagine a circumstance in which analysis of human milk for these chemicals would be clinically useful outside of research.

Most professional organizations, including the AAP, that have considered the issue of pollutants in human milk continue to recommend breastfeeding and do not recommend testing of breast milk.[15]

▌ Regulations

There are no regulations for human milk. Although it is tempting to apply the numbers used for infant formula, the risk benefit situation is not comparable. The alternative to contaminated formula is uncontaminated formula. There likely is no such thing as uncontaminated human milk. The most difficult situation is encountered with the persistent fat-soluble agents, because their levels in human milk have been at or near the upper regulatory allowances for formula or infant foods. For the other environmental contaminants, allowances in human milk are relatively low.

Health departments in states in which PCBs have been a problem, such as New York and the Great Lakes states, issue advisories about fish consumption and have had experience dealing with PCBs. The EPA has issued guidance for states in developing fish advisories for PCBs and other persistent contaminants.

The most important action is to eliminate exposure to persistent bioaccumulating toxic chemicals. The manufacture and use of DDT, all the cyclodienes (ie, dieldrin), and most PCBs have been stopped in the United States, but not in many other parts of the world. Since 25% of the US food supply is imported, global action is necessary.

▌ Frequently Asked Questions

Q *Should I get my breast milk tested for chemical pollutants?*
A No. Residue levels of many chemicals can be found in milk; quantitating them is difficult, and there are no programs to promote quality assurance. Even if a very good laboratory generates a result, there are no accepted normal or safe values to evaluate the results.

Q *Might an illness occurring in a breastfed child be due to a contaminant in milk?*
A Nursing infants have been poisoned by contaminant chemicals in breast milk, although in most cases the mother herself was also ill. Investigating such a case would be research and the phenomenon is so rare for environmental chemicals that it would be reportable.

Q *Would dieting during lactation increase the levels of contaminants, since the same amount of contaminants would be dissolved in a smaller amount of fat? Or would weight loss mobilize the contaminants out of fat and allow them to be excreted?*
A Very few women lose fat successfully during lactation. A weight loss of several kilograms, which might be perhaps one-third or less fat loss, would be a small change in the total amount of body fat and would not be expected to increase levels detectably. There is no evidence for the mobilization phenomenon.

■ References

1. Rogan WJ. Pollutants in breast milk. *Arch Pediatr Adolesc Med.* 1996;150: 981-990

2. Jensen AA. Chemical contaminants in human milk. *Residue Rev.* 1983;89:1-128

3. Niessen KH, Ramolla J, Binder M, Brugmann G, Hofmann U. Chlorinated hydrocarbons in adipose tissue of infants and toddlers: inventory and studies on their association with intake of mothers' milk. *Eur J Pediatr.* 1984;142:238-243

4. Kelce WR, Stone CR, Laws SC, Gray LE, Kemppainen JA, Wilson EM. Persistent DDT metabolite p,p¹-DDE is a potent androgen receptor agonist. *Nature.* 1995;375:581-585

5. Rogan WJ, Gladen BC, McKinney JD, et al. Polychlorinated biphenyls (PCBs) and dichlorodiphenyl dichloroethene (DDE) in human milk: effects on growth, morbidity, and duration of lactation. *Am J Public Health.* 1987;77: 1294-1297

6. Gladen BC, Rogan WJ. DDE and shortened duration of lactation in a northern Mexican town. *Am J Public Health.* 1995;85:504-508

7. Koopman-Esseboom C, Morse DC, Weisglas-Kuperus N, et al. Effects of dioxins and polychlorinated biphenyls on thyroid hormone status of pregnant women and their infants. *Pediatr Res.* 1994;36:468-473

8. Rogan WJ, Gladen BC, Hung K-L, et al. Congenital poisoning by polychlorinated biphenyls and their contaminants in Taiwan. *Science.* 1988;241:334-336

9. Taguchi S, Yakushiji T. Influence of termite treatment in the home on the chlordane concentration in human milk. *Arch Environ Contam Toxicol.* 1988;17:65-71

10. Cripps DJ, Peters HA, Gocmen A, Dogramaci I. Porphyria turcica due to hexachlorobenzene: a 20 to 30 year follow-up study on 204 patients. *Br J Dermatol.* 1984;111:413-422

11. Bagnell PC, Ellenberger HA. Obstructive jaundice due to a chlorinated hydrocarbon in breast milk. *Can Med Assoc J.* 1977;117:1047-1048

12. Pellizari ED, Hartwell TD, Harris BS, Waddell RD, Whitaker DA, Erickson MD. Purgeable organic compounds in mothers' milk. *Bull Environ Contam Toxicol.* 1982;28:322-328

13. Carella A. On lead poisoning in infants due to lead nipple shields used by wet nurses. *Nuovi Ann Ig Microbiol.* 1967;18:445-455

14. Myers GJ, Marsh DO, Davidson PW, et al. Main neurodevelopmental study of Seychellois children following in utero exposure to methyl mercury from a maternal fish diet: outcome at 6 months. *Neurotoxicity.* 1995;16:653-664

15. American Academy of Pediatrics, Committee on Environmental Health. PCBs in breast milk. *Pediatrics.* 1994;94:122-123

17 Nitrates and Nitrites in Water

N itrogen, an essential nutrient, is absorbed and incorporated by plants from nitrate or ammonium in soil. The use of nitrogen fertilizer for improved crop yields has been increasing dramatically both in the United States and globally. Diffuse nitrate contamination of ground and surface water is one of the most serious environmental consequences of modern agricultural activity. Nitrate levels in drinking water have been increasing commensurate with the increased use of nitrogenous fertilizers. Intensive livestock operations that produce large amounts of animal waste, substandard human septic systems, and municipal waste streams each contribute to increasing nitrate contamination of ground water. Shallow and poorly constructed wells in rural areas are at greatest risk of nitrate contamination.

Nitrate poisoning is a preventable cause of methemoglobinemia in infants. The first case of fatal methemoglobinemia in an infant resulting from contaminated drinking water was reported in 1945.[1] There have now been approximately 2000 cases of acquired methemoglobinemia with an estimated case fatality rate of 10%.[2] The most common cause of methemoglobinemia in children is ingestion of water contaminated with nitrates from agricultural fertilizers, barnyard runoff, or septic system leachate. Young infants fed formula reconstituted with well water that contains nitrates are at the greatest risk.

The current US Environmental Protection Agency (EPA) drinking water standard limits nitrate concentrations to 10 mg/L (10 ppm) and nitrite concentrations to 1 mg/L (1 ppm).[3] This health advisory level was set to prevent methemoglobinemia in infants.[4] Results from a national survey indicate that approximately 1.2% of community water wells and 2.4% of private wells exceed the health advisory level.[5] It is estimated that about 1.5 million people, including 22 500 infants served by private wells, and another 3 million people, including 43 500 infants served by public community wells, are exposed to nitrate in drinking water in excess of the health advisory level.[6]

A survey of 686 private wells in rural Iowa revealed 18.3% of wells had nitrate levels that exceeded 10 mg/L.[7] Twenty-eight percent of 104 wells in Kansas exceeded the health advisory level.[8] During a 2-year period (1991-1992), the American Association of Poison Control Centers reported that 542 children younger than 6 years experienced overexposure to nitrates or nitrites.[9,10]

■ Routes of Exposure

Drinking water is the main source of nitrate in infants.[9] In breastfed infants, there is little or no evidence for increased risk of methemoglobinemia from maternal ingestion of nitrate-contaminated water.[11] It is uncertain whether transplacental transfer of nitrates occurs or whether breastmilk transfers nitrates to infants. Vegetables are the main dietary source of nitrate, contributing more than 70% of total dietary nitrate in adults and older children. Spinach, carrots, celery, and cabbage are high in nitrates and should not be fed to children younger than 4 months. The greatest risk appears to result from either homemade or poorly refrigerated baby foods made from these vegetables (see Table 17.1).[12,13] An ethyl nitrite folk remedy called 'sweet spirits of nitre' has caused fatalities.[14]

Transdermal absorption is higher in infants than in adults. Methemoglobinemia may result from such subtle exposures as diapers marked with aniline-containing laundry inks or rinsed in oxidizing agents, and leather colored with aniline dyes.[15,16] Similarly, use of topical anesthetic agents and silver nitrate burn creams can cause methemoglobinemia in children. Inadvertent use of nitrite salts has resulted in numerous outbreaks of methemoglobinemia.[17,18] An outbreak was reported in a New Jersey elementary school from soup made with tap water that had a nitrite additive used in boilers and hot water tanks.[19] Deliberate abuse of volatile nitrites (amyl, butyl, and isobutyl nitrites) as psychedelics or aphrodisiacs has produced methemoglobinemia. Although rare, methemoglobinemia may be hereditary.

Table 17.1. Reported Inducers of Methemoglobinemia*

Agent	Source
Inorganic Nitrate/Nitrite	Contaminated well water
	Meat preservatives
	Vegetables (carrots, spinach)
	Silver nitrate burn cream
	Industrial salts
	Cold packs - anticorrosives
Organic Nitrate/Nitrite	
Amyl/sodium nitrite	Inhalants
Butyl/isobutyl nitrite	Room deodorizers
Nitroglycerin	Pharmaceuticals
Animal waste	Contaminated well water
Aniline	Laundry ink
Nitrobenzene	Industrial solvents
Local anesthetics	Benzocaine, lidocaine, etc
Sulfonamides	Antibiotics
Phenazopyridine	Pyridium
Antimalarials	Chloroquine, primaquine
Sulfones	Dapsone
Naphthalene	Mothballs
Others	
Copper sulfate	Fungicide
Chlorates	Explosives
Nitrogen oxides	Diesel fuel or welding gases

* Reprinted with permission from *Emergcare*. 1990:6:65-88.

∎ Clinical Effects

Nitrate is rapidly absorbed from the proximal small intestine. Approximately 70% of ingested nitrate is found in urine within 24 hours. Ordinarily most ingested nitrate is metabolized and excreted unless conditions favor reduction to nitrite. Nitrates do not cause methemoglobinemia, but can be converted to nitrites by gut flora. In turn, nitrites convert ferrous (Fe^{+2}) iron in hemoglobin to ferric (Fe^{+3}) iron resulting in methemoglobin, an abnormal hemoglobin incapable of carrying oxygen.

Infants younger than 4 months are at the greatest risk for methemoglobinemia. The gastric pH of infants is higher than that in older children and adults with resultant proliferation of intestinal bacteria that reduce ingested nitrates to more reactive nitrites. Fetal hemoglobin (hemoglobin F), the predominant form in infants up to 3 months, is more readily oxidized to methemoglobin by nitrite than is adult hemoglobin (hemoglobin A). The system responsible for reduction of induced methemoglobin to normal ferrous hemoglobin has only about half the activity in infants as in adults.

Methemoglobinemia generally presents with few clinical signs other than cyanosis. Methemoglobin is dark brown and results in obvious cyanosis at levels as low as 3%. Symptoms are generally minimal until methemoglobin levels exceed 20% (see Table 17.2). Usually cyanosis is manifest well before other symptoms appear unless exposure is intense.

The mucous membranes of infants with methemoglobinemia-induced cyanosis tend to have a brownish (rather than blue) cast. The

Table 17.2. Signs and Symptoms Associated With Increasing Methemoglobinemia

Asymptomatic 3% to 10%	Mild Toxicity 10% to 30%	Moderate Toxicity 30% to 50%	Severe Toxicity Over 50%
Cyanosis	Headache	Headache	Stupor
	Fatigue	Weakness	Bradycardia
		Tachypnea	Respiratory depression
		Tachycardia	
		Possible vasodilatation	Acidosis
			Seizures

brown discoloration increases with the level of methemoglobin as does irritability, tachypnea, altered mental status, and complaints of headache in older children. The oxidative stress of nitrates may result in oxidation of hemoglobin protein, causing Heinz body hemolytic anemia. In addition, several of the compounds that cause methemoglobinemia may also cause sulfhemoglobinemia, which may worsen the appearance of cyanosis. The patient may be dehydrated, as gastroenteritis or diarrhea frequently occurs with and predisposes the patient to methemoglobinemia. In large dosages nitrates and nitrites especially are potent vasodilators and may cause hypotension and shock. Systolic flow murmurs may be noted on auscultation as a result of vasodilatation. After inhalation of volatile nitrites, T-wave inversions, ST segment changes, and arrhythmias may be noted on an electrocardiogram. In the absence of respiratory symptoms, history of cardiovascular disease, abnormal pulse, or abnormal oximetry, a diagnosis of methemoglobinemia should be considered in a child who becomes acutely cyanotic and unresponsive to oxygen administration. Initial screening tests for methemoglobinemia include placing a drop of blood on white filter paper. Blood with a level of methemoglobin greater than 15% dries a deep brown or slate gray. Similarly, a blood sample in an anticoagulant tube appears chocolate brown and does not turn red upon shaking to mix with air in the tube. In the presence of methemoglobin, PO_2 levels from arterial blood gases are normal. The definitive test is the measured proportion of methemoglobin to hemoglobin. In general, levels of methemoglobin less than 20% are very well tolerated, those greater than 50% are serious, and those greater than 70% are often fatal. Nitrate levels may be assayed in blood, urine, or saliva but are not as clinically helpful as methemoglobin levels.

▋ Treatment

Health professionals who suspect that a child has methemoglobinemia are advised to consult with the local poison control center or a toxicologist to help guide management. An asymptomatic child with cyanosis who has a methemoglobin level of less than 20% usually requires no treatment other than identifying and eliminating the source of exposure. Depending on the route and severity of exposure, it may be necessary to remove the child's contaminated clothing, wash the skin, and administer activated charcoal and cathartics. If toxicity is moderate to severe, administering 100% oxygen saturates the normal hemoglobin. For levels greater than 30% or if symptoms persist despite supplemental oxygen, intravenous methylene blue should be administered as a 1% solution in saline at a dosage of 1 to 2 mg/kg over 5 to 10 minutes. Oxidized methylene blue acts as a cofactor for methemoglobin reductase and results in rapid conversion of ferric iron in methemoglobin to ferrous iron with normalization of oxygen binding. The total dose of methylene blue, by any route, should not exceed 7 mg/kg of body weight (4 mg/kg in newborns). Treatment with methylene blue should be avoided in patients with known glucose-6-phosphate dehydrogenase deficiency because it may result in hemolytic crisis. In cases of severe methemoglobinemia and/or when treatment with methylene blue is contraindicated, hyperbaric oxygenation and exchange transfusion should be considered. Careful, longitudinal follow-up of neurodevelopment is advised.

■ Prevention

As in other toxicologic conditions, clinical treatment alone for methemoglobinemia is not sufficient. It is critical to identify and eliminate the sources of exposure. Assessment of potential nitrate exposure includes questions about family residence, occupation (toxicants may be brought home by workers), drinking water, foods ingested, and use of topical medications or folk remedies. Prenatal and newborn care for patients with private wells should include a recommendation for testing well water for nitrate contamination. Water with elevated nitrate levels should not be ingested by infants or used in preparation of infant formula. Boiling water prior to mixing formula, although a good measure for prevention of microbial contamination, is not a safe practice with nitrate-contaminated water because boiling tends to increase nitrate concentrations. Boiling water for 1 minute is sufficient to kill microorganisms such as *Cryptosporidium* without overconcentrating nitrates. Alternative sources of water include drilling new and deeper wells, monitored public water supplies, or bottled water free of nitrates. Newer effective systems for treating nitrate contamination, such as ion-exchange resins and reverse osmosis, are available but expensive. Water testing for nitrate can be obtained from any reference or public health laboratory utilizing approved EPA laboratory methods. Care must be taken to interpret the results correctly as the units of measure are not uniform across laboratories. Concentrations may be reported as either total nitrate or as nitrogen derived from nitrates.

▌ Frequently Asked Questions

Q *Are available commercial treatment systems sufficient for protection against nitrate contamination?*
A Water softeners and charcoal filters do not significantly affect nitrate concentrations. The two technologies that remove nitrates, reverse osmosis and ion exchange resins, are expensive.

Q *Is low-grade nitrate contamination a risk for cancer?*
A Exposure to the nitrate concentrations found in drinking water in the United States is unlikely to contribute to risk of cancer.

Q *Are the current Health Advisory Levels sufficiently strict to protect the population?*
A The vast majority of the population is protected from methemoglobinemia or other potential adverse effects of nitrates at current health advisory levels.[20] The EPA's current standards for nitrate at 10 mg/L and nitrite at 1 mg/L are designed to protect the health even of persons who are considered hypersusceptible. These standards, however, only apply to public water supplies.

Q *Should I have my well water tested? How often?*
A Individuals with private wells should have them tested quarterly for at least 1 year to determine whether episodic elevations of nitrate or bacterial coliforms occur. If those levels are all acceptable, yearly follow-up is recommended.

▌ References

1. Comly HH. Cyanosis in infants caused by nitrates in well water. *JAMA.* 1945;129:112-116

2. Plumb D, Morrisette M. *Nitrates and Groundwater, a Public Health Concern.* Navarre, Minn: Freshwater Foundation; 1988

3. US Environmental Protection Agency. National Primary Drinking Water Regulations: Final Rule, 40. CFR Parts 141, 142, and 143. *Federal Register.* 1991;3526-97

4. National Academy of Sciences, National Research Council. *Drinking Water and Health.* Washington, DC: National Academy of Sciences; 1977

5. *National Pesticide Survey: Project Summary.* Washington, DC: Office of Drinking Water, US Environmental Protection Agency; 1990

6. *Another Look: National Pesticide Survey: Phase II Report.* Washington, DC: US Environmental Protection Agency; 1992

7. Kross BC, Hallberg GR, Bruner DR, Cherryholmes K. The nitrate contamination of private well water in Iowa. *Am J Public Health.* 1993;83:270-272

8. Koellike J, Steichen J, Yearout R, Heiman H. *Identification of Factors Affecting Farmstead Well Water Quality in Kansas.* Manhattan, Kan: Kansas Water Resources Research Institute, Kansas State University; 1987, Report GI226-02

9. Litovitz TL, Holm KC, Bailey KM, Schmitz BF. 1992 Annual report of the American Association of Poison Control Centers National Data Collecting System. *Am J Emerg Med.* 1993;11:494-555

10. Litovitz TL, Holm KC, Bailey KM, Schmitz BF. 1991 Annual report of the American Association of Poison Control Centers National Data Collecting System. *Am J Emerg Med.* 1992;10:452-505

11. Hartman PE. Nitrates and nitrites: ingestion, pharmacodynamics and toxicology. In: de Serres, Hollaender, eds. *Chemical Mutagens.* 1982;7:211-294

12. Dagan R, Zaltzstein E, Gorodischer R. Methemoglobinemia in young infants with diarrhoea. *Eur J Pediatr.* 1988;147:87-89

13. Kay MA, O'Brien W, Kessler B. Transient organic aciduria and methemoglobinaemia with acute gastroenteritis. *Pediatrics.* 1990;85:589-592

14. Kross BC, Ayebo A. *Nitrate/nitrite toxicity. Case Studies in Environmental Medicine, Number 16.* Atlanta, GA: Agency for Toxic Substances and Disease Registry, US Department of Health and Human Services. October 1991.

15. Graubarth J, Bloom CJ, Coleman FC, Solomon HN. Dye Poisoning in the nursery: a review of seventeen cases. *JAMA.* 1945;128:1155-1157

16. Howarth BE. Epidemic of aniline methaemoglobinaemia in nursery babies. *Lancet.* 1951;1:934-935

17. Roueche B. Eleven blue men. In: Rouche B, ed. *Eleven Blue Men.* New York, NY: Berkely Publishing Co; 1953:87-99

18. Kaplan A, Smith C, Promnitz DA. Methemoglobinaemia due to accidental sodium nitrite poisoning. *S Afr Med J.* 1990;77:300-301

19. Askew GL, Finelli L, Genese CA, et al. Boilerbaisse: an outbreak of methemoglobinemia in New Jersey in 1992. *Pediatrics.* 1994;94:381-384

20. National Research Council. *Nitrate and Nitrite in Drinking Water.* Washington, DC: 1995:49

18 | Noise

Noise is undesirable sound. Sound is vibration in a medium, usually air, and has frequency (pitch), intensity (loudness), periodicity, and duration. The frequency of sound is measured in cycles per second and is expressed in hertz (Hz) (1 Hz = 60 cycles per second). People respond to frequencies ranging from 20 to 20 000 Hz, but are most sensitive to the sounds in the range of 500 to 3000 Hz, the band of frequencies that includes human speech.

The loudness of sound is measured in terms of pascals (Pa) or decibels (dB). The range of sound limits in human hearing is 0.00002 (the weakest sound that a keen human adult ear can detect under quiet conditions) to 200 Pa (the pressure causing pain in the adult ear). The decibel is a method of compressing this range by expressing the ratio of one sound energy level to another. The unit most commonly used is dB SPL, indicating that the ratio of sound pressure levels is being used. Human speech is approximately 50 dB SPL.

The perceived loudness of sound varies with the frequency. For example, to match the perceived loudness of a 1000-Hz 40-dB SPL tone requires more than 80 dB SPL at 50 Hz and more than 60 dB SPL at 10 000 Hz. This 40-dB SPL equivalency curve is used to determine the measure of sound intensity, referred to as the decibel weighted by the A scale, dBA. Periodicity refers to either continuous sound or impulse sound. Duration is the total length of time of exposure to sound.

Few studies have been done to estimate children's exposure to noise. From available data it is likely that children are routinely exposed to more noise than the 24-hour equivalent noise exposures (Leq24) of 70 dbA recommended as an upper limit by the US Environmental Protection Agency (EPA) in 1974.[1] A longitudinal study of hearing in suburban and rural Ohio children aged 6 to 18 years found that Leq24 varied from 77 to 84 dB, and exposures were higher in boys than girls.[2]

■ Routes of Exposure

Sound waves enter the ear through the external auditory canal and vibrate the eardrum. This vibration in turn travels through the three ossicles of the middle ear (the malleus, incus, and stapes), where the stapes vibrates through the oval window, vibrating the fluid of the inner ear, the cochlea. Within the cochlea, the basilar membrane covers the organ of Corti, which is composed of the hair cells. Each hair cell responds to a specific frequency of the vibration and converts this signal to a nerve impulse. The impulses, transmitted by auditory nerve, are interpreted as sound or noise by the brain. Loss of hearing originating in the external auditory canal, eardrum, ossicles, or middle ear is called conductive hearing loss and is usually treatable.

Although sound vibration may also be transmitted to the body directly through the skin, it is not discussed here.

■ Clinical Effects

Noise affects hearing and results in several adverse physiologic and psychologic effects.[3]

Susceptibility to noise-induced hearing loss (NIHL) is highly variable; while some individuals are able to tolerate high noise levels for prolonged periods of time, other persons in the same conditions may lose some hearing.[4] Trauma to the hair cells of the cochlea results in hearing loss. Prolonged exposure to sounds louder than 85 dBA is potentially injurious.[5] Continuous exposure to hazardous levels of noise tends to have its maximum effect in the high-frequency regions of the cochlea. NIHL is usually most severe around 4000 Hz, with downward extension toward speech frequencies with prolonged exposure. This pattern of loss of frequency perception is true regardless of the frequency of the noise exposure. Impulse noise is more harmful than continuous noise because it bypasses the body's natural protective reaction to noise, the dampening of the ossicles mediated by the facial nerve.[6]

Exposure to loud noise may result in a temporary decrease in the sensitivity of hearing and tinnitus. This condition, called *temporary threshold shift*, lasts for several hours depending on the degree of exposure.

Little evidence is available to suggest that the organs of hearing are more sensitive to NIHL in children than in adults. Children are at increased risk of increased exposure to noise related to their behaviors. Older children play with firecrackers and cap pistols, and teenagers attend loud concerts. Infants cannot remove themselves from noxious noise.

Evidence is available that suggests that exposure to excessive noise during pregnancy may result in high-frequency hearing loss in newborns and may be associated with prematurity and intrauterine growth retardation.[7] Incorporation of individualized environmental care (including reduction of noise) to the management of premature infants decreases time on the ventilator and in oxygen.[8,9]

Physiologic Effects of Noise

Noise causes a stress response. For people, the hypothalamic-pituitary-adrenal axis is sensitive to noise as low as 65 dBA, resulting in a 53% increase in plasma 17-OH-corticosteroid levels.[10] Increased excretion of adrenaline and noradrenaline has been demonstrated in humans exposed to noise at 90 dBA for 30 minutes.[11]

Noise contributes to sleep deprivation.[12,13] Noise levels at 40 to 45 dBA result in a 10% to 20% increase in awakening or electroencephalogram (EEG) arousal changes. Noise levels at 50 dBA resulted in a 25% probability of arousal features on the EEG.[14]

Noise has undesirable cardiovascular effects. Exposure to noise levels greater than 70 dBA causes increases in vasoconstriction, heart rate, and blood pressure.

Psychological Effects of Noise

Exposure to moderate levels of noise can cause psychological stress.[15] Annoyance, including feelings of bother, interference with activity, and symptoms such as headache, tiredness, and irritability are common psychological reactions to noise. The degree of annoyance is related to the nature of the sound and individual tolerance. Intense noise can cause personality changes and a reduced ability to cope. Sudden, unexpected noise can cause a startle reaction, which may provoke physiological stress responses.

Work performance can be affected by noise. At low levels it can improve performance of simple tasks. However, noise may impair intellectual function and performance of complex tasks.

A stress response consisting of acute terror and panic has been described in children both in Labrador, Canada, and in Germany upon exposure to sonic booms.[16] Biochemical evidence of the stress response was found in elevated urinary cortisol levels. Hypertension accompanied a 30-minute exposure to 100 dBA in 60 children aged 11 to 16 years.

❚ Diagnosis

The typical finding in NIHL is a dip in hearing threshold around 4000 Hz on an audiogram. Physicians in facilities that are unable to provide pure tone audiograms should refer their patients for evaluation. Audiologic evaluation, including pure tone audiometry, should be performed to determine NIHL in children who have no evidence of acute or serous otitis media but have a history of:

- *in utero* exposure to excessive noise by maternal occupation or recreation
- excessive environmental noise exposure, such as prolonged exposure to cap pistols or "boom boxes"
- poor school performance
- short attention span
- complaining of ringing in the ears, a feeling of fullness in the ears, muffling of hearing, or difficulty in understanding speech.

The American Academy of Pediatrics currently recommends objective hearing screening for high-risk newborns and at 4, 5, 10, 12, and 18 years of age.[7,17,18]

❚ Treatment of Clinical Symptoms

There is no known treatment for NIHL.

∎ Prevention of Exposure

Questions addressed to parents and their children about noise exposure should be part of the routine health supervision visits.

Reduce noise exposure.[3] Encourage parents and children to:

- avoid loud noises, especially loud impulse noise whenever possible
- avoid toys that make loud noise, especially cap pistols
- avoid the use of firecrackers
- reduce the volume on televisions, computers, radios
- turn off televisions, computers, and radios when not in use
- use headphones with caution. The volume level of the radio should be low enough so that normal conversation can still be heard.
- create a "stimulus haven," the quietest room in the house for play and interactions.[19]

See Table 18.1 for common exposures to noise.

When noise reduction is not possible, hearing protectors need to be worn, such as during occupational exposures, use of power lawn mowers, recreational exposures such as loud concerts, and other situational noise exposures. There are two types of hearing protectors—earplugs or earmuffs. Earplugs should fit properly; a slight tug required to remove them indicates correct fit. They are available in most drug stores. Earplugs should be checked while chewing because jaw motion may loosen them. Earmuffs are the most effective type of ear protector and are available at most hardware stores. They have cups lined with sound-absorbing material that are held against the head with a spring band or oil-filled ring that provides a tight seal.

Unfortunately, environmental noise often cannot be controlled, which makes noise reduction or hearing protection difficult. Government regulations are needed to protect parents and children from these noises. The standard for the workplace is no more than 8 hours of exposure to 90 dBA, 4 hours at 95 dBA, and 2 hours to 100 dBA, with no exposure allowed to continuous noise above 115 dBA or impulse noise above 140 dBA. In nonoccupational settings, environmental noise is expressed as a day-night average sound level (DNL). For the protection of public health, the US EPA proposed a DNL of 55 dB during waking hours and 45 dB during sleeping hours

Table 18.1. Decibel Ranges and Effects of Common Sounds

Example	Sound Pressure, dBA	Effect From Exposure
Breathing	0–10	Threshold of hearing
Whisper, rustling leaves	20	Very quiet
Quiet rural area at night	30	
Library, soft background music	40	
Quiet suburb (daytime), conversation in living room	50	Quiet
Conversation in restaurant or average office, background music, chirping bird	60	Intrusive
Freeway traffic at 15 meters, vacuum cleaner, noisy office or party, TV audio	70	Annoying
Garbage disposal, clothes washer, average factory, freight train at 15 meters, food blender, dishwasher, arcade games	80	Possible hearing damage
Busy urban street, diesel truck	90	Hearing damage (8-h exposure), speech interference
Jet takeoff (305 meters away), subway, outboard motor, power lawn mower, power lawn mower, motorcycle at 8 meters, farm tractor, printing plant, jack hammer, garbage truck	100	
Steel mill, riveting, automobile horn at 1 meter, boombox stereo held close to ear	110	
Thunderclap, textile loom, live rock music, jet takeoff (161 meters away), siren, chain saw, stereo in cars	120	Human pain threshold
Armored personnel carrier, jet takeoff (100 meters away), earphones at loud level	130	
Aircraft carrier deck	140	
Jet takeoff (25 meters away), toy cap pistol, firecracker	150	Eardrum rupture

in neighborhoods, and 45 dB in daytime and 35 dB at night in hospitals. In 1972, Congress passed the Noise Control Act, giving the EPA a mandate to regulate environmental noise. The Act placed the EPA in charge of all federal noise activities and ordered other agencies to help develop noise-reduction plans. The EPA's Office of Noise Abatement and Control supported research on noise, established noise standards for new trucks and motorcycles, proposed regulations for tractors, buses, lawn mowers, and jackhammers, and started a program to rate the sound levels of consumer products and developed a "buy quiet" program to encourage federal and state agencies to purchase quiet products. This office was closed in 1982, and no effort is being made to enforce the noise regulations that have been established.

∎ Frequently Asked Questions

Q *We live near an airport and the jets fly directly over our house as they take off and land. Will this be harmful to my newborn baby?*

A If the noise is causing discomfort to the parents' ears, it may be causing pain to the infant. The infant should be observed for sleep disturbances and response to the noise. Short of moving, parents may be able to muffle the sound by placing a hat that covers the infant's ears.

Q *Are there unique hazards to the use of headphones?*

A There are several reports of hearing loss secondary to the use of headphones. Children and teenagers should be educated about the potential danger of loud music, whether heard in concert halls or through headphones.

∎ Resource

US Environmental Protection Agency, Office of Air and Radiation at 202/260-7400; fax: 202/260-5155.

■ References

1. De Joy DM. Environmental noise and children: review of recent findings. *J Auditory Res.* 1983;23:181-194

2. Roche AF, Chumleawc RM, Siervogel RM. *Longitudinal Study of Human Hearing, Its Relationship to Noise and Other Factors. III. Results From the First 5 Years.* Washington, DC: US Environmental Protection Agency/Aerospace Medical Research Lab. Report No., AFAMRL-TR-82-68; 1982

3. Swift D, Molon T. Disorders of the ear and hearing. In: Brooks S, ed. *Environmental Medicine.* St Louis, Mo: CV Mosby Co; 1995

4. Henderson D, Hamernik RP. Biologic bases of noise-induced hearing loss. *Occup Med.* 1995;10:513-534

5. Thompson DA. Ergonomics and the prevention of occupational injuries. In: LaDou J, ed. *Occupational Medicine.* Norwalk, CT: Appleton and Lange; 1990:54

6. Jackler RK, Schindler DN. Occupational hearing loss. In: LaDou J, ed. *Occupational Medicine.* Norwalk, CT: Appleton and Lange; 1990:99-101

7. American Academy of Pediatrics, Committee on Environmental Health. Noise: a hazard to the fetus and newborn. *Pediatrics.* 1997;100:724-727

8. Als H, Lawhon G, Brown E, et al. Individualized behavioral and environmental care for the very low birth weight preterm infant at high risk for bronchopulmonary dysplasia; neonatal intensive care unit and developmental outcome. *Pediatrics.* 1986;78:1123-1132

9. Buehler DM, Als H, Duffy FH, McAnulty GB, Liederman J. Effectiveness of individualized developmental care for low-risk preterm infants: behavioral and electrophysiologic evidence. *Pediatrics.* 1995;96:923-932

10. Henkin RI, Knigge KM. Effect of sound on hypothalamic pituitary-adrenal axis. *Am J Physiol.* 1963;204:701-704

11. Frankenshaeuser M, Lundberg U. Immediate and delayed effects of noise on performance and arousal. *Biol Psychol.* 1974;2:127-133

12. Falk SA, Woods NF. Hospital noise—levels and potential health hazards. *N Engl J Med.* 1973;289:774-781

13. Hilton BA. Quantity and quality of patients' sleep and sleep-disturbing factors in a respiratory intensive care unit. *J Adv Nurs.* 1976;1:453-468

14. Thiessen GJ. Disturbance of sleep by noise. *J Acoustic Soc Am.* 1978;64:216-222

15. Kam PC, Kam AC, Thompson JF. Noise pollution in the anesthetic and intensive care environment. *Anesthesia.* 1994;49:982-986

16. Rosenberg J. Jets over Labrador and Quebec: noise effects on human health. *Can Med Assoc J.* 1991;144:869-875

17. American Academy of Pediatrics, Committee on Psychosocial Aspects of Child and Family Health, *Guidelines for Health Supervision III.* Elk Grove Village, Ill: American Academy of Pediatrics; 1997

18. American Academy of Pediatrics, Joint Committee on Infant Hearing. Joint Committee on Infant Hearing 1990 Position Statement. *AAP News.* 1991;7:6-14

19. Wachs TD. Nature of relations between the physical and social microenvironment of the two-year-old child. *Early Dev Parenting.* 1993;2:81-87

19 Outdoor Air Pollutants

ndividual outdoor air pollutants typically exist as part of a complex mixture of multiple pollutants. In the United States and many other countries, however, only a few air pollutants are regularly monitored to assess air quality. The 1970 Clean Air Act required the US Environmental Protection Agency (EPA) to establish national ambient (outdoor) air quality standards for six criteria pollutants: ozone (O_3), respirable particulate matter (PM_{10}), lead, sulfur dioxide (SO_2), carbon monoxide (CO), and nitrogen oxides (NO_x).[1] The act also required the identification of all air pollutants believed to place the public health in danger. Specific populations, most notably those that included persons with asthma and emphysema, were noted to have increased sensitivity to environmental pollutants.

∎ Ozone

Ozone is one of the most pervasive outdoor air pollutants. Ozone and other photochemical oxidants (such as peroxyacetylnitrate [PAN]) are secondary pollutants formed in the atmosphere from a chemical reaction between volatile organic compounds (VOCs) and NO_xs in the presence of sunlight. The primary sources of these precursor compounds include motor vehicle exhausts and power plants, although hydrocarbon emissions from trees and evaporative emissions from gasoline can also contribute to their formation. Ozone is the principal component of urban smog. Levels of ozone are generally highest on hot summer days, and increase to maximum levels in the late afternoon. Indoor concentrations of ozone can vary from 10% to 80% of outdoor levels, depending on the amount of fresh air entering the building.

■ Particulate Matter

Particulate matter refers to a variety of outdoor air pollutants of varying size and composition. Solid particulate matter, including soot and smoke, results from the incomplete combustion of organic matter. Particulate matter also can include dusts that have been generated from the mechanical breakdown of solid matter (such as rocks, soil, and dust).

Particle size is the primary determinant of where the particles will be deposited in the respiratory system. Particles larger than 10 μm in diameter are too large to be inhaled beyond the nasal passages. Children, however, frequently breathe through their mouths, thus bypassing the nasal clearance mechanism. Particles smaller than 5 μm are able to penetrate deep into the lungs. Automotive exhaust generates particles smaller than 10 μm that remain suspended in the atmosphere for longer periods of time and are more likely to be inhaled. The concentration of particulates smaller than 10 μm in air is called PM_{10} and the concentration of particulates smaller than 2.5 μm is called $PM_{2.5}$.

■ Lead

While paint and soil are generally the most common sources of lead exposure for children (see Chapter 14), industrial operations such as battery recycling can generate potentially harmful air emissions of lead. Before the introduction of unleaded gasoline in the United States, the use of leaded gasoline in motor vehicles was an important source of lead exposure for children. In many other countries, particularly developing countries, use of leaded gasoline continues. Together with the absence of stringent controls on automotive emissions and the volume of traffic, the use of leaded gasoline in some major cities of the developing world creates the potential for serious risks to children from mobile sources of lead exposure.[2]

▮ Sulfur Compounds

Sulfur-containing compounds include SO_2, sulfuric acid aerosol (H_2SO_4), sulfate particles, and hydrogen sulfide (H_2S). The primary source of SO_2 is from burning coal; thus, major emitters of SO_2 include coal-fired power plants, smelters, and pulp and paper mills. Sulfuric acid aerosol is formed in the atmosphere from the oxidation of SO_2 in the presence of moisture. Facilities that either manufacture or use acids also can emit H_2SO_4.

Hydrogen sulfide is emitted from a variety of industrial processes, including oil refining, wood pulp production and waste water treatment, as well as from the operation of geothermal plants and landfills. Hydrogen sulfide, which has an odor similar to that of rotten eggs, can be detected at levels far below those associated with physiological effects.

▮ Carbon Monoxide and Nitrogen Dioxide

In addition to fine particles and photochemical pollution, motor vehicle emissions also contribute to outdoor levels of CO and NO_2. Indoor sources of CO and NO_2 can generate higher levels of exposure indoors than those typically measured outdoors (see Chapters 7 and 13).

▮ Volatile Organic Compounds

Volatile organic compounds (VOCs) include compounds such as benzene, xylene, styrene, and various chlorinated and brominated compounds. Indoor concentrations of 11 prevalent VOCs often exceed outdoor concentrations, and obvious industrial sources (such as chemical plants) contribute a relatively small proportion to the average person's total exposure to these substances (see Chapter 13).

▮ Routes of Exposure

The primary route of exposure to air pollution is through inhalation. Substances released into the atmosphere, however, can enter the hydrologic cycle as a result of atmospheric dispersion and precipitation. Similarly, deposition of suspended particulate matter occurs. Thus, material that was originally released into the atmosphere can be ingested as a result of the subsequent contamination of water, soil, or vegetation.

▌Systems Affected

Most of the common outdoor air pollutants are recognized irritants to the respiratory system, with ozone being the most potent irritant. Some toxic air pollutants are known to have other systemic effects (eg, impairment of neurological development from lead), and the specific health risks of many of these toxic compounds (lead, mercury, carbon dioxide, dioxins, VOCs) are addressed in other chapters.

▌Clinical Effects

Children are considered especially vulnerable to outdoor air pollution for several reasons. Because children tend to spend more time outside than adults, often while being physically active, they have a greater opportunity for exposure to pollutants. While playing or at rest, children breathe more rapidly and inhale more pollutants per pound of body weight than do adults. In addition, because airway passages in children are narrower than those in adults, irritation caused by air pollution can result in proportionally greater airway obstruction. Unlike adults, children may not cease vigorous outdoor activities when bronchospasm occurs.

Because children with asthma have increased airway reactivity, the effects of air pollution on the respiratory system can be more serious for them. Some evidence suggests that exposure to ozone can enhance a person's responsiveness to inhaled allergens.[3,4] In addition, children with asthma whose condition is not well managed and who may have exposures to other pollutants can also be more vulnerable to asthma attacks because of poor air quality.

From the viewpoint of toxicity, the key distinguishing features of outdoor air pollutants are their chemical and physical characteristics and concentration. It is common for air pollutants to occur together; for example, on days when ozone levels are high, outdoor air levels of fine particles and acid aerosols may also be high. The combined effects of multiple pollutants are not completely understood but could produce synergistic effects.

In children, acute health effects associated with outdoor air pollution include increased respiratory symptoms, such as wheezing and cough, transient decrements in lung function, more serious lower respiratory tract infections, and exacerbations of asthma.[5] Increases in the number of hospital emergency department admissions have been observed when air pollution levels are elevated, which commonly occurs in major urban areas.[6,7] Historically, episodes of very heavy air pollution (such as the London Smog of 1952) have been linked with increased death rates among adults and children.[8]

The effects of repeated or long-term exposure to outdoor air pollution on the developing lungs of children are not well understood.[9] Most of the acute respiratory effects of outdoor air pollution such as symptoms of cough, shortness of breath, or decrements in lung function are thought to be reversible, but some residual damage over time following repeated exposures also seems probable.[10] Some of the increases in the prevalence of chronic obstructive lung disease in adults who live in more polluted areas could be the result of exposures that occurred during childhood. Evidence from experimental studies using animals and autopsy studies of young adults revealed the presence of lesions that could be early signs of airway disease following long-term exposure to ozone.

∎ Treatment of Clinical Symptoms

The treatment of symptoms and the use of medication should be based on the usual clinical indications. A therapeutic regimen should not be changed in response to periods of poor air quality unless there is a clear indication of a change in a patient's respiratory symptoms or function. However, it might be advisable to recommend restriction of strenuous physical activity during periods of poor air quality.

∎ Prevention of Exposure

Under the Clean Air Act, the EPA has the authority to set standards for air pollutants that protect the health of people with specific sensitivities, including children and those with asthma. The current US national ambient air quality standards are shown in Table 19.1. Although ambient concentrations of these six pollutants have decreased over the last decade, large numbers of people are still exposed to potentially unhealthful levels of these pollutants.

In November 1996, the EPA proposed revisions to the national ambient air quality standards for both particulate matter and ozone, citing health risks to children as a major reason. For particulate matter, the new standard retains the current annual PM_{10} standard of 50 $\mu g/m^3$ but establishes a new annual standard for fine particulate matter ($PM_{2.5}$) of 15 $\mu g/m^3$ and a new 24-hour standard (air measurement made for 24 hours) for $PM_{2.5}$ of 65 $\mu g/m^3$. For ozone, the new standard replaced the former 1-hour standard of 0.12 parts per million (ppm) with an 8-hour standard of 0.08 ppm. It should be noted that there are different measuring times used for each pollutant. Final standards were adopted in 1997, following a public comment period and hearings.

Emission standards were developed for only a few of the hazardous air pollutants prior to the passage of the Clean Air Act Amendments of 1990. These amendments gave the EPA the authority to develop technology-based emission standards for an initial list of 189 hazardous air pollutants. Although these standards are also designed to protect public health, they are based on the available technology to control emissions.

Table 19.1. National Ambient Air Quality Standards (NAAQS) - 1997

Pollutant	Ambient Air Limit	Averaging Time
Ozone	0.08 ppm	8 h avg
PM_{10}	50 $\mu g/m^3$	Annual arithmetic mean
	150 $\mu g/m^3$	24 h
$PM_{2.5}$	15 $\mu g/m^3$	Annual arithmetic mean
	65 $\mu g/m^3$	24 h
Sulfur dioxide	0.03 ppm	Annual arithmetic mean
	0.14 ppm	24 h
Nitrogen dioxide	0.053 ppm	Annual arithmetic mean
Carbon monoxide	9 ppm	8 h
	35 ppm	1 h
Lead	1.5 $\mu g/m^3$	24 h

∎ Frequently Asked Questions

Q *How can I find out about the levels of air pollution in my community?*

A Most large metropolitan areas are required to regularly monitor air quality for one or more of the national ambient (outdoor) air quality standards. Often, the result of air quality monitoring is expressed as the Pollutant Standards Index (PSI). The PSI converts the concentrations of five specific pollutants (CO, ozone, NO_2, SO_2, and particulate matter) into one number, scaled from 0 to 500. The index PSI value of 100 corresponds to the short-term national ambient air quality standard. Thus, a PSI value above 100 indicates that the concentration of one or more pollutants exceeds its national standard. The descriptor terms associated with different PSI values are as follows: 0 to 50, "good"; above 50, "moderate"; above 100, "unhealthful"; 200 to 299, "very unhealthful"; 300 and above, "hazardous." Table 19.2 gives additional information about the PSI.

Information about the air quality in a community often is made available through local news media. Parents can contact their state department of environmental protection or the nearest EPA regional office for more information about air quality measurements in their community.

Q *What can be done to protect my children from outdoor air pollution when they want and need to be able to play outdoors?*

A The potential harm posed by outdoor air pollution depends on the concentration of pollutants, which can vary from day to day and even during the course of a day. While exposure to outdoor air pollutants cannot be entirely prevented, it can be reduced by restricting the amount of time that children spend outdoors during periods of poor air quality, especially time spent engaged in strenuous physical activity. For example, ozone levels during the summer tend to be highest in the middle to late afternoon. On days when ozone levels are expected or reported to be high, outdoor activities could be restricted during the afternoon or rescheduled to the morning, particularly for children who have exhibited sensitivity to high levels of air pollution. In many areas, local radio stations, television news programs, and newspapers regularly provide information on air quality conditions.

Table 19.2. Comparison of Pollutant Standards Index (PSI) Values with Pollutant Concentrations, Descriptor Words, General Health Effects, and Cautionary Statements

Index Value	Air Quality Level	Pollutant Level				
		PM (24-h) µg/m^3	SO$_2$ (24-h) µg/m^3	CO (8-h) ppm	O$_3$ (1-h) ppm	NO$_2$ (1-h) ppm
500	Significant harm	600	2620	50	0.6	2.0
400	Emergency	500	2100	40	0.5	1.6
300	Warning	420	1600	30	0.4	1.2
200	Alert	350	800	15	0.2	0.6
100	NAAQS	150	365	9	0.12	*
50	50% of NAAQS	50	80†	4.5	0.06	*
0		0	0	0	0	*

Continued on next page

* No index values reported at concentration levels below those specified by "Alert Level" criteria.

† Annual primary national ambient air quality standard (NAAQS).

Health Effect Descriptor	General Health Effects	Cautionary Statements
Very hazardous	Premature death of ill and elderly. Healthy people will experience adverse symptoms that affect their normal activity.	All persons should remain indoors, keeping windows and doors closed. All persons should minimize physical exertion.
Hazardous	Premature onset of certain diseases in addition to significant aggravation of symptoms and decreased exercise tolerance in healthy persons.	Elderly and persons with existing diseases should stay indoors and avoid physical exertion. General population should avoid outdoor activity.
Very unhealthful	Significant aggravation of symptoms and decreased exercise tolerance in persons with heart or lung disease, with widespread symptoms in the healthy population.	Elderly and persons with existing heart or lung disease should stay indoors and reduce physical activity.
Unhealthful	Mild aggravation of symptoms in susceptible persons, with irritation symptoms in the healthy population.	Persons with existing heart or respiratory ailments should reduce physical exertion and outdoor activity.
Moderate		
Good		

Q *My family lives in an area that places them at risk for exposure to increased levels of outdoor air pollution. How can I help my child with asthma?*

A Asthma is a multifactorial disease and the indoor environment could be contributing more to a child's asthma than outdoor air pollution. A child's regular exposure to dust mites, cockroaches, animal danders, molds, and environmental tobacco smoke in the home may be causing more harm than exposure to outdoor air pollution. Improved medical management of the child's asthma and control of exposure to allergens and irritants in the child's home could be more beneficial than physically relocating the child to a less polluted area.

Q *Would face dust masks be effective for protecting my children when air pollution levels are high?*

A Dust masks and other forms of respiratory protection, which are sized for adults and not children, are not recommended for protection against outdoor air pollution. Not only do poor fit and uncertain compliance limit any potential benefits, but most simple dust masks do not include the materials needed to filter out harmful VOCs or ozone.

Q *What is the relationship between ozone in urban smog and stratospheric ozone?*

A These issues are unrelated. Ozone in the troposphere, or ground level, is a major component of urban smog and a health hazard. The formation of ground level ozone is independent of ozone in the upper atmosphere, or stratosphere. Stratospheric ozone provides a protective shield absorbing harmful ultraviolet radiation. Too little stratospheric ozone increases the risk of skin cancer and eye damage from ultraviolet rays.

Q *Why is asthma on the increase?*

A Many scientists are puzzled by the apparent increase in the prevalence of asthma. The increase seems to be related to a variety of factors, including increased diagnosis of the disease, increased exposure to environmental allergens and irritants indoors, increased exposure of infants to parental tobacco smoke, and psychosocial and socioeconomic factors. No studies have linked outdoor air pollution with the increase in asthma prevalence.

■ Resources

American Lung Association, local associations: (800-LUNG USA)

Centers for Disease Control and Prevention, Air Pollution and Respiratory Health Branch: 770/488-7320

US Environmental Protection Agency, Public Information Center, 401 M Street, SW, Washington, DC 20460; telephone, 202/260-3059; fax, 202/260-6257; EPA Clean Air Act, 202/382-7548; and 10 regional offices. EPA web site on the Internet: www.epa.gov/oar/oaqps

■ References

1. US Environmental Protection Agency. *National Air Quality and Emissions Trends Report*, 1994. EPA 454/R95-014. Research Triangle Park, NC: Office of Air Quality Planning and Standards; 1995

2. World Health Organization and United Nations Environment Programme. *Urban Air Pollution in Megacities of the World*. Cambridge, Mass: Blackwell Publishers; 1992

3. Molfino NA, Wright SC, Katz I, et al. Effects of low concentrations of ozone on inhaled allergen responses in asthmatic subjects. *Lancet*. 1991;338: 199-203

4. Hanania NA, Tarlo SM, Silverman F, et al. Effect of exposure to low levels of ozone on the responses to inhaled allergen in allergic asthmatic patients. *Chest*. 1998;114: 752-756

5. Bates DV. The effects of air pollution on children. *Environ Health Perspect*. 1995;103(suppl 6):49-53

6. Committee of the Environmental and Occupational Health Assembly of the American Thoracic Society. Health effects of outdoor air pollution. *Am J Respir Crit Care Med*. 1996;153:3-50

7. White MC, Etzel RA, Wilcox WD, Lloyd C. Exacerbations of childhood asthma and ozone pollution in Atlanta. *Environ Res*. 1994;65:56-68

8. Dockery DW, Pope CA. Acute respiratory effects of particulate air pollution. *Annu Rev Public Health*. 1994;15:107-132

9. American Academy of Pediatrics, Committee on Environmental Health. Ambient air pollution: respiratory hazards to children. *Pediatrics*. 1993;91: 1210-1213

10. Lippman NM. Health effects of tropospheric ozone: review of recent research findings and their implications to ambient air quality standards. *J Expo Anal Environ Epidemiol*. 1993;3:103-129

20 | Pesticides

More than 600 chemicals are registered in the United States as pesticides, including insecticides, herbicides, fungicides, rodenticides, fumigants, and insect repellents. Use of pesticides in the United States doubled from the 1960s to the 1980s to more than 1 billion pounds per year. A survey in 1990 by the US Environmental Protection Agency (EPA) estimated that 84% of American households used pesticides, most commonly insecticides.[1]

Pesticides have numerous beneficial effects. When used appropriately for control of insects and rodents, pesticides can assist in the prevention of the spread of disease. Pesticides can have a positive impact on crop yields. These compounds, however, can also be toxic to people. Because they are present in food, medications, homes, schools, and parks, people may frequently be exposed. Children at increased risk of pesticide exposure include those whose parents are farmers or farm workers, pesticide applicators or landscapers, or those who live adjacent to agricultural areas. Children and teenagers may work or play near their parents in the fields, which may expose them to pesticides. People who work with pesticides may use these agricultural-strength chemicals at home.[2] Inappropriate applications may cause illness and death.

This chapter focuses on hazards from acute exposures to pesticides and on prevention of these hazards. For a discussion about the effects of smaller doses of pesticides, see Chapter 12.

■ Insecticides

The major classes of insecticides are organophosphates, carbamates, organochlorines, and pyrethrum and synthetic pyrethroids.

*   **Organophosphates** are responsible for most acute pesticide poisonings. Toxicity ratings of pesticides are based on estimated fatal dose. Children are more likely to be exposed to organophosphates classified as mildly or moderately toxic (eg, malathion, chlorpyrifos, diazinon, and dichlorvos) in the home or garden setting.[3]

    Table 20.1 lists common organophosphate insecticides with toxicity information.

*   **Carbamates** are similar to organophosphates. The most toxic carbamate is Aldicarb. Carbaryl, bendiocarb, and propoxur are more commonly found in household use and are moderately toxic. Table 20.2 lists common carbamate insecticides with toxicity information.

*   **Organochlorines.** Halogenated hydrocarbons were developed in the 1940s for use as insecticides, fungicides, and herbicides. Organochlorines are lipid soluble, have low molecular weight, and persist in the environment. Dichlorodiphenyltrichloroethane (DDT), chlordane, and others were enormously successful due to their efficacy and low acute toxicity. Production of DDT and most other organochlorine compounds was banned in the United States in the 1970s because of concern about their persistence, bioaccumulation in the food chain, possible long-term carcinogenicity, and increasing resistance of the targeted pests.

    Chlordane, DDT, and its metabolite DDE, although no longer used in the United States, can remain in soil for more than 20 years, possibly resulting in human exposure. People may be exposed by eating crops grown in contaminated soil, eating fish from contaminated waters, or breathing air or touching soil near buildings treated for termites. Infants can be exposed through drinking breast milk (see Chapter 16). Organochlorines continue to be used in developing countries, including those exporting food to the United States. Lindane (Kwell) continues to be prescribed for lice and scabies, although safer preparations are available. Lindane poses a serious risk of poisoning if accidentally ingested or misused topically. A recent change in labeling for Lindane indicates that it is to be used only in patients who have failed to respond to adequate doses of other approved agents.

Table 20.1. Examples of Common Organophosphate Insecticides

Chemical Name	Trade (Brand) Name*	EFD, mg/kg†
Agricultural Products: 25% to 50% formulations, highly toxic		
Azinphos-methyl	Guthion	10.0
Coumaphos	Co-ral	15.0
Disulfoton‡	Di-Syston	12.0
DPN	. . .	14.0
EPN	. . .	14.0
Fonofos	Dyfonate	. . .
Mevinphos	Phosdrin	3.7
Methamidophos	Monitor	Delayed neuropathy
Parathion	Thiophos	3.0
Ethyl parathion	Parathion	14.0
Methyl parathion	Dalf, Penncap-M	14.0
Phorate	Thimet	1.1
Terbufos	Counter	. . .
Tetraethyl pyrophosphate	TEPP, Tetron, Bladen	1.0
Animal Insecticides: moderately toxic		
Chlorfenvinphos	Supona, Dermaton (tick dip)	. . .
DEF	DeGreen	325.0
Dichlorvos§	DDVP, Vapona	56.0
Dimethoate	Cygon, De-fend	315.0
Phosmet	Imidon	. . .
Trichlorfon	Dylox	. .
Household/Garden Pest Control: 1% to 2% formulations, low toxicity		
Acephate	Orthene	. . .
Chlorpyrifos‖	Lorsban, Dursban	. . .
2-4 DEP	. . .	850.0
Diazinon	Spectracide, Dimpylate	466
Dichlorvos ‖	DDVP, Vapona (plastic strip)	. . .
Malathion	Cythion, Karbolas	1375.0
Merphos	Folex	2500.0
Temephos	Abate, abathion	2000.0

*The trade (brand) name gives no information about the active ingredient in a product. For example, there are over 100 products named "Spectracide"and many products named "orthene."

†EFD indicates estimated fatal dose. Note: Pesticides contain solvent carriers such as toluene and xylene labeled as inert ingredients but which may produce toxic effects.

‡The water solubility of these agents allows them to be absorbed by the plants and fruits.

§Found in flea collars and No-pest strips.

‖Some classify these as moderately toxic.

Table 20.2. Examples of Common Carbamate Insecticides

Chemical Name	Trade (Brand) Name*	EFD, mg/kg†
Highly Toxic		
Aldicarb	Temik	0.9
Oxyamyl	Vydate	. . .
Isolan	Isolan	12.0
Carbofuran	Furadan	11.0
Methomyl	Lannate, Nudrin	17.0
Methiocarb	Mesurol	. . .
Moderately Toxic		
Propoxur	Baygon, Unden	95.0
Bendiocarb	Ficam	. . .
Befencarb	Bux	. . .
Methiocarb	Mesurol, Draza	. . .
Primicarb	Aphox, Rapid	. . .
Mildly Toxic		
Carbaryl	Sevin	500
Fenethcarb	. . .	. . .
Ambenonium	. . .	. . .
Benzpyrinium	. . .	. . .
Demarcarium	. . .	. . .

*The trade (brand) name gives no information about the active ingredient in a product. Products with the same trade name may have different active ingredients.

†EFD indicates estimated fatal dose.

- **Pyrethrum and Synthetic Pyrethroids.** Pyrethrum, an extract of dried chrysanthemum flowers, refers to a composite of six insecticidal ingredients known as pyrethrins. Natural pyrethrins are used mainly for indoor bug bombs and aerosols due to their instability in light and heat. Anti-lice shampoos such as A200 and Rid contain pyrethrins. Pyrethroids, synthetic chemicals based on the structure and biologic activity of pyrethrum, are modified to increase their stability. Pyrethroids are used in agriculture and gardening for control of structural pests (eg, termites) and against lice and scabies (as permethrin, eg, Elimite). Both pyrethrum and pyrethroids rapidly penetrate insects and paralyze them.

▌Herbicides

Herbicides kill unwanted plants in agriculture, in homes, on lawns and gardens, in parks, on school grounds, and along roadways where children walk, play, and ride bicycles. Herbicides are used in about 14 million households annually.

- **Glyphosate** (Roundup, Rodeo) is a broad-spectrum herbicide used to kill unwanted plants both in agriculture and landscapes.
- **Bipyridyls.** The bipyridyls paraquat and diquat are nonselective plant-killing agents preferred in agriculture because they become inactive on contact with soil. These are widely used by municipal and industrial entities.
- **Chlorophenoxy Herbicides** include 2,4-dichlorophenoxyacetic acid (2,4-D or Weedone, Weed-be-gone); 2,4,5-trichlorophenoxy-acetic acid (2,4,5-T or Kuron, Kurosal); 2,4,5-trichlorophenoxy propionic acid (2,4,5 fenoprop or Silvex) and 4-chloro-2-methyl-phenoxyproponic acid (Mecoprop). The 50:50 mixture of n-butyl esters of 2,4 dichloro (2,4-D) and 2,4,5 trichlorophenoxyacetic acid (2,4,5-T) was used heavily in South Vietnam and Cambodia for defoliation by the US Armed Forces. The mixture was contaminated with a small amount of a specific highly toxic dioxin 2,3,7,8-tetrachlorodibenzo-p-dioxin (TCDD), which is carcinogenic and teratogenic in animals. Its danger to humans is debated. The mixture was known as Agent Orange (named after the color of the drum). Since 1969, the use of 2,4,5-T and its derivatives has been banned. 2,4-D, which is used in more than 1000 pesticide products worldwide, is not contaminated with TCDD.

▌Fungicides

Fungicides include carbamates, organophosphates, and miscellaneous compounds such as captan, captofol, iprodione, and elemental sulfur.[4]

▌Wood Preservatives

Wood preservatives include copper chromium arsenate and penta-chlorophenol. These preservatives were banned from materials other than wood by the EPA in 1987.

∎ Rodenticides

Rodenticides commonly used in US homes are usually anticoagulants or cholecalciferol. Anticoagulants interfere with the activation of vitamin K-dependent factors (II, VII, IX, X). Examples include warfarins, the tenfold more potent indanediones, and superwarfarins (eg, brodifacoum), approximately 100 times more potent than the warfarins. Yellow phosphorus, strychnine, and arsenic rodenticides are no longer registered but may be in use from existing stored supplies.

∎ Insect Repellents

Diethyltoluamide (DEET) is the active ingredient in many insect repellent products. DEET is used to repel insects, such as mosquitoes, and ticks that may carry Lyme disease. Marketed in the United States since 1956 and used by about one third of the US population each year, DEET is available in many commercial products as an aerosol, liquid, lotion, or stick and in impregnated materials such as wristbands. Commercial products registered for direct application to human skin contain from 4% to 99.9% DEET.

Products containing citronella, sold as insect repellents, are not as effective as DEET and therefore not recommended when concern exists about arthropod-borne disease. Permethrin (Permanone, Duranon) is marketed as a spray for tents and clothing, but not for direct application to the skin.[5]

∎ Routes of Exposure

Children may be exposed to pesticides through ingestion, inhalation, and dermal absorption.

Ingestion
Ingestion of pesticides may result in acute poisoning. Pesticides stored in food containers (eg, soft drink bottles) pose a special hazard for children. An EPA survey reported that nearly half of US households with a child younger than 5 years had a pesticide stored within the reach of children.[1]

Infants and children may be exposed through their diets to trace amounts of pesticides applied to food crops (see Chapter 12). Pesticides are found in some water supplies: a 1990 EPA survey found that 10.4% of community water system wells and 4.2% of rural domestic wells contained one or more pesticides that were not removed by standard water treatment technologies (see Chapter 24).[6]

Inhalation
Pesticides applied as dusts, mists, sprays, or gases may reach the alveoli, where they are absorbed into the bloodstream. Where suburban neighborhoods are interspersed with agricultural lands, chemicals from aerial spraying may drift into residential areas.

Dermal Absorption
Many pesticides are readily absorbed through the skin, possibly producing systemic effects. Dermal absorption of organochlorines is variable; Lindane (Kwell, for topical scabies and lice treatment) is efficiently absorbed. DEET is absorbed through the skin. The potential for dermal exposures in children is high because of their relatively large body surface area and extensive contact with lawns, gardens, and floors by crawling and playing on the ground.

▌ Systems Affected and Clinical Effects

Organophosphates

Acute
Organophosphates phosphorylate the active site of the enzyme acetylcholinesterase (AChE) at the nerve ending, irreversibly inhibiting this enzyme. The signs and symptoms of acute organophosphate poisoning result from the accumulation of acetylcholine at cholinergic receptors (muscarinic effects), as well as at voluntary muscle and autonomic ganglia (nicotinic effects). Accumulation of acetylcholine in the brain causes sensory and behavioral disturbances, impaired coordination, depressed cognition, and coma.

Organophosphates are rapidly distributed throughout the body. Symptoms usually develop within 4 hours of exposure, but may be delayed up to 12 hours with dermal exposure. Initial symptoms may include headache, dizziness, nausea, and abdominal pain. Anxiety and restlessness may be prominent. With worsening, muscle twitching, weakness, bradycardia, and hypersecretion (sweating, salivation, rhinorrhea, bronchorrhea) may develop. Miosis is a helpful sign but may lead to the assumption of a drug ingestion, and it may be absent in 20% or more of cases.[7] Central nervous system effects include headache, blurred vision, anxiety, confusion, emotional lability, ataxia, toxic psychosis, vertigo, convulsions, and coma. Cranial nerve palsies have been noted.[8]

Later more severe intoxications result in sympathetic and nicotinic manifestations with muscle weakness and fasciculations including twitching (particularly in eyelids), tachycardia, cramps in muscles, hypertension, and sweating. Finally, paralysis of respiratory and skeletal muscles and convulsions may develop.[4,7]

Chronic
Chronic neurobehavioral or neurologic effects have been reported in a small proportion of poisonings. Symptoms reported to persist for months or years include headaches, visual difficulties, problems with memory and concentration, confusion, unusual fatigue, irritability, and depression.[9,10] In serious poisonings with some organophosphates, there have been reports of organophosphate-induced delayed polyneuropathy associated with paralysis in the legs, sensory disturbances, and weakness.[11]

Carbamates
Carbamates act similarly to organophosphates in binding AChE, but the bonds are more readily reversible. The symptoms produced are not easily clinically differentiated from those of organophosphate poisoning. While AChE may be low in organophosphate poisoning, it is usually normal in carbamate poisoning.[8] Carbamates may be highly toxic, although the effects of exposure are more short-lived, with some cases abating within 6 to 8 hours.

Organochlorines
The toxic action of organochlorines is primarily on the nervous system. By interfering with the flux of cations across nerve cell membranes, organochlorines produce abnormal nerve function and irritability, which may result in seizures. Disturbances of sensation, coordination, and mental function are characteristic. Symptoms may begin with tremor, myoclonic jerks, slurred speech, weakness, and change in mental status and may progress to seizures, coma, and res-

piratory depression. Lindane poisoning presents with nausea, vomiting, and CNS stimulation or generalized seizures.

Pyrethrum and Synthetic Pyrethroids

Pyrethrum and synthetic pyrethroids are absorbed from the gastrointestinal and respiratory tracts but only very slightly through the skin. Because pyrethrins are very rapidly metabolized by the liver and most metabolites are promptly excreted by the kidneys, they have low toxicity when ingested. Most problematic are allergic reactions, which have occurred in the form of contact dermatitis, anaphylaxis, or asthma.[4] Paresthesias described as stinging, burning, itching, or numbness may occur when liquid or volatile compounds contact the skin, but rarely persist more than 24 hours.[8] Extraordinary absorbed doses may rarely cause incoordination, dizziness, headaches, nausea, and diarrhea.

The active ingredient is usually formulated (mixed with carriers, solvents, or synergists) with "inert ingredients" that may be toxic. For example, xylene (an inert ingredient in some pyrethroid formulations) is a CNS depressant and reproductive toxicant. Synergists (chemicals that inhibit the detoxification process) such as piperonyl butoxide and sulfoxide are of low toxicity. Organophosphates and carbamates are often combined with pyrethroids and may have significant toxicity.

Herbicides

Glyphosate

At usual exposure levels, glyphosate has a low level of toxicity. Ingestions of 3/4 cup or more (usually as an attempted suicide) have been fatal.[12,13] Symptoms include abdominal pain, vomiting, pulmonary edema, kidney damage, and renal failure. More commonly, lower levels cause skin and eye irritation. The surfactant polyethoxylated tallowamine, added to improve product application, is more toxic than the active ingredient glyphosate. The two mixed together (Roundup) show a synergistic increase in toxicity.

Bipyridyls (eg, Paraquat and Diquat)

Bipyridyl toxicity is thought to involve the production of free radical oxygen and, secondarily, interference of NADP and NADPH. Paraquat and diquat are corrosive to the tissues they contact directly. Initially, local effects of paraquat result in caustic burns to the mucosa of the mouth, esophagus, and upper gastrointestinal tract. This is followed by a period of multisystem injury with damage to the liver, kidney, myocardium, and skeletal muscle. Two to 14 days following exposure, progressive pulmonary failure occurs due to irreversible alveolar fibrosis. Diquat is less damaging to the skin and does not concentrate in the lungs. Intense nausea, vomiting, and diarrhea may be followed by hypertension, dehydration, renal failure, and shock.

Death has occurred after ingestion of as little as 10 mL of a 20% concentrate of paraquat in an adult and is common in ingestions exceeding 40 mg/kg. Sufficient amounts of paraquat may be absorbed dermally to produce systemic toxicity and death.

Chlorophenoxy Herbicides
Chlorophenoxy herbicides are primarily irritants, causing cough, nausea, and emesis. Few cases of large ingestions have been reported. Symptoms include coma, myosis, fever, hypertension, muscle rigidity, and tachycardia. Pulmonary edema, respiratory failure, and rhabdomyolysis may occur.[8,11,14]

Fungicides
Because a large variety of compounds are used in fungicides, the systems affected and clinical effects vary with each compound.

Rodenticides

Anticoagulants
Anticoagulants may produce bleeding. However, data reported by the American Association of Poison Control Centers showed no fatalities after anticoagulant ingestion.[15,16]

Cholecalciferol
Cholecalciferol produces persistent hypercalcemia that induces vasoconstriction resulting in renal dysfunction and a reduced glomerular filtration rate and renal plasma flow. Typically, 2 or 3 days pass between ingestion and the onset of clinical manifestations of hypercalcemia. Calcium levels of 11.5 to 12 mg/dL may produce anorexia, muscle weakness (due to decreased neuromuscular activity), apathy, nausea, vomiting, constipation, and headache. Levels greater than 13 mg/dL may produce bone pain, ectopic calcification, polyuria, hypertension, renal failure, nephrocalcinosis, and cardiac

dysrhythmias. Moderately severe hypercalcemia may interrupt bone growth for 6 months.

■ Insect Repellents

DEET

Occasionally, persons who use DEET experience adverse reactions, generally consisting of temporary irritation to the skin and eyes. A portion of dermally applied DEET is absorbed systemically.[17] In 1961, a case of encephalitis linked to DEET was reported.[18] Since that time, additional reports of adverse reactions included rashes, fevers, seizures, and death (mostly in children; one child had a rare inborn error of metabolism, ornithine transcarbamylase deficiency).[19,20,21] The relationship between exposure to DEET and reported neurologic symptoms is inconclusive. Most of the cases of toxicity involved the use of DEET from 10% to 50% and were related to overdose and misuse. Clinicians evaluating children with unexplained encephalopathy or seizures should consider the possibility of exposure to DEET.[5,22,23]

■ Long-term Effects of Pesticides

More research is needed to define the short- and long-term effects of pesticides accurately. Epidemiologic studies have found associations between certain childhood cancers (eg, all brain cancers and leukemia) and pesticide exposure. Results of studies have been inconsistent.[24] A statistical simulation by a committee of the National Academy of Sciences suggested that for some pesticides, the reference dose (the dose of a non-cancer toxicant at which no health effects are likely) may be exceeded by thousands of children daily. Some children may display mild symptoms of inattention and gastrointestinal, flu-like symptoms related to dietary pesticides.[25] Multiple exposures from a variety of sources (ie, food, yard, school) may be cumulative.[26]

■ Diagnostic Methods

The history of exposure is of particular importance. In a recent review of 190 acute pesticide poisonings, laboratory tests were not often found to be diagnostically helpful.[3] In addition, symptoms of pesticide exposure are likely to be nonspecific.

■ Treatment

When a poisoning has occurred, the label of the chemical should be obtained whenever possible. Many pesticides have confusingly similar names. Many active ingredients are sold using the same trade names. Therefore it is important to ascertain the exact ingredients for any product of concern. The EPA-mandated label contains concise information on specific treatment guidelines, symptoms and signs, and a toll-free telephone number for manufacturer assistance.

Regional poison control centers can help with patient evaluation and management and have a medical toxicologist available for consultation. The National Pesticide Telecommunications Network can help answer questions about pesticide identification, toxicology, acute and chronic symptoms, and treatment (see Resources section).

Serious poisonings should be managed with guidance from a medical toxicologist and/or a regional poison control center. In an agricultural exposure, the county cooperative extension service agent can provide invaluable knowledge of the local crops, chemical usage patterns, and modes of application.

Care should be taken to identify other children or adults who may have had similar exposure and need evaluation and treatment. Eliminating a source of contamination may prevent future exposures.[14]

Insecticides

Organophosphates

Patients who are asymptomatic or have only minor symptoms should be closely observed. With symptoms, a test dose of atropine, which helps alleviate the muscarinic effects of organophosphates, should be administered. If the test dose confirms cholinergic excess by **not** producing signs of atropinization (dilation of pupils, dry mouth, flushing of skin, tachycardia, or fever), treatment with additional doses to dry the secretions is indicated. The most reliable end point of adequate atropinization is control of bronchorrhea (drying of the secretions and clear lungs). Tachycardia before administration of atropine is not a contraindication to administration.

Pralidoxime (2-Pam, Protopam) breaks the bond in the AChE-phosphate complex and should be used as an antidote for most clinically significant organophosphate poisonings. Pralidoxime affects both nicotinic and muscarinic effects of organophosphates. A blood sample for cholinesterase activity should be obtained prior to administering pralidoxime, as it quickly reactivates the enzyme.[27]

Carbamates

Treatment with atropine for carbamate poisoning is the same as for organophosphates. Pralidoxime therapy is generally unnecessary and in some cases severe reactions and sudden death have occurred with its use.[28] In mixed poisonings involving organophosphates and carbamates or unidentified agents, cautious use of pralidoxime should be considered.

Organochlorines

There is no specific antidote for poisoning from organochlorines. Treatment is symptomatic, with use of anticonvulsants for seizures and general supportive measures. Epinephrine is not advised for poisoning from organochlorines because of increased myocardial susceptibility to catecholamines and life-threatening dysrhythmias.

Pyrethrum and Synthetic Pyrethroids

Generally, ingestion represents little risk. In extremely large ingestions, intubation and lavage may be advised.

Herbicides

Glyphosate

There is no specific antidote for glyphosate poisoning. Treatment is supportive.

Bipyridyl Herbicides (Paraquat and Diquat)

Hemoperfusion has been shown to be ineffective in reducing mortality. In paraquat poisoning, supplemental oxygen may increase lung damage and should be avoided if possible. Renal status should be closely monitored, particularly with diquat, as dialysis may be required.

Chlorophenoxy Herbicides

There is no specific antidote for poisoning from chlorophenoxy herbicides. The patient should be monitored for seizures and signs of multiple organ dysfunction (eg, gastrointestinal irritation, liver, kidney, and muscle damage). Alkalinization of the urine may enhance clearance.

Fungicides
Treatment for fungicide poisoning is guided by the specific compound ingested.

Rodenticides

Anticoagulants
Consulting with a poison control center can assist in determining the significance of the ingestion. More significant ingestions should be managed with the help of a toxicologist. In general, for one-time ingestions of warfarin-related or superwarfarin-related rodenticides in children younger than 6 years, no hospital visits, decontamination, or prothrombin time determinations are needed. The child should be observed at home and a physician should be notified if bleeding or bruising occurs.

Insect Repellents

DEET
Treatment for poisoning from DEET is supportive. There is no specific antidote.

❚ Prevention: Reduction of Pesticide-Related Risks

With the exception of poison baits, as little as 1% of pesticides applied indoors reach the targeted pest. The rest may contaminate surfaces and air in the treated building. Outdoor pesticides may fall on nontargeted organisms, plants, animals, and outdoor furniture and play areas. They may contaminate groundwater, rivers, or wells. Biomagnification of long-lasting compounds may result in exposures to animals (including humans) at the top of the food chain at concentrations tens of thousands of times greater than those at the bottom of the food chain.

Pest resurgence occurs when, along with the targeted pest, its predators and pathogens are killed. The remaining pest population then multiplies with fewer restraints, resulting in an infestation worse than the original.

Natural enemies to other potential pests may also be killed or drastically reduced in number. Thus, a secondary pest may rapidly multiply in the absence of former competitors, parasites, and predators. More than 600 pest insects, weeds, and plant pathogens are now resistant to one or more pesticides. Once a pest has developed resistance to one class of chemicals, often it will develop resistance to others.

▌ Integrated Pest Management

Integrated pest management is an increasingly useful approach to minimizing pesticide use while providing long-term pest control. It integrates both chemical and non-chemical methods to provide the least toxic alternative for pest control. Integrated pest management utilizes regular monitoring to determine if and when treatments are needed. Management tactics include physical (eg, barriers, caulking), mechanical (eg, vacuuming up white flies), cultural (eg, choosing plants well suited to the site), biological (using predators, pathogens such as *Bacillus thuringiensis*, and naturally occurring bacteria that kill insects), and educational (eg, cleaning up ant-attracting foods in the kitchen). Treatments are not made based on a predetermined schedule, but rather when monitoring indicates that the pest will cause unacceptable economic, medical or aesthetic damage. Treatments are chosen and timed to be most effective and least hazardous to nontargeted organisms and the general environment.

Integrated pest management programs have been successfully adopted by school systems, cities, and counties (for parks and roadways), and farms across the United States and have often resulted in substantial cost savings. The national Parent Teacher Association passed a resolution to work toward pesticide-free schools.

▌ Frequently Asked Questions

Q *I am having pest problems in my lawn and garden. Should I get regular preventive applications by a professional service?*

A Regular lawn treatment exposes people to pesticides unnecessarily. It also may kill insects that are beneficial in controlling the pest population, thereby requiring the use of more chemicals. If a professional lawn service is used, its personnel should (1) regularly monitor the lawn for pests and treat the lawn only when pests exist; (2) provide possible alternatives to the standard treatment; (3) give advance warning (including neighbors) before applying any pesticides (this allows time to cover outdoor furniture and remove toys and pet food dishes); (4) be trained and certified; (5) give advance notification of the types of chemicals to be used and information on their effects on health; and (6) avoid applications under adverse weather conditions (eg, high winds).

Simple steps that may reduce the need for pesticides include:

1. Growing plant varieties that grow well in the area. A county extension agent or personnel in a nursery may have advice.

2. Timing the watering and fertilizing of the plants according to their needs.

3. Following recommendations given for mowing and pruning grass and plants.

4. Deciding what degree of damage from weeds, insects, and diseases can be tolerated and not taking control measures unless that degree is reached.

5. Considering nonchemical options first when controls are needed. For example, determine whether weeds can be removed by hoeing or pulling.

Q *Is an insect repellent containing DEET safe for use on my children?*
A DEET is the active ingredient in most insect repellents. While it is generally used without any problems, there have been rare reports of side effects. Usually, these problems have occurred with excessive use. DEET should be used in areas where there is concern about illness from insect bites. It can also be used when insects are likely to be a nuisance such as at barbecues or at the beach.

No definitive studies exist in the scientific literature about what concentration of DEET is safe for children. The efficacy of DEET plateaus at a concentration of 30%. A cautious approach is to use a low concentration, 10% or less, on children.

Precautions when using DEET:

1. Read and carefully follow all directions before using the product. Young children should not apply DEET to themselves.

2. Wear long sleeves and pants when possible and apply repellent to clothing - a long sleeved shirt with snug collar and cuffs is best. The shirt should be tucked in at the waist. Socks should be tucked over pants, hiking shoes, or boots.

3. Apply DEET sparingly only to exposed skin. Do not use DEET underneath clothing.

4. Do not use DEET on the hands of young children. Avoid the eye and mouth areas.

5. Do not apply DEET over cuts, wounds, or irritated skin.

6. Wash treated skin with soap and water upon returning indoors. Wash treated clothing.

7. Avoid using sprays in enclosed areas. Do not use DEET near food.

8. Wash the exposed area if an allergic reaction is suspected.

Q *We have rodents in and around our home. How can we safely get rid of them?*

A Most pesticides for controlling rats (rodenticides) available for home use today are the anticoagulants warfarin or superwarfarin (coumarins) or indanediones. They kill the rodents by causing internal bleeding. These anticoagulants also can cause bleeding in children if ingested and therefore must be used carefully. Each year, more than 10 000 children are exposed to these products, making anticoagulant baits one of the most common pesticide ingestions in children younger than 6 years. Poisoning can be avoided by following the product label and using common sense. Fortunately, the amounts usually eaten by young children rarely cause serious injury. Contact your physician, poison center, or the emergency department of the nearest hospital immediately if it is suspected that a child may have ingested a product containing anticoagulants.

> The following measures may reduce the danger of exposure:
> 1. Place all rodenticides out of the reach of children and non-target animals or in tamper-proof bait boxes. Outdoors, place bait inside the entrance of a burrow and then collapse the entrance over the bait.
> 2. Securely lock or fasten shut the lids of all bait boxes.
> 3. Place bait in the baffle-protected feeding chamber, never in the runway of the box.
> 4. Always use sanitation measures in conjunction with pesticides to limit rodent access to food and hiding places. Work with neighbors to secure the neighborhood. If baiting alone is used without sanitation measures, the rodent population will rebound each time the baiting stops. Measures include using rat-proof garbage cans and food storage precautions (including keeping food in the refrigerator), and frequently raking up garden waste (including fallen fruit).
> 5. Modify the habitat by rat-proofing buildings and changing landscaping to eliminate hiding places.
> 6. Continue to monitor periodically to ensure that rats are not recolonizing.

Q *What is the best way to treat my roach problem?*

A Hygiene measures are key. Cockroaches are found where there is water and food. Eating should be discouraged in areas other than in the kitchen. All foodstuffs should be stored in closed containers. Water sources should be eliminated by caulking cracks around faucets and pipe fittings. Cracks and crevices where cockroaches can enter the home should be sealed.

A prudent approach is to minimize exposure to sprays whenever possible. Individual bait stations are recommended. If possible, baiting should be done outside the home as well. Boric acid, formulated for use as a pesticide, can be used in cracks and crevices in areas inaccessible to children.

If these measures are not successful, the family should consult a professional exterminator. If professional extermination is to be done, the family should find out what insecticide will be used and its possible toxic effects. After application of the insecticide, young children and pregnant women should stay out of the area for as long as possible. The room should be well ventilated for several hours before people and pets return. Crawling babies should not be allowed in the area until it has been well vacuumed or mopped and the resident can be certain that the pesticide was not applied in an area where the infant can reach. For example, if the pesticide is applied to the wall, a crawling infant could hold onto the wall or wipe his hands and sustain a significant exposure.

Families should avoid using over-the-counter bug sprays and bug bombs.

Q *How do citronella and Skin So Soft compare to DEET as insect repellents?*

A Both citronella and Skin So Soft have mild repellent properties. DEET is significantly more effective. Therefore, when repellent is being used to prevent insect-borne infection (eg, Lyme disease or anthropoid-borne encephalitis), DEET should be used.

Q *I recently bought a product containing DEET combined with a sunscreen. Is it safe to use?*

A Sunscreen preparations are usually applied liberally to exposed areas, and reapplied frequently to minimize sun exposure. This kind of application may result in overexposure to DEET, which should be applied sparingly. The EPA is studying the effects of these products.

∎ Resources

ATSDR Methyl Parathion Hotline: 800/447-1544

EPA Office of Pesticide Programs, Communication Services Branch 800/535-PEST (National Pesticide Hotline): 703/305-5017, http:/www. epa.gov/pesticides (general information)

EPA pamphlets:

Our Citizen's Guide to Pest Control and Pesticide Safety

Pest Control in the School Environment

Healthy Lawn, Healthy Environment

Fact Sheets on lawn care, pesticide labels, and pesticide safety. Available free from the National Center for Environmental Assessment Publications and Information, PO Box 42419, Cincinnati, OH 45242-2419 (513/489-8190).

National Campaign for Pesticide Policy Reform: 202/547-9009

National Pesticide Telecommunications Network (The telephone number for health professionals is 800/858-7377; for the general public, 800/858-7378). Internet address: http://ace/orst.edu/info/nptn

Pesticide Educational Center: 415/391-8511

Extoxnet, an internet site, is a cooperative effort among the University of California at Davis, Oregon State University, Michigan State University, and Cornell University that provides updated pesticide information in understandable terms. It includes toxicology briefs and information on carcinogenicity, testing, and exposure assessment. Internet address: http://ace.ace.orst.edu/info/extoxnet.

∎ References

1. Whitmore RW, Kelly JE, Reading PL. *National Home and Garden Pesticide Survey: Final Report, Volume 1*. Research Triangle Institute NC: RTI\5100. 17-01F, Research Triangle Park, NC; 1992

2. Reigart JR. Pesticides and children. *Pediatr Ann.* 1995;24:663-668

3. Lessenger JE, Estock MD, Younglove T. An analysis of 190 cases of suspected pesticide illness. *J Am Board Fam Pract.* 1995;8:278-282

4. Ellenhorn MJ, Schonwald S, Ordog G, Wasserberger J. Pesticides. In: *Ellenhorn's Medical Toxicology: Diagnosis and Treatment of Human Poisoning.* Second ed. Williams and Wilkins, Baltimore, MD;1997:1614-1663

5. Brown M, Hebert AA. Insect repellents: an overview. *J Am Acad Dermatol.* 1997;36:243-249

6. Offfice of Water, Office of Pesticides and Toxic Substances. *National Survey of Pesticides in Drinking Water Wells. Phase 1.* Washington, DC: US Environmental Protection Agency. Report, EPA 570/9-90-015.

7. Zwiener RJ, Ginsburg CM. Organophosphate and carbamate poisoning in infants and children. *Pediatrics.* 1988;81:121-126

8. Reigart JR, Roberts JR. *Recognition and Management of Pesticide Poisonings.* 5th ed. Washington, DC: Environmental Protection Agency; 1999

9. Savage EP, Keefe TJ, Mounce LM, Heaton RK, Lewis JA, Burcar PJ. Chronic neurological sequelae of acute organophosphate pesticide poisoning. *Arch Environ Health*. 1988;43:38-45

10. Steenland K, Jenkins B, Ames R, O'Malley M, Chrislip D, Russo J. Chronic neurological sequelae to organophosphate pesticide poisoning. *Am J Public Health*. 1994;84:731-736

11. O'Malley M. Clinical evaluation of pesticide exposure and poisonings. *Lancet*. 1997;349:1161-1166

12. Menkes DB, Temple WA, Edwards IR Intentional self-poisoning with glyphosate-containing herbicides. *Hum Exp Toxicol*. 1991;10:103-107

13. Talbot AR, Shiaw M, Huang JS, et al. Acute poisoning with a glyphosate-surfacant herbicide (Roundup): a review of 93 cases. *Hum Exp Toxicol*. 1991;10:1-8

14. Rodgers GC, Jr, Matyunas NJ, eds. *Handbook of Common Poisonings in Children*. 3rd ed. Elk Grove Village, Ill: American Academy of Pediatrics; 1994

15. Litovitz T, Manoguerra A. Comparison of pediatric poisoning hazards: An analysis of 3.8 million exposure incidents. *Pediatrics*. 1992;89:999-1006

16. Litovitz TL, Klein-Schwartz W, Dyer KS, Shannon M, Lee S, Powers M. 1997 annual report of the American Association of Poison Control Centers Toxic Exposure Surveillance System. *Am J Emerg Med*. 1998;16:443-497

17. Selim S, Hartnagel RE Jr, Osimitz TG, Gabriel KL, Schoenig GP. Absorption, metabolism, and excretion of N,N-diethyl-m-toluamide following dermal application to human volunteers. *Fundam Appl Toxicol*. 1995:95-100

18. Gryboski J, Weinstein D, Ordway N. Toxic encephalopathy apparently related to the use of an insect repellent. *N Engl J Med*. 1961;264:289-291

19. Centers for Disease Control. Seizures temporally associated with the use of DEET insect repellent: New York and Connecticut. *MMWR Morb Mortal Wkly Rep*. 1989;38/39;678-680

20. Veltri JC, Osimitz TG, Bradford DC, Page BC. Retrospective analysis of calls to poison control centers resulting from exposure to the insect repellent N,N-diethyl-m-toluamide (DEET) from 1985-1989. *J Toxicol Clin Toxicol*. 1994; 32:1-16

21. Heick HM, Shipman RT, Norman MG, James W. Reye-like syndrome associated with use of insect repellent in a presumed heterozygote for ornithine carbamyl transferase deficiency. *J Pediatr*. 1980;97:471-473

22. Osimitz TG, Murphy JV. Neurological effects associated with use of the insect repellent N,N-diethyl-m-toluamide. *J Toxicol Clin Toxicol*. 1997;35: 435-441

23. Garrettson L. Commentary-DEET: Caution for children still needed. *J Toxicol Clin Toxicol*. 1997;35:443-445.

24. Zahm SH, Ward MH. Pesticides and childhood cancer. *Environ Health Perspect*. 1998;106:893-908

25. National Research Council. *Pesticides in the Diet of Infants and Children*. Washington, DC: National Academy Press; 1993

26. Needleman H, Landrigan P. *Raising Children Toxic Free.* Farrar, Straus and Giroux; 1994

27. Wagner S, ed. Cholinesterase-inhibiting pesticide toxicity. In: *Case Studies in Environmental Medicine.* Atlanta, GA: Agency for Toxic Substances and Disease Registry; September 1993

28. Kurtz PH. Pralidoxime in the treatment of carbamate intoxication. *Am J Emerg Med.* 1990;8:68-70

21 Polychlorinated Biphenyls, Dibenzofurans, and Dibenzodioxins

P olychlorinated biphenyls (PCBs) are compounds with two linked phenyl rings and variable degrees of chlorination. They are clear, nonvolatile, hydrophobic oils that cannot be metabolized by most organisms and persist in the environment. About 1.5 million metric tons were produced from the 1930s until their production was banned and many uses phased out under the Toxic Substances Control Act of 1977. Much of what was made is still somewhere in the environment. The PCBs were used primarily in the electrical industry as insulators and dielectrics, especially for applications in which a fire hazard was present, such as in heavy transformers. Their optical and solvent properties led to such uses as a component of carbonless copy paper, as microscope immersion oil, and as a vehicle for paint and pesticides. During the 1960s, analytical chemists interested in dichlorodiphenyltrichlorethane (DDT) residues in the tissues of pelagic birds began identifying background peaks in their chromatograms as PCBs. Since then, numerous studies throughout the world have shown detectable levels of PCBs in human tissue and human milk; except for DDT and its analogues, PCBs are the most dispersed of the halogenated hydrocarbon pollutant chemicals.[1]

Polychlorinated dibenzofurans (PCDFs) are partially oxidized PCBs. They were not made intentionally but appear as contaminants in PCBs that have undergone high temperature applications or have been in fires or explosions. Polychlorinated dibenzodioxins

(PCDDs), commonly referred to as dioxins, also are contaminants. These compounds were formed during the manufacture of hexachlorophene, pentachlorophenol, and the phenoxyacid herbicides 2,4,5-T (a component of Agent Orange) and silvex, under what would now be considered poorly controlled conditions. They are also formed, albeit at very low yield, during paper bleaching and waste incineration. One dioxin congener, 2,3,7,8-tetrachlorodibenzo-p-dioxin (TCDD), may be the most toxic synthetic chemical known: if the toxicity of a chemical is ranked by the minimal lethal dose in moles per kilogram in the most susceptible species, TCDD in guinea pigs at 3.1×10^{-9} is exceeded only by botulinum, tetanus, and diphtheria toxins in mice.[2]

■ Routes of Exposure

A middle aged person in the United States has had dermal contact with these agents, some of which they absorbed and stored. Now that immersion oil and carbonless copy paper, among other things, no longer contain PCBs, the current source of exposure for most people is contaminated food. The PCBs are "unavoidable" contaminants because, unlike pesticides, regulations cannot prevent contamination by preventing application. The concentration of PCBs in commercial food must be below the tolerances set by the Food and Drug Administration for food in commerce. However, because the chemicals are not metabolized or excreted, even very small daily doses accumulate to measurable amounts over years. The most concentrated dietary source is usually fish, since the residues bioconcentrate and fish is the food at the highest trophic level regularly consumed by humans. Bioconcentration also increases exposure for the Arctic Inuit who eat blubber of sea mammals who themselves are fish eaters,[3] and, to a lesser extent, for anglers who consume their own catch from contaminated waters. In areas where PCB contamination has been a problem, state and local health departments have issued advisories that recommend limiting the consumption of contaminated fish.

The major dietary source of PCBs for young children is human milk, from which they absorb and store these chemicals (see Chapter 16).

Predictable occupational exposure to these agents is now rare and would be most likely for those involved in the cleanup of hazardous waste sites or maintenance work for electrical utilities. Heavy electrical equipment produced decades ago is still in service, and transformers may leak or become damaged during fires or explosions, thus exposing workers and the environment to PCBs or PCDFs. Substantial quantities of PCBs are still present in older industrial facilities other than electric utilities, such as railroads, and in military equipment. Modern herbicides are not contaminated with PCDDs. There is exposure from waste incineration and paper bleaching, but the amounts are minuscule.

Two episodes of mass poisoning have occurred in Asia in which PCBs that were heat degraded, and thus heavily contaminated with PCDFs, were the causative agents. In 1968, an epidemic of acne among residents of Kyushu province in Japan was traced to the use of cooking oil that had been contaminated by heat-degraded PCBs during processing. More than 1000 people were eventually given the diagnosis of "Yusho" (oil disease).[4] An extraordinarily similar outbreak occurred in Taiwan in 1979, involving contaminated rice oil.[5] To our knowledge, there has not been an episode in which people were exposed only to PCDFs; background exposure probably comes mostly from fish consumption.

A chemical plant explosion released kilogram quantities of TCDD in Seveso, Italy, in 1975. The highest recorded serum levels of TCDD in humans occurred in children in the most heavily exposed areas in this incident.[6] In Vietnam, spraying with Agent Orange has left a legacy of TCDD contamination still detectable in breast milk.[7] Older members of the general population were exposed to TCDD through contaminated herbicides, wood treatments, and perhaps antiseptics during the 1960s and 1970s, and TCDD residues are detectable in most people if the analytical method is sensitive enough.

∎ Systems Affected and Clinical Effects

At background exposures, these agents have been associated with delay on developmental tests, including subtle delays in psychomotor development from the newborn period through 2 years of age, defects in short-term memory in 7-month-olds and 4-year-olds, and lowered IQs in 11-year-olds.[8] For the most part, prenatal exposure to PCBs from the mother's body burden, rather than exposure through human milk, seems to account for the findings. There may also be subclinical effects on thyroid function in the newborn. The results of studies on birth weight and low-dose exposure have been inconsistent.

Severe disease occurred in the children of the poisoned Taiwanese and Japanese. In Japan in 1968, among 13 women who were pregnant around the time of exposure, one of the children was stillborn and was deeply and diffusely pigmented (a "cola-colored" baby). Some of the live born children were small, hyperbilirubinemic, and pigmented and had conjunctival swelling with dilatation of the sebaceous glands of the eyelid. Follow-up of children up to 9 years later showed apathy, lethargy, and soft neurologic signs. The growth deficit apparent at birth resolved by about 4 years of age.

In Taiwan, 117 children who were born during or after the food contamination in 1979 and thus exposed to their mothers' body burden of PCBs and PCDFs were examined in 1985 and have since been followed up.[9] They have a variety of ectodermal defects, such as excess pigmentation, carious teeth, poor nail formation, and short stature. They show more poor conduct and hyperactive behavior and have persistent developmental delay, on the average about 5 to 8 points on standard IQ scales. Furthermore, the delay is as severe in children born up to 6 years after exposure as it is those born in 1979.[10]

Despite the extreme toxicity of TCDD in the laboratory and its wide distribution, there are few documented instances of symptomatic TCDD poisoning in children. Children in the area near the explosion that released TCDD in Seveso, Italy, had chloracne, most pronounced on areas unprotected by clothing,[11] and some had liver function abnormalities noted on clinical laboratory testing.[12] Hemorrhagic cystitis developed in a Missouri girl who played in an exercise yard for horses that had been sprayed with waste oil contaminated with TCDD.[13] There are anecdotal reports of toxicity in the children who were born in areas sprayed with Agent Orange, a herbicide contaminated with TCDD, during the Vietnam War, but no systematic study has been reported. The offspring of male Vietnam veterans, who may have had exposure from Agent Orange, show no clear excess of malformations[14]; no data are available on the offspring of female veterans. The results of studies about effects of exposure to these substances on children is summarized in Table 21.1.

Table 21.1. Reported Signs and Symptoms by Age at Occurrence

Prenatal exposure to low levels of PCBs:

• Newborns: decrease in birth weight (inconsistent)

• Infants: motor delay detectable from newborn period to 2 years

• 7-month-olds: defects in visual recognition memory

• 4-year-olds: defects in visual recognition memory

• 11-year-olds: delays in cognitive development

Prenatal exposure to high levels of PCBs and PCDFs

• Newborns: low birth weight, conjunctivitis, natal teeth, pigmentation

• Infant through school age: delays on all cognitive domains tested; behavior disorders; growth retardation; abnormal development of hair, nails, and teeth; pigmentation; increased risk of bronchitis

• Puberty: small penis but normal development in boys; growth delay but normal development in girls

Direct ingestion of high doses of PCBs and PCDFs

• Any age: chloracne, keratoses, and hyperpigmentation; mixed peripheral neuropathy; gastritis

Dermal exposure to high levels of TCDD

• Children: probably higher absorbed dose for a given exposure than adults; chloracne; liver function test abnormalities

▌ Diagnostic Methods

The idea of measuring these compounds arises most frequently in discussions about breastfeeding. Although many laboratories can measure PCBs, there are no agreed-upon methods, quality assurance programs, or reference values available, and no laboratory is licensed to measure these chemicals for diagnostic or therapeutic use. Thus, any measurement would have to be regarded as research and would be interpretable only within a research project. Any reasonably sensitive method will detect PCBs in most samples of human milk. The PCDFs and PCDDs are much more difficult to measure, and no clinical interpretation is available if the measurement is done. Thus far, all expert bodies, including the American Academy of Pediatrics, that have considered this topic recommend breastfeeding and do not recommend testing of milk. More information is included in Chapter 16.

Treatment

No regimen is known to lower body burden of these compounds. In Asia, treatments that have been tried include cholestyramine, sauna bathing, and fasting, none of which work. Theoretically, a woman might be counseled not to attempt weight reduction during lactation, since the compounds would be passed into the breast milk, but in the United States, at least, women tend not to lose more than a kilogram or so during lactation, and that amount should not matter.

Regulation

PCBs are banned from new production throughout the world. They are unavoidable contaminants of foods, and so have "temporary tolerances," which are levels that, if found in a food in commerce, result in a requirement from the Food and Drug Administration that the food be removed from the market. For infant and junior foods, the tolerance is 1.5 ppm fat basis for PCBs; for fish, it is 5 ppm fat basis. There are no tolerances for PCDFs or PCDDs.

There are also "allowable daily intakes," set by the Food and Agriculture Organization and the World Health Organization. These are amounts of chemical, expressed as a microgram of chemical per kilogram of consumer, that are believed to be safe. For PCBs, the allowable daily intake is 6 µg/kg per day, which is about the median for a fully breastfed 5-kg infant. There are no allowable daily intakes for dioxin or PCDFs. There is a "tolerable daily intake" (reflecting greater uncertainty in the data) of $1 \times 10^{-5} \times$ µg/kg per day for dioxin. The median daily intake of a 5-kg breastfed infant is about 70% of the tolerable daily intake.

Any waste substance, commonly waste oils, with more than 50 ppm of PCBs must be handled as a hazardous substance and disposed of as a hazardous waste.

Alternatives

PCBs have been replaced mostly by mineral oils, which are less toxic but can explode and burn more readily. Dioxins and PCDFs were never made deliberately, and no product is now contaminated at the levels seen during the 1960s.

∎ Frequently Asked Question

Q *Should I be concerned about dioxins in coffee filters?*
A Paper products are usually bleached by using chlorine bleaches. The reaction between the chlorine and the lignins in the wood fiber produces many complex chlorinated organic compounds, among them TCDD. The amounts are minuscule; on the other hand, it is difficult to see the benefit of a white coffee filter compared with a tan filter.

∎ Resources

Health departments in states in which PCBs have been a problem, such as New York and the Great Lakes states, issue advisories about fish consumption and have had experience dealing with PCBs. The Environmental Protection Agency has issued guidelines for states for the development of fish advisories for PCBs and other persistent contaminants. See http://www.epa.gov/OST/fish/.

∎ References

1. International Programme on Chemical Safety. *Polychlorinated biphenyls and terphenyls.* Environmental Health Criteria, 140 ed. Geneva: World Health Organization; 1993

2. Anonymous. Dioxin's lethality compared to other poisons. *Chemical and Engineering News.* June 6, 1983;45

3. Dewailly E, Nantel A, Weber JP, Meyer F. High levels of PCBs in breast milk of Inuit women from arctic Quebec. *Bull Environ Contam Toxicol.* 1989;43:641-646

4. Kuratsune M. Yusho. In: T*opics in Environmental Health.* 2nd ed. Amsterdam, the Netherlands: Elsevier; 1989:381-400. Kimbrough RD, Jensen AA, eds. *Halogenated Biphenyls, Terphenyls, Naphthalenes, Dibenzodioxins, and Related Products;* vol 4

5. Hsu ST, Ma CI, Hsu SK, et al. Discovery and epidemiology of PCB poisoning in Taiwan: a four-year follow-up. *Environ Health Perspect.* 1985;59:5-10

6. Mocarelli P, Needham LL, Morocchi A, et al. Serum concentrations of 2,3,7,8-tetrachlorodibenzo-*p*-dioxin and test results from selected residents of Seveso, Italy. *J Toxicol Environ Health.* 1991;32:357-366

7. Schecter A, Dai LC, Thuy LT, et al. Agent Orange and the Vietnamese: the persistence of elevated dioxin levels in human tissues. *Am J Public Health.* 1995;85:516-522

8. Jacobson JL, Jacobson SW. Intellectual impairment in children exposed to polychlorinated biphenyls in utero. *N Engl J Med.* 1996;335:783-789

9. Rogan WJ, Gladen BC, Hung KL, et al. Congenital poisoning by polychlorinated biphenyls and their contaminants in Taiwan. *Science.* 1988;241:334-336

10. Chen YC, Yu ML, Rogan WJ, Gladen BC, Hsu CC. A 6-year follow-up of behavior and activity disorders in the Taiwan Yu-cheng children. *Am J Public Health.* 1994;84:415-421

11. Caramaschi F, del Corno G, Favaretti C, Giambelluca SE, Montesarchio E, Fara GM. Chloracne following environmental contamination by TCDD in Seveso, Italy. *Int J Epidemiol.* 1981;10:135-143

12. Mocarelli P, Marocchi A, Brambilla P, Gerthoux PM, Young DS, Mantel N. Clinical laboratory manifestations of exposure to dioxin in children. A six-year study of the effects of an environmental disaster near Seveso, Italy. *JAMA.* 1986;256:2687-2695

13. Carter CD, Kimbrough RD, Liddle JA, et al. Tetrachlorodibenzodioxin: An accidental poisoning episode in horse arenas. *Science.* 1975;188:738-740

14. Erickson JD, Mulinare J, McClain PW. Vietnam verterans' risks for fathering babies with birth defects. *JAMA.* 1984;252:903-912

22 Ionizing Radiation (Including Radon)

R adiation includes energy transmitted by waves through space or some type of medium, such as light seen as colors, infrared rays perceived as heat, and audible radiowaves amplified through radio and television. We cannot similarly perceive radiation with shorter wavelengths: ultraviolet rays, x-rays, and gamma rays. Radiation with the shortest wavelengths, x-rays and gamma rays, possess immense quantities of energy and penetrate solid objects. This energy may cause ionization in tissue, which drives outer electrons from their orbits around atoms. The free electrons created can react with other molecules in living organisms and cause tissue damage.

■ Sources of Exposure

Exposures to radiation can be from external sources (radon and x-ray machines) or from internal emitters (radioactive fallout, ingested or inhaled, or medical radioisotopes). The transfer of energy in sufficient doses from the environment to individuals can adversely affect their health.[1] X-rays transfer energy along thin paths, whereas neutrons have greater mass and transfer energy along wider paths. The units of measure of energy absorbed by x-rays and gamma rays were the rad (radiation absorbed dose) and the rem (roentgen equivalent man), with the latter measurement based on the greater relative biological effectiveness (RBE) of doses from particulate radiation, such

223

as neutrons (Fig 1). Thus, rem = (rad) × (RBE). The RBE of gamma radiation is 1, and, if the RBE of neutrons is 10, exposure to 100 rad of each is (100 × 1) + (100 × 10) = 1100 rem. The rad and rem have been replaced by the Gray (1 Gy = 100 rad), and the Sievert (1 Sv = 100 rem), so the example becomes (1 Gy × 1) + (1 Gy × 10) = 11 Sv.

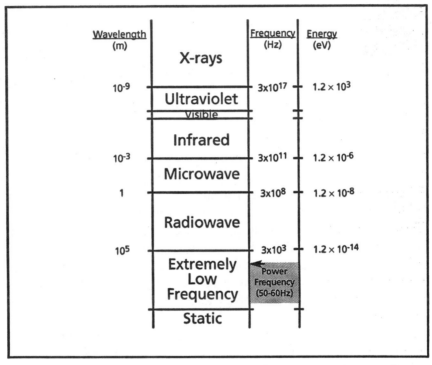

Fig 1. Approximate ranges of wavelength, frequency, and energy for different types of electromagnetic radiation or fields.

On average, the annual effective dose equivalent of ionizing radiation to a person in the United States is 0.0036 Sv (0.36 rem), 55% of which is from radon, 27% from other natural sources, 11% from medical x-rays, and 7% from other man-made sources (Fig 2).[2] Doses to children from diagnostic radiation are shown in Table 22.1. Note that the exposure for a newborn from fluoroscopy for 1 minute is 1000 times greater than that from a chest film; exposure from radiographic determination of scoliosis in a small child is ten times greater than exposure from a chest film.

Radiation exposure may be instantaneous (atomic bomb), chronic (uranium miners), fractionated (radiotherapy), or partial-body. For a given dose, whole-body exposure is more harmful than partial-body exposures. Radioisotopes decay with time into stable elements, and have physical half-lives of various lengths, from fractions of a second to millions of years. They also have biological half-lives related to the rate at which they are excreted from the body.

▋ Biological Processes and Clinical Effects

Atoms or molecules that become ionized attain stability again by forming substances that may alter molecular processes within a cell or its environment. Ionizing radiation, in colliding with a cell, can cause changes in its constituents, including DNA. Such damage, if unrepaired, may disable or kill the cell.

Ionizing radiation produces the same reactions regardless of the type of particle or ray emitted. Differences are quantitative, not qualitative. Prompt effects of overexposure include acute radiation sickness (nausea, vomiting, diarrhea, declining white blood count, and thrombocytopenia), epilation (loss of hair), and death.

Delayed effects are largely due to teratogenesis, carcinogenesis, and mutagenesis. The smaller the exposure, the less likely that late effects will be found. In evaluating the feasibility of studying the off-

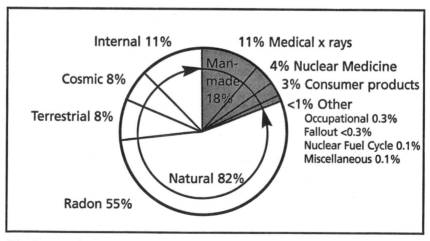

Fig 2. Population exposure to ionizing radiation in the United States (average annual effective equivalent dose).

225

Table 22.1. Some diagnostic radiation exposures of children at Minneapolis Children's Medical Center in 1996.*

Procedure	Age	Entrance Skin Exposure, mR†
Chest, recumbent position	NB	4
	3-6 y	6
	14 y	14
Abdomen, upright position	NB-6 mo	6
	2-6 y	9
	14 y	50
Cervical spine (no grid)	NB	6
	5-10 y	10
	12 y	15
Thoracic spine (AP)	Small	10
	Medium	15
	Large	20
Lumbar spine (AP)	8 y	35
	10 y	50
	16 y	70
Pelvis	5 y	20
	12 y	50
Skull, lateral	NB	5
	12 y	15
Scoliosis (AP)	Small	50
	Medium	70
	Large	100
Abdomen, with barium	NB	15
	3-6 y	20
	8-12 y	30
Portable chest	NB (AP)	4
	NB (lateral)	6
Wrist/ankle	6-10 y	5
Fluoroscopy	Maximum	4.5-9.4 R/min‡
Computed tomography scan	Head	3.6 R/study
	Body	1.3 R/study

* Table was provided by Shashikant Sane, MD, Minneapolis Children's Medical Center. Measurements by J.T. Payne, PhD.

† Abbreviations: mR, milliroentgens; NB, newborn; AP, anteroposterior; R, roentgen.

‡ Maximum exposure from four machines at table top or patient entrance.

spring of military veterans, an expert committee of the Institute of Medicine noted that exposures of fathers to fallout from weapons tests, as in the South Pacific, seldom exceeded 0.5 rem.[3] The Committee noted that at the maximum relative risk (0.2% increase in adverse reproductive outcomes), a sample size of 212 000 000 exposed children would be needed to detect a statistically significant excess as compared with unexposed children. Or, the frequency of such effects among the 500 000 children of atomic veterans would have to be increased 150-fold to be detected.[3] In general, the best estimates of dose-related delayed effects of ionizing radiation come from studies of the Japanese atomic bomb survivors who experienced a single, instantaneous whole-body exposure, possibly affected by other adverse influences such as malnutrition in war-torn Japan.

Teratogenesis

Intrauterine exposure to ionizing radiation may cause small head size alone or with severe mental retardation. Susceptibility to severe mental retardation is greatest at 8 to 15 weeks of gestational age, with some occurring during the 16th to 25th week. The lowest dose that caused severe mental retardation from atomic bomb exposure was 0.6 Sv, far above diagnostic exposures in medical radiology. The lowest dose that caused small head size without mental retardation was 0.10 to 0.19 Sv among conceptuses exposed at 4 to 17 weeks of gestational age. Mental retardation is apparently due to interruption in the proliferation and migration of neurons from near the cerebral ventricles to the cortex.[4]

Carcinogenesis

Diagnostic Radiation

In a series of reports from 1956 to 1975, Stewart and associates described and expanded on their report of a 1.5-fold excess of almost every type of cancer in children younger than 10 years after maternal exposure to diagnostic abdominal x-rays during pregnancy.[5] The biological plausibility of the same relative risk for so many neoplasms has been questioned.[6] Among them was lymphoma, which has not been linked to radiation exposure at any age. It is reasonable to believe that leukemia, other than the chronic lymphocytic form, can be radiation induced by *in utero* exposure because leukemia can be induced at any age.

227

Atomic Bomb Exposure

Among the 807 Japanese atomic bomb survivors exposed *in utero*, no excess of childhood cancer was observed.[7] As the cohort, now 55 years old, grows older and the risk of cancer increases, an excess is expected of the types of cancer previously observed among atomic bomb survivors exposed as children or adults. Because the increase in the number of cases of leukemia after childhood exposure lasted for about 30 years, more cases are unlikely among the *in utero* cohort. An excess in breast cancer after childhood exposure, however, was not found until the cohort reached about age 30 years, which is the age at which breast cancer may begin to occur. No cases have been observed yet among the *in utero* group. An excess of thyroid cancer occurred in children exposed to the atomic bomb beginning at 11 years of age, but because of its rarity, no cases are expected among the group exposed *in utero*.

Prenatal or childhood radiation exposures rarely lead to an increase in cancers before age 15, but increased frequencies of cancers in adults are expected if the exposure and sample size are large enough. Among all atomic bomb survivors, excess of cancer was very difficult to assess when exposures were under 0.20 Sv, a level rarely experienced from medical exposures in the United States. Intrauterine exposures to as little as 0.01 Gy for medical diagnosis during pregnancy have been the basis of litigation concerning children with severe mental retardation or parental fear of cancer in the child—well below the minimal carcinogenic dose detectable epidemiologically.

Radon

The US population is constantly exposed to radon, which accounts for 55% of background radiation (average exposure, 0.002 Sv [0.2 rem] per person per year). Radon gas comes from radioactive decay of radium, a product of ubiquitous uranium deposits in rocks and soil. When inhaled, radon decay products (also known as radon daughters or radon progeny), caused an increase in rates of lung cancer in uranium miners. No excess of other cancers has been detected. Radon enters homes through cracks in the foundation, porous cinderblocks, and granite walls. Thus, radiation exposures in basements may be higher than those on the first-floor level. Extrapolation downward from the dose-response curve for lung cancer among uranium miners indicates that about 10% of lung cancer in the United States is attributable to radon exposure.[8] The vast majority of these cancers occur in cigarette smokers. Until recently there were insufficient data to detect an increased risk of lung cancer after life-long residential radon exposure. A summary analysis (meta-analysis) has now been made of eight epidemiologic studies, the results of which are consistent with low-dose effects found in other studies of humans and animals.[9] These results indicate a linear dose-response relationship detectable down to 4 pCi/L, the level at which remedial action should be taken, according to the US Environmental Protection Agency (EPA) and the US Department of Health and Human Services.

Mutagenesis

Ionizing radiation is a germ-cell mutagen in plants and experimental animals, and is assumed to affect humans too. Studies of children who were conceived after one or both parents were exposed to the atomic bomb have as yet shown no excess of genetic effects. The studies started with clinical observations, and then included cytogenetic, biochemical, and molecular studies as soon as laboratory procedures were developed. Two-dimensional electrophoresis examination of 30 serum and erythrocyte proteins from about 16 000 children were made. Among 1.2 million locus tests, three apparent mutations were observed in the parent-exposed group and four mutations were observed in the (one-third smaller) unexposed group.[10] DNA studies are now in progress in the search for germline mutations through study of stored samples on the child and both parents.

Ionizing radiation causes chromosome breaks in somatic cells (eg, lymphocytes and skin fibroblasts) that are detectable decades after exposure,[11] and presumably account for the increased rates of cancer observed after exposure in childhood or adulthood. In the studies of atomic bomb survivors, differential color staining of four chromosomes was initiated as soon as it was developed, and staining of all 23 chromosome pairs, as recently reported, greatly improves detection of small translocations.

▌ Special Susceptibility and Epidemics

Special Susceptibility

Children with ataxia-telangiectasia (AT) are prone to the development of lymphoma, and, when treated with conventional doses of radiotherapy, suffer an acute radiation reaction that may result in death.[12] A DNA repair defect in patients with AT interferes with repair of cells damaged by radiation. This catastrophic reaction has been seen when AT was not diagnosed before radiotherapy because some young children had only ataxia. Ocular telangiectasia, which develops at about age 6 years, was not yet apparent.

Epidemics

Gamma rays (external radiation) and radioisotopes (internal emitters) in fallout have caused epidemics of delayed radiation effects after *in utero* or childhood exposure: 1) developmental effects and cancer were caused by exposure to the atomic bomb; 2) thyroid ablation in two infants and thyroid neoplasia in the Marshall Islanders were due to fallout from nuclear weapons tests; and 3) hundreds of cases of thyroid cancer in children in Ukraine and Belarus were attributed to fallout from the Chernobyl accident. A small cluster of cases of leukemia and lymphoma in children near the Sellafield nuclear facility in England was ascribed to paternal radiation exposure during the 6 months before conception. Expert re-evaluation of the study has led to the conclusion that the paternal exposure was not to blame.[13]

❚ Diagnostic Methods

Radiation-induced diseases are indistinguishable from those that occur in the general population. The role of radiation can be implicated only by epidemiologic studies that show a dose-response effect, alternative explanations are excluded (eg, heritable disorders), and a link between exposure and the suspected effect is biologically plausible. Biological dosimetry can estimate exposures above 0.2 Gy by such methods as painting chromosomes for the detection of recognized chromosomal translocations, and by the glycophorin A test for somatic-cell mutations of red blood cells.

❚ Treatment of Clinical Symptoms

For acute radiation sickness caused by the Chernobyl accident, blood counts of those affected were sustained through the use of combined treatment with cytokines, such as stem-cell factors and colony-stimulating factors that produce both rapid and delayed hematopoietic responses from surviving progenitor cells.[14] Otherwise the treatment was symptomatic. For delayed radiation effects, treatment of the disease was the same as that when radiation exposure was not involved.

▌ Prevention of Exposure

External Radiation
The risk of cancer associated with most diagnostic radiation is low, and use of radiation should not be restricted when needed for correct diagnosis.[15] Any medical procedure has a risk and diagnostic radiography is no exception. Limitation of radiation, shielding sensitive body parts like the thyroid, and assuring a nonpregnant state, are all components of good medical practice. Therapeutic doses should only be used when the indications are unmistakable and the risk justified, as in the treatment of malignant tumors.

Special populations, such as extremely low birth weight infants, may undergo multiple radiologic examinations during a short period. In particular, computed tomography should be used sparingly for premature infants, particularly when other imaging techniques are available.

Radon
The US EPA recommends that homes be tested for radon. Radon can be measured by two methods: (1) α-track detectors can be placed in the home for at least 3 months to obtain a time-integrated measurement of the radon level, or (2) charcoal canisters can be exposed to the air in the home for 4 days.[16] These canisters are extremely sensitive and humidity dependent but are appropriate as a screening device. However, the α-track detector, used for a long period, gives a better estimate of exposure than does the charcoal canister because the former device averages out daily fluctuations in indoor radon levels.

Radon exposure can be reduced by increasing ventilation and by reducing the influx of radon in the home. Several methods of reducing exposure include sealing cracks in the foundation, creating negative pressure under the basement floor, and prohibiting the use of building materials containing excessive radium. When levels of radon higher than 4 pCi/L are found, repairs should be made to reduce the radon level. Pediatricians should advise families about the hazards of radon exposure and should point out that cigarette smoking multiplies the radon-induced risk of lung cancer.

Table 22.2. Regional Radon Contacts

Region 1 (Maine, Vermont, New Hampshire, Massachusetts, Connecticut, Rhode Island):
US EPA
JFK Federal Building, Boston, MA 02203 617/565-3234

Region 2 (New York, New Jersey)
US EPA
290 Broadway, 28th Floor, New York, NY 10007-1866 212/637-4010

Region 3 (Pennsylvania, Delaware, Maryland, District of Columbia, West Virginia, Virginia):
US EPA
841 Chestnut, Building 3AT32, Philadelphia, PA 19107 215/566-2086

Region 4 (Kentucky, Tennessee, North Carolina, South Carolina, Georgia, Alabama, Mississippi, Florida):
US EPA
100 Alabama St, SW, Atlanta, GA 30303-3104 404/562-9145

Region 5 (Michigan, Ohio, Indiana, Illinois, Wisconsin, Minnesota):
US EPA
77 W Jackson Blvd, AE-17J, Chicago, IL 60604 312/353-6686

Region 6 (Arkansas, Louisiana, Oklahoma, Texas, New Mexico):
US EPA
1445 Ross Ave (6PD-T), Dallas, TX 75202-2733 214/665-7550

Region 7 (Iowa, Missouri, Kansas, Nebraska):
US EPA
726 Minnesota Ave., Kansas City, KS 66101 913/551-7605

Region 8 (North Dakota, South Dakota, Montana, Wyoming, Colorado, Utah):
US EPA
999 18th St, Suite 500 (P2-TX), Denver, CO 80202-2466 303/312-6147

Region 9 (California, Arizona, Nevada, Hawaii):
US EPA
75 Hawthorn St (AIR6), San Francisco, CA 94105 415/744-1046

Region 10 (Washington, Oregon, Idaho, Alaska):
US EPA
1200 Sixth Ave (OAQ-107), Seattle, WA 98101 206/553-7299

Water may also be a source of exposure to radon. In a limited number of studies, radon exposure has been linked to gastrointestinal cancers, although this is not yet proven.

Fallout (Internal Emitters)

The radioisotopes can be inhaled or ingested. People in exposed areas should avoid drinking fresh milk in particular. Instead, foods made before the event causing fallout occurred should be eaten. Potassium iodide should be administered promptly to protect the thyroid from radioiodines. Foil-wrapped tablets available for adults (130 mg, 1 per day) should be split to provide the appropriate dose for children. If potassium iodide is not available, a drop a day of tincture of iodine should be administered. This should be continued daily until the public health authorities report that it is safe to stop.

Regulations

Recommendations concerning radiation protection are made by the National Commission on Radiation Protection and Measurements and the International Commission on Radiological Protection. The Nuclear Regulatory Commission regulates and monitors nuclear facilities and the medical/research uses of radioisotopes.

∎ Frequently Asked Questions

Q *Should I test for radon in my home?*
A The EPA recommends that all homes be checked. An inexpensive home-testing kit should be used and the sample obtained should be sent to a certified laboratory for analysis. If the level of radon exceeds 4 pCi/L, the cracks through which radon enters the house, as in the basement, should be sealed. Further information can be obtained from the booklet, *Radon Reduction Methods: A Homeowner's Guide,* published by the EPA. See the Resources section on page 234 for the hotline telephone number.

Q *How many x-rays are safe for my child?*
A As many as your physicians think necessary for diagnosis and follow-up, taking into account the benefit weighed against the (very small) risk.

Q *Will x-ray examinations of my child affect future grandchildren?*
A No. No genetic effects of radiation from the atomic bombs in Japan have been demonstrable in series of studies, most recently involving effects on DNA. Mutations must have occurred, as in all living organisms, but have not as yet been demonstrated in survivors.

Q *Is my child's (chronic) illness due to past radiation exposures?*
A There is no way to determine this for an individual patient. Illnesses induced by radiation cannot be distinguished from illnesses in the general population. The relationship can only be established by large epidemiologic studies showing a higher incidence in a radiated group (such as atomic bomb survivors) supported by other evidence.

∎ Resources

For radiation protection: National Council on Radiation Protection, 7910 Woodmont Ave, Suite 800, Bethesda, MD 20814-3095; telephone: 301/657-2652; fax: 301/907-8768.

For radiation effects: Radiation Epidemiology Branch, National Cancer Institute, EPS-7048, Bethesda, MD 20892-7238; telephone: 301/496-6600; fax: 301/402-0207.

For radon testing: EPA Radon Hotline: 800/767-7236.

EPA Office of Radon Programs: 202/475-9605 (National Information Line).

∎ References

1. Mettler FA Jr, Upton AC. *Medical Effects of Ionizing Radiation.* 2nd ed. Philadelphia, Pa: WB Saunders Co; 1995

2. Committee on the Biological Effects of Ionizing Radiation (BEIR V). *Health Effects of Exposure to Low Levels of Ionizing Radiation.* Washington, DC: National Academy Press. 1990;355-359

3. Committee to Study the Feasibility of, and Need for, Epidemiologic Studies of Adverse Reproductive Outcomes in Families of Atomic Veterans. *Adverse*

Reproductive Outcomes in Families of Atomic Veterans: The Feasibility of Epidemiologic Studies. Washington, DC: National Academy Press; 1995

4. Miller RW. Delayed effects of external radiation exposure: a brief history. *Radiat Res.* 1995;144:160-169

5. Bithell JF, Stewart AM. Pre-natal irradiation and childhood malignancy: a review of British data from the Oxford survey. *Br J Cancer.* 1975;31:271-287

6. Boice JD Jr, Miller RW. Childhood and adult cancer after intrauterine exposure to ionizing radiation. *Teratology* 1999;59:227-233

7. Miller RW, Boice JD Jr. Cancer after intrauterine exposure to the atomic bomb. *Radiat Res.* 1997;147:396-397

8. Committee on Biological Effects of Ionizing Radiation, National Research Council: *Health Risks of Radon and Other Internally Deposited Alpha-Emitters.* Washington, DC, National Academy Press; 1988

9. Lubin JH, Boice JD, Jr. Lung cancer risk from residential radon: meta-analysis of eight epidemiologic studies. *J Natl Cancer Inst.* 1997;89:49-57

10. Neel JV, Schull WJ, Awa AA, et al. The children of parents exposed to atomic bombs: estimates of the genetic doubling dose of radiation for humans. *Am J Hum Genet.* 1990;46:1053-1072

11. Ohtaki K, Sposto R, Kodama Y, Nakano M, Awa AA. Aneuploidy in somatic cells of *in utero* exposed atomic bomb survivors in Hiroshima. *Mutation Res.* 1994;316:49-58

12. Cunlift PR, Mann JR, Cameron AH, Roberts KD, Ward HN. Radiosensitivity in ataxia-telangiectasia. *Br J Radiol.* 1975;48:374-376

13. Doll R, Evans HJ, Darby SC. Paternal exposure not to blame. *Nature.* 1994;367:678-680

14. Harrison JR. Casualties of Chernobyl. *Radiol Protect Bull.* 1996; 173:24-27

15. American Academy of Pediatrics, Committee on Environmental Health. Risk of ionizing radiation exposure to children: a subject review. *Pediatrics.* 1998;101:717-719

16. American Academy of Pediatrics, Committee on Environmental Hazards. Radon exposure: a hazard to children. *Pediatrics.* 1989;83:799-802

23 Ultraviolet Light

S unlight is divided into visible light, ranging from 400 nm (violet) to 700 nm (red); longer infrared, "above red" or more than 700 nm, also called heat; and shorter ultraviolet (UV) radiation (UVR), "below violet" or less than 400 nm. Ultraviolet radiation is divided into UV-A (320 to 400 nm), also called black (invisible) light; UV-B (290 to 320 nm), which is more skin penetrating; and UV-C (<290 nm). UV-B constitutes less than 0.5% of sunlight but is responsible for most of the acute and chronic sun damage to normal skin. Most UVR is absorbed by stratospheric ozone. UV-B is more intense during summer than during winter, at midday compared with early morning or late afternoon, in places closer to the equator than in temperate zones, and at high altitudes. Sand, snow, concrete, and water can reflect up to 85% of sunlight, providing greater exposure.[1]

Exposure to UVR during childhood can result in substantial morbidity and even mortality later in life.

■ Routes of Exposure

Individuals are exposed to UVR when they are outdoors in the sunlight and when they use sunlamps and sunbeds.

■ Systems Affected

The skin, eyes, and immune system are affected.

■ Clinical Effects

Erythema and Sunburn

Exposure to solar radiation causes vasodilatation and an increase in the volume of blood in the dermis, resulting in erythema. The minimal erythemal dose depends on factors such as skin type and thickness, the amount of melanin in the epidermis and the capacity of the epidermis to produce melanin after sun exposure, and the intensity of the radiation. Six sun-reactive skin classifications have been developed (see Table 23.1).

Nonmelanoma Skin Cancer

Cumulative sunlight exposure over a prolonged period is important in the development of nonmelanoma skin cancer (NMSC), basal cell and squamous cell carcinoma. In the US adult population, NMSC is by far the most common malignant neoplasm (approximately 1 million cases per year). It is rarely fatal unless left untreated. In general, NMSC occurs in maximally sun-exposed areas of fair-skinned persons and is uncommon in blacks; NMSC is extremely rare in children in the absence of predisposing conditions.[2]

Table 23.1. Classification of Sun-Reactive Skin Types

Skin Type	History of Sunburning or Tanning
I	Always burns easily, never tans
II	Always burns easily, tans minimally
III	Burns moderately, tans gradually and uniformly (light brown)
IV	Burns minimally, always tans well (moderate brown)
V	Rarely burns, tans profusely (dark brown)
VI	Never burns, deeply pigmented (black)

Cutaneous Malignant Melanoma

Exposure to large amounts of sunlight that is episodic and relatively infrequent is important in the pathogenesis of cutaneous malignant melanoma (referred to hereafter as melanoma). Although much less common than NMSC, melanoma is a serious public health issue. The incidence rates of melanoma in the United States have risen more rapidly than any other cancer except lung cancer in women. The lifetime risk of melanoma was 1 in 1500 in 1930, 1 in 250 in 1980, 1 in 120 in 1987, and, in 1996, was projected to reach 1 in 75 by 2000.[3] More than 7300 melanoma deaths occurred during 1996. The American Cancer Society states that melanoma would have developed in more than 40 000 Americans in 1998, making this the sixth most frequent cancer in males and the seventh most frequent cancer in females. Although melanoma is potentially curable if detected in the early stages, melanoma that has metastasized has a grave prognosis. Thus, efforts have been directed toward prevention and early detection.

The exact cause of the increase in the incidence of melanoma is unknown. It most likely represents a combination of effects, including stratospheric ozone depletion, resulting in more intense UVR reaching the earth's surfaces and changes in dress favoring more skin exposure. Other factors, yet to be determined, are most likely involved.

Several factors implicate sunlight in the pathogenesis of most, but not all, cases of melanoma:

1. Latitude: There is an inverse relationship between latitude and the incidence and mortality rates of melanoma in whites, with higher rates found closer to the equator (where the amount of sunlight is greater).[4]

2. Race and pigmentation: Melanoma occurs predominantly in whites with an incidence approximately 10 times greater for white men and women than for blacks. The mortality rate among whites is five times greater than for blacks. There is, in general, an inverse correlation between incidence and the skin pigmentation of people in various countries in the world. Melanin decreases the transmission of UVR. This may protect melanocytes from sunlight-induced changes that lead to their malignant transformation.[5]

3. Childhood exposure: Episodic high exposures sufficient to cause sunburn, particularly during childhood and adolescence, increase

the risk of melanoma.[6-8] In a study, blistering sunburns at 15 to 20 years of age (but not after age 30) were significantly associated with increased risk (relative risk of 2.2 for more than 5 sunburns vs none).[9] Migration studies indicate that high exposure to sunlight during childhood sets the stage for high rates of melanoma in adulthood.[10]

Approximately 80% of lifetime sun exposure occurs before the age of 18.[11] In childhood and adolescence, melanocytes may be more sensitive to the sun, resulting in alteration of their DNA, possibly leading to the formation of unstable moles that may become malignant. Sunlight exposure and blistering sunburns during youth may be more intense than later in life because of child and adolescent behavior patterns. Passing through critical stages of carcinogenesis early in life may increase the chance of completing the remaining stages. One of these stages may involve the formation of nevi (moles), particularly dysplastic nevi.

4. Nevi: Acute sun exposure is implicated in the development of nevi in children. The number of nevi increases with increasing age[12]; nevi occur with more frequency on sun-exposed areas; and the number of nevi on exposed areas increases with the total cumulative sun exposure during childhood and adolescence.[5,13] Children with light skin who tend to burn rather than tan have more nevi at all ages, and children who have more severe sunburns have more nevi.[12]

There is a relationship between the number and type of melanocytic nevi and the development of melanoma. Dysplastic melanocytic nevi, which may represent a reaction to solar injury, are considered precursor lesions that increase risk.[14] The presence of congenital nevi greater than 1.5 cm in diameter also increases risk.[5]

The familial dysplastic nevus syndrome is a disorder with the following features: (1) a distinctive appearance of abnormal melanocytic nevi; (2) unique histologic features of the nevi; (3) autosomal dominant pattern of inheritance; and (4) hypermutability of fibroblasts and lymphoblasts. Fibroblasts and lymphoblasts from patients with this syndrome are abnormally sensitive to UV damage, and persons with this syndrome are at markedly higher risk for the development of melanoma.[14]

5. Xeroderma pigmentosum (XP): Melanomas are frequently found in persons with XP and related disorders in which there is a genet-

ically determined defect in the repair of DNA damaged by UVR and a high risk of NMSC.[15]

Exposure to sunbeds and sunlamps, which produce primarily UV-A, is associated with increased risk.[16]

Phototoxicity and Photoallergy

Chemical photosensitivity refers to an adverse cutaneous reaction that occurs when certain chemicals or drugs are applied topically or taken systemically at the same time that a person is exposed to UV or visible radiation. Phototoxicity is a form of chemical photosensitivity that does not depend on an immunologic response, as the reaction can occur on the person's first exposure to the offending agent. Most phototoxic agents are activated in the UV-A range (320 to 400 nm). Photoallergy is an acquired altered reactivity of the skin that is dependent on antigen-antibody or cell-mediated hypersensitivity.[17]

Persons who take medications or use topical agents that are sensitizing should avoid all sun exposure, if possible, and completely avoid all UV-A from artificial sources. The consequences of exposure can be uncomfortable, serious, or life-threatening.[17] Sensitizing medications include sulfonamides, tretinoin, tetracyclines, and thiazides.

Skin Aging

Long-term exposure to sunlight without sunscreen protection starting in childhood causes wrinkles and varying degrees of skin thickening and thinning. The cumulative effects of excessive unprotected sun exposure weaken the skin's elasticity, leading to sagging cheeks, deeper facial wrinkles, and skin discoloration later in life.[18]

Effects on the Eye

In adults, more than 90% of UVR is absorbed by the anterior structure of the eye. UVR can contribute to the development of age-related cataracts, pterygium, photodermatitis, and cancer of the skin around the eye.[19]

Melanoma of the uveal tract, the most common primary intraocular malignant neoplasm in adults, is associated with a tendency to sunburn and with intense exposure to UVR.[20] Infants and children under age 10 may be at increased risk for retinal injury because the transmissibility of the lens to damaging visible blue and UV light is greatest during this period. Cataract formation seems to be positively correlated with decreasing latitude and increasing UV-B and total sunlight exposure.[17]

Effects on the Immune System

In mice, contact hypersensitivity and delayed-type hypersensitivity can be suppressed by exposure to UVR. Immune suppression is thought to play an important role in the growth of skin cancer, in progression of certain infections, and in vaccine response. In humans, exposure to UVR doses achieved at midday in the summer sun causes suppression of contact hypersensitivity similar to that demonstrated in mice.[21]

Research needs in this area have been identified by the Environmental Protection Agency and the World Health Organization. These include the study of the effects of UVR on the effectiveness of immunizations against measles, hepatitis, and bacille Calmette-Guérin (BCG). Research needs were identified in clarifying the role of UVR in allergy, asthma, and autoimmune disease.[21]

■ Treatment of Clinical Syndromes

Pediatricians will rarely encounter patients with NMSC or melanoma. Patients at high risk, including children with XP and related disorders and those with a large number of nevi and a family history of melanoma, should be treated in collaboration with a dermatologist.

Sunburns should be treated with cool compresses and analgesics; 1% hydrocortisone cream can be applied to small areas of first-degree burn. Instruction about preventing future sunburns should be given at the time of the burn.

■ Prevention of Exposure

Although other major risk factors (eg, precursor lesions, age, race, previous melanoma, and family history) are more closely associated with melanoma than are sunburns, solar radiation is the only risk factor that is avoidable. Estimates are that effective sun protection during the first 18 years of life would reduce the number of lifetime skin cancers by almost 80%.[11]

Pediatricians have an important role in education beginning in infancy, and later when developmental stages result in new patterns of sun exposure (eg, when the child begins to walk, before starting school, and before entering adolescence).[22] Preteens and teens may need special reinforcement as they are often susceptible to societal notions of beauty and health. Teen counseling should include warnings about using sunbeds and sunlamps.

All parents and children should receive advice about sun protection. Not all children sunburn easily, but people of all skin types can experience skin cancer, skin aging, and sun-related damage to the immune system. Children who should be especially targeted include those with XP, who must avoid all UVR, and those with familial dysplastic nevus syndrome, with excessive numbers of nevi, or with two or more family members with melanoma. Children showing signs of excessive sun exposure (eg, freckles) should also receive special instruction.

There is no evidence that even rigorous sun protection through use of protective clothing and screens interferes with maintenance of normal serum levels of vitamin D.[23]

Avoiding exposure
Infants under 6 months of age should be kept out of direct sunlight. They should be dressed in cool, comfortable clothing and wear hats with brims. Children's activities should be planned to avoid peak-intensity midday sun.

Clothes
Clothes offer the simplest and often most practical means of sun protection. The factors that determine the sun protection provided by a fabric are its material, structure, color and thickness; the most important factor affecting the UV-B transmission is the structure, or weave, of the material. Children can be protected by wearing long-sleeved shirts and pants and brimmed hats.[24]

Window Glass
Window glass blocks virtually all UV-B and at least half of all UV-A energy.

Sunscreens
There are no data from clinical trials to demonstrate the efficacy of using sunscreens in preventing skin cancer. The American College of

Preventive Medicine and others have questioned the use of sunscreen in preventing cancer.[25] The American Cancer Society and the American Academy of Dermatology continue to recommend sunscreen use as part of a program of sun avoidance.[26] Sunscreens reduce the intensity of UVR affecting the epidermis. Opaque sunscreens, including zinc oxide and titanium dioxide, do not selectively absorb UVR, but reflect and scatter all light. They are useful for patients with photosensitivity and other disorders who require protection from full-spectrum UVR, but may be cosmetically unacceptable.[1] Chemical UV absorbent agents are the most commonly used in sunscreens. "Normal UV-B absorbers" have maximal UV-B absorption but permit transmission of all radiation above 320 nm. "Broad-spectrum absorbers" absorb UV-A and UV-B. Early sunscreen preparations incorporated one type of chemical agent, whereas more recent formulations combine UV absorbers to provide a higher degree of protection. They are usually colorless and, therefore, cosmetically acceptable. PABA (p-aminobenzoic acid) and its esters, the most widely used sunscreen chemicals, absorb mainly within the UV-B range. They are useful in preventing sunburn but minimally effective for photosensitivity disorders. Other chemical sunscreens containing benzophenones or anthranilates protect against UV-A radiation. Sunscreen effectiveness has been tested.[27]

The sun protection factor (SPF) indicates the degree of protection provided; the higher the SPF, the greater the protection. For example, a person who would normally experience a sunburn in 10 minutes can be protected up to about 150 minutes (10×15) with an SPF-15 sunscreen. Sunscreens with an SPF of 15 or more theoretically filter more than 92% of the UVR responsible for erythema; sunscreens with an SPF of 30 filter out about 97% of the UVR. In actual use, the SPF is often substantially lower than expected because the amount used is less than half the recommended amount.[1,28] An SPF of 15 should be adequate in most cases.

Sunscreens should be used when a child might sunburn. Although there are no data showing that sunscreens prevent melanoma, there is no benefit in burning and it should be avoided. It is also likely that preventing sun exposure might prevent or delay skin aging, keratoses, and nonmelanoma skin cancer.

The issue of whether sunscreen is safe for infants under the age of 6 months is controversial. There are concerns that human skin under 6 months may have different absorptive characteristics and that biologic systems that metabolize and excrete drugs may not be fully developed.[29] The Australian Cancer Society concluded that there is no evidence to suggest that using sunscreen on small areas of a baby's skin is associated with any long-term effects. They recommend that sunscreen be used when physical protection, such as clothing, hats, and shade is not adequate.[30] On the basis of available evidence, it is reasonable to tell parents what is known about the safety of sunscreens in infants younger than 6 months and to emphasize the importance of avoiding high-risk exposure. In situations where the infant's skin is not protected adequately by clothing, it may be reasonable to apply sunscreen to small areas, such as the face and the back of the hands.[31]

The UV Index

The UV index, developed by the National Weather Service, predicts the intensity of UV light. It is based on the sun's position, cloud movements, altitude, ozone data, and other factors. It is conservatively calculated based on effects on skin types that burn easily. Higher numbers predict more intense UV light during midday of the following day (see Table 23.2). The index, available in 58 cities, is printed in the weather section of many daily newspapers.[32]

Table 23.2. Exposure Levels Predicted by the UV Index*

Index Value	Exposure Level	Time in the Sun Needed for Burn
0-2	Minimal	1 h
3-4	Low	30-60 min
5-6	Moderate	20-30 min
7-9	High	13-20 min
10-15	Very high	<13 min

*These UV effects are on unprotected skin type II, which always burns easily and tans minimally.

Protection for the Eyes

Wearing a hat with a brim can reduce UV-B exposure to the eyes by 50%. Sunglasses should be worn whenever the child may be in the sun long enough to get a sunburn or tan. Sunglasses should be chosen to block 99% of the sun's rays.[33]

Changes in Knowledge and Attitudes

Pediatricians alone cannot change social concepts in which a suntan is equated with health and beauty. School programs and public education campaigns must address this issue. Australia, which has the world's highest incidence of melanoma, has mounted a long sun-safety campaign directed toward children and teenagers. Melanoma mortality, which had been rising steadily, peaked in 1985 and subsequently plateaued overall; the mortality rate has fallen in women.[34]

Some encouraging trends have been noted in the depiction of tans among models in American fashion magazines.[35] Public health campaigns promoting sun protection have been mounted in the United States. This includes the SunWise Program sponsored by the EPA, which targets elementary school children.

❚ Frequently Asked Questions

Q *Why is a baby at special risk from sunburn?*
A A baby's skin is thinner than an adult's and burns more easily. Even dark-skinned babies may be sunburned. Babies cannot tell you if they are too hot or beginning to burn and cannot get out of the sun without an adult's help. Babies also need an adult to dress them properly and to apply sunscreen.

Q *What can I do to protect my child?*
A Babies younger than 6 months should be kept out of direct sunlight because of the risk of heat stroke. They should be moved under a tree, umbrella, or stroller canopy, although on reflective surfaces an umbrella or canopy may reduce UVR exposure by only 50%.

Q *How should I apply sunscreen to my baby?*
A Sunscreen should be tested on the baby's wrist for a reaction before applying it all over. The sunscreen needs to be applied

around the eyes, avoiding the eyelids. If the baby cries or complains that the sunscreen burns the eyes, the parent should try a different brand or try a sunscreen stick or sunblock with titanium dioxide or zinc oxide. If a rash develops, the pediatrician can make another suggestion.

When choosing a sunscreen, parents should look for the words "broad-spectrum" on the label—it means that the sunscreen will screen out the ultraviolet B (UV-B) and ultraviolet A (UV-A) rays. A sun protection factor (SPF) of 15 should be adequate in most cases.

Parents should apply sunscreen liberally and rub it in well 30 minutes before going outdoors, making sure to cover all exposed areas, especially the baby's face, nose, ears, feet, and hands, and even the backs of the knees. Sunscreen should be used even on cloudy days, because the sun's rays can penetrate through the clouds. Zinc oxide, a very effective sunblock, can be used as extra protection on the nose, cheeks, tops of the ears, and the shoulders. Zinc oxide should not be blended into the skin. Sunscreens should be used for sun protection and not as a reason to stay in the sun longer.

Q *Why are some sunscreens labeled "PABA-free"?*
A PABA is a common ingredient used in many sunscreens. Some persons have a rash or a burning sensation when using preparations containing PABA, and some PABA preparations can cause a yellow discoloration on clothing.

Q *How do I choose sunglasses for my child?*
A Sunglasses that absorb 99% to 100% of the full UV spectrum are recommended.

Parents should look for a label that indicates sufficient UV blocking capacity such as: "Blocks 99% of ultraviolet rays," "special purpose," or "meets ANSI [American National Standards Institute] UV requirements." Because labeling is not uniform, labels that are marked only "blocks harmful UV" may not provide enough protection.

Lens color has nothing to do with UV protection.

It is never too early for a child, even an infant, to wear sunglasses. Larger lenses, well-fitted and close to the surface of the eye, provide the best protection.

∎ Resource

The American Academy of Pediatrics provides a patient education pamphlet, *Fun in the Sun*, available from the Division of Consumer Education.

∎ References

1. Gilcrest BA. Actinic injury. *Ann Rev Med.* 1990;41:199-210

2. Sasson M, Mallory SB. Malignant primary skin tumors in children. *Curr Opin Pediatr.* 1996;8:373-377

3. Rigel DS, Friedman RJ, Kopf AW. The incidence of malignant melanoma in the United States: issues as we approach the 21st century. *J Am Acad Dermatol.* 1996;34:839-847

4. Kopf AW, Krioke ML, Stern RS. Sun and malignant melanoma. *J Am Acad Dermatol.* 1984;11:674-684

5. Kopf AW, Bart RS, Hennessey P. Congenital nevocytic nevi and malignant melanoma. *J Am Acad Dermatol.* 1979; 1:123-130

6. Marks R. Prevention and control of melanoma: the public health approach. *CA.* 1996;46:199-216

7. Lew RA, Sober AJ, Cook N, Marvell R, Fitzpatrick TB. Sun exposure habits in patients with cutaneous melanoma: a case-control study. *J Dermatol Surg Oncol.* 1983;9:981-986

8. Cress RD, Holly EA, Ahn DK. Cutaneous melanoma in women. V. Characteristics of those who tan and those who burn when exposed to summer sun. *Epidemiology.* 1995;6:538-543

9. Weinstock MA, Colditz GA, Willett WC, et al. Nonfamilial cutaneous melanoma incidence in women associated with sun exposure before 20 years of age. *Pediatrics.* 1989;84:199-204

10. Khlat M, Vail A, Parkin M, Green A. Mortality from melanoma in migrants to Australia: variation by age at arrival and duration of stay. *Am J Epidemiol.* 1992;135:1103-1113

11. Stern RS, Weinstein MC, Baker SG. Risk reduction for nonmelanoma skin cancer with childhood sunscreen use. *Arch Dermatol.* 1986;122:538-545

12. Gallagher RP, McLean DI, Yang CP, et al. Suntan, sunburn, and pigmentation factors and the frequency of acquired melanocytic nevi in children: similarities to melanoma: the Vancouver Mole Study. *Arch Dermatol.* 1990;126:770-776

13. Holman CD, Armstrong BK. Pigmentary traits, ethnic origin, benign nevi, and family history as risk factors for cutaneous malignant melanoma. *J Natl Cancer Inst.* 1984;72:257-266

14. Clark WH. The dysplastic nevus syndrome. *Arch Dermatol.* 1988;124: 1207-1210

15. Taylor AMR, McCorville CM, Boyd PJ. Cancer and DNA processing disorders. *Br Med Bull.* 1994;50:708-717

16. Westerdal J, Olsson H, Masback A, et al. Use of sunbeds or sunlamps and malignant melanoma in southern Sweden. *Am J Epidemiol.* 1994;140:691-699

17. American Medical Association Council on Scientific Affairs. Harmful effects of ultraviolet radiation. *JAMA.* 1989;262:380-384

18. Gilmore GD. Sunscreens: a review of the skin cancer protection value and educational opportunities. *J School Health.* 1989;59:210-213

19. The National Society to Prevent Blindness. The American Optometric Association, the American Academy of Ophthalmology. Statement on ocular ultraviolet radiation hazards in sunlight. November 10, 1993

20. Holly EA, Aston DA, Char DH, Kristiansen JJ, Ahn DK. Uveal melanoma in relation to ultraviolet light exposure and host factors. *Cancer Res.* 1990;50:5773-5777

21. Selgrade MK, Repacholi MH, Koren HS. Ultraviolet radiation-induced immune modulation: potential consequences for infectious, allergic, and autoimmune disease. *Environ Health Perspect.* 1997;105:332-334

22. Williams ML, Sagebiel RW. Sunburn, melanoma, and the pediatrician. *Pediatrics.* 1989;84:381-382

23. Sollitto RB, Kraemer KH, DiGiovanna JJ. Normal vitamin D levels can be maintained despite rigorous photoprotection: six years experience with xeroderma pigmentosum. *J Am Acad Dermatol.* 1997;37:942-947

24. Welsh C, Duffey B. The protection against solar actinic radiation afforded by common clothing fabrics. *Clin Exp Dermatol.* 1981;6:577-582

25. Hill L, Ferrini RL. Skin cancer prevention and screening: a summary of the American College of Preventive Medicine's practice policy statements. *CA Cancer J Clin.* 1998;45:232-235

26. McDonald CJ. Society perspective on the American College of Preventive Medicine's policy statements on skin cancer prevention and screening. *CA Cancer J Clin* 1998;45:229-231

27. Putting sunscreens to the test. *Consumer Reports.* 1995;60:334-339

28. Sunscreens: are they safe and effective? *Med Lett Drugs Ther* 1999;41:43-44

29. Sunscreen drug products for over-the counter human use: tentative final monograph. *Federal Register.* May 12, 1993;58:28194

30. Australian Cancer Society. *Policy statement: babies and sunscreen.* Sydney Australia; 1998

31. American Academy of Pediatrics Committee on Environmental Health. Ultraviolet light: a hazard to children. *Pediatrics.* 1999;104:328-333

32. Environmental Protection Agency. *The Federal experimental ultraviolet index: what you need to know.* Washington, DC: United States Environmental Protection Agency; 1994. EPA publication 430-F-94-016

33. Wagner RS. Why children must wear sunglasses. *Contemp Pediatr.* 1995;12:27-37

34. Giles GG, Armstrong BK, Burton RC, Staples MP, Thursfield VJ. Has mortality from melanoma stopped rising? Analysis of trends between 1931 and 1994. *BMJ.* 1996;312:1121-1125

35. Pierre MG, Kuskowski M, Schmidt C. Trends in photoprotection in American fashion magazines, 1983-1993. *J Am Acad Dermatol.* 1996;34:424-428

24 Water Pollutants

A lthough 70% of the earth is covered by water, only 3% of the earth's water is fresh. Of that 3%, two thirds is frozen in glaciers and ice caps, leaving only 1% available for human use. Fresh water is classified as either ground water, such as underground aquifers (0.7%), or surface water, such as lakes and rivers (0.3%), but less than half of the nonfrozen fresh water in the world is readily accessible.[1] Water pollution results from sources of contamination termed either point or nonpoint. Point sources of pollution include municipal wastewater treatment plant discharges and industrial wastewater discharges into surface waters. Nonpoint sources of pollution include agricultural runoff, urban runoff, soil contamination, and atmospheric deposition that contaminate surface waters directly and seep into underground aquifers to contaminate ground water as well. In the United States, approximately half of the drinking water comes from ground water, with the other half coming from either surface water or mixed surface and ground water sources.[2] Preserving the quality of fresh water is essential to public health and ecological integrity but is threatened by increasing population pressure and industrial and agricultural growth.

Water pollutants can be categorized as biological agents, chemicals, or radionuclides (see Table 24.1). Hundreds of biological agents and thousands of chemical agents can be found in water. For many water pollutants, little is known of their long-term health effects. Federal regulations were not mandated until passage of the Safe Drinking Water Act of 1974, and as yet only exist for a small per-

251

Table 24.1. Examples of Some Water Pollutants, Common Sources and Systems Affected

Pollutant Category (Specific Examples)	Common Source	Systems Affected
Biological agents		
Bacterial		
Campylobacter species	Feces: human, animal	Gastrointestinal
Escherichia coli	Feces: human, animal	Gastrointestinal
Salmonella species	Feces: human, animal	Gastrointestinal
Shigella coli	Feces: human	Gastrointestinal
Vibrio species	Feces: human, animal	Gastrointestinal
Viruses		
Calicivirus	Feces: human	Gastrointestinal
Enterovirus	Feces: human	Gastrointestinal, neurologic
Hepatitis A virus	Feces: human	Gastrointestinal (liver)
Rotavirus	Feces: human	Gastrointestinal
Parasites		
Balantidium coli	Feces: human, animal	Gastrointestinal
Cryptosporidium parvum	Feces: human, animal	Gastrointestinal
Entamoeba histolytica	Feces: human	Gastrointestinal
Giardia lamblia	Feces: human, animal	Gastrointestinal
Chemicals		
Metals and metalloids		
Arsenic	Smelting, coal burning, pesticides	All systems, lung and skin cancer
Lead	Pipes, solder, soil	Neurologic, hematologic
Mercury	Bioaccumulation	Neurologic

Continued on next page

Table 24.1. Continued

Pollutant Category (Specific Examples)	Common Source	Systems Affected
Natural Toxins		
Microcystins	Cyanobacteria	Gastrointestinal, neurologic
Pfiesteria toxins	*Pfiesteria piscicida*	Neurologic, dermatologic
Organic chemicals		
Methyl tertiary butyl ether	Leaking gasoline storage tanks	Unknown
Pesticides	Agriculture and urban runoff	Multiple
Polychlorinated biphenyls	Transformers, industry	Neurologic, hormonal
Trichloroethylene	Degreasing, dry cleaning, solvents	Animal cancers
Chlorination by-products		
Trihalomethanes Bromoform	Water chlorination	Animal cancers
Carbon tetrachloride		
Chloroform		
Inorganic ions		
Nitrates	Nitrogen fertilizers	Hematologic
Radionuclides		
Radon	Natural uranium	Pulmonary, gastrointestinal

centage of the contaminants present in water. These standards apply to community water supplies serving 25 or more customers, but not to smaller suppliers or private wells. Modern water treatment facilities have made the water supply in the United States among the safest in the world, eliminating the majority of waterborne bacterial illnesses. Nonetheless, about 30 waterborne disease outbreaks are reported each year in the United States.[3]

The discussion in this chapter will be limited to a few representative examples of each of the categories of water pollution. While biological contamination of drinking water represents the largest threat to human health worldwide, it will not be extensively discussed in this chapter. See AAP's *Red Book*[4] for information about infectious diarrheal diseases. Details on specific pollutants can be found in other chapters in this book.

■ Chemical Contaminants in Water

Water and sediments in water are the ultimate sinks for most chemicals produced and used by humans. There are more than 15 000 high volume production (production of more than 10 000 pounds per year) man-made chemicals in use, and hundreds of new chemicals are introduced into use each year. More than half of these chemicals have not been tested for toxic effects on humans.[5] Thousands of synthetic organic chemicals are used in agricultural and industrial processes.

Metals and Metalloids

Arsenic
Arsenic is ubiquitous. Human activities, such as smelting, coal burning, wood preservation, pesticide distribution, and other industrial processes produce at least three times more arsenic than natural processes.[6] Arsenic can be found in the environment in organic and inorganic states and in valence states of 0, 3, and 5. The toxicity of arsenic to humans depends on the form, with organic being less toxic than inorganic and pentavalent being less toxic than trivalent. Except in electronics, industrial uses of arsenicals are decreasing. Drinking water and food represent the major sources of arsenic for humans.

Lead
Drinking water represents a potential route of exposure to lead. In the past two decades, expanded regulations and monitoring of drinking water have made most large municipal water supplies safe from

exposure to lead. Nevertheless, some homes in the United States have lead levels in water above acceptable levels. Chicago, Boston, and other cities historically used 100% lead piping to connect water mains to homes. Millions of these lead connectors still exist. In addition, lead solder, used to connect copper pipes, was widely used until the late 1980s. Drinking water, particularly that which is soft (ie, low in calcium or magnesium), or below a neutral pH, causes lead to leach from lead connector pipes or soldered joints (see Chapter 14).

Mercury
Mercury in fish originates from combustion sources that release mercury into the air, such as coal-fired power plants used for generating electrical energy and municipal waste incinerators that burn garbage.[7] Atmospheric mercury is ultimately deposited into lakes and rivers by dustfall, rain, and snow. In the aquatic environment, mercury is converted by sediment bacteria into methyl mercury, which becomes concentrated in the muscle tissues of fish by direct absorption from the water and by biomagnification up though the aquatic food chain (see Chapter 15).

Natural Toxins
Water from ponds and lakes, as well as municipal and recreational waters, may contain cyanobacteria (blue-green algae), including *Microcystis aeruginosa*. These bacteria produce cyanotoxins such as microcystins, which are hepatotoxic and neurotoxic compounds.[8] Water from the rivers flowing into the Chesapeake Bay on the Eastern shore of the United States may be contaminated with *Pfiesteria piscicida,* a dinoflagellate which can produce neurotoxins.[9]

Organic Chemicals

Methyl Tertiary Butyl Ether
Methyl tertiary butyl ether (MTBE) is used in medicine to dissolve gallstones and in industry as a gasoline additive in reformulated gasoline. (It replaces lead as an octane enhancer in unleaded gasoline.) MTBE has a characteristic, very strong odor. This odor can herald a leak from an underground gasoline storage tank that has leached into local ground water.

Pesticides
Pesticides may not be removed by conventional drinking water treatment. As detection technologies have improved, increasingly low

concentrations of common insecticides, herbicides, and fungicides have been documented in the drinking water.

Some of the older pesticides were designed to be persistent in the environment for years, and can be found distributed worldwide in water and soil. Newer pesticides degrade more quickly, but still contaminate water. Concentrations in water often correlate with growing seasons in agricultural areas and rainy seasons in more urban settings.

Chemical contamination of ground water in municipal and private wells has been found in the past two decades. Private wells may become contaminated with agricultural pesticides. During the late 1970s and early 1980s, aldicarb, a carbamate pesticide, was found in private wells in New York, California, Maine, and Florida. In Wisconsin, where aldicarb was used to treat potatoes, about 300 private wells were found to be contaminated.[10] Environmental analyses revealed that the water-soluble pesticide leached through the sandy soils often favored for the growing of potatoes and other crops (see Chapter 20).

Polychlorinated Biphenyls (PCBs)

Polychlorinated biphenyls (PCBs) have very low solubility in water. They are a problem because they readily bioaccumulate in the fat of wildlife, are very resistant to biological degradation, and remain in the environment for decades. The sediments of many lakes and rivers are contaminated with PCBs. Contaminated sediments, a nonpoint source, are still the major source of PCBs found in fish and wildlife (see Chapter 21).

Chlorination By-products

In the 1970s, chlorination of waters having high natural organic content (eg, humic and tannic acids) were found to cause the formation of chloroform and other chlorinated compounds called trihalomethanes (THMs).

Inorganic Ions

Nitrates

Nitrates enter the water supply from urban and agricultural runoff of nitrogen fertilizers. They may also be produced by bacterial action on animal waste runoff (see Chapter 17).

Radionuclides

Radon

Radon gas is a product of the radioactive decay of uranium. It enters the water supply naturally and becomes aerosolized during use of tap water. Radon further breaks down into radon daughters (see Chapter 22). Radon in water is important because during showering, radon may be inhaled.

■ Routes of Exposure

Drinking water can be contaminated, as well as water used for the irrigation of foods often eaten raw such as carrots, lettuce, and tomatoes. Fish and shellfish harvested from polluted fresh and marine waters are also important sources of exposure to water pollutants.[11] Recreational exposure via the skin as well as ingestion and inhalation can result in illness if waters are contaminated.

The fetus may also be exposed to pollutants when a pregnant woman ingests water or food in which water pollutants have bioaccumulated. Adverse fetal effects may be associated with chronic exposures from materials prior to pregnancy as well. Lead, mercury, and PCBs accumulate in the body and are not readily excreted. These toxicants may be found in the body years after exposure has ceased.

■ Clinical Effects

Biological Agents
Waterborne illness is usually mild gastroenteritis with diarrhea. Even when water systems are in compliance with federal and local regulations, sporadic and epidemic illnesses occur.[12] This is of particular concern for infants and immunocompromised persons exposed to pathogens such as *Cryptosporidium* despite state-of-the-art water treatment. It is rare to have serious dysentery or enteric fever due to *Vibrio cholerae* and *Salmonella typhi* except in areas where water quality is compromised.

Chemicals
Metals and Metalloids
Arsenic. Arsenic exists in a number of valence states and in both organic and inorganic forms. In its trivalent form, it is a sulfhydryl-containing enzyme poison. In the pentavalent arsenate form, it competitively substitutes for phosphate, leading to rapid hydrolysis of the

high-energy bonds in adenosine triphosphate. Because it is an enzyme poison, it affects almost all organ systems.

Among the important health effects of low-level, chronic ingestion of arsenic are skin cancer, peripheral vascular disease, peripheral neuropathy, portal hypertension, renal insufficiency, and bone marrow suppression.[13]

Lead. Clinical effects of lead exposure are discussed in Chapter 14.

Mercury. An important source of mercury exposure is ingestion of fish harvested from waters contaminated with mercury. The devastating neurological effects of cerebral palsy, mental retardation, and deafness documented in children from the maternal consumption of mercury-contaminated fish in Japan provide powerful testimony to the potent neurological effects of mercury on the fetus.[14] Although the human body can eliminate some mercury, large amounts cannot be eliminated and accumulate in maternal and fetal tissues. Epidemiologic studies specifically examining neurologic development in children of mothers who eat a lot of fish containing mercury are currently in progress (see Chapter 15).

Natural Toxins

Microcystins produced by cyanobacteria have been linked to liver failure and death in patients who underwent hemodialysis at a dialysis center supplied by untreated water from a lake with massive growth of blue-green algae.[15] Chronic, daily exposure to waterways contain toxin-producing *Pfiesteria* dinoflagellates has been associated with learning and memory difficulties in a small sample of adults in Maryland.[9]

Organic Chemicals

MTBE. Exposure to MTBE in oxygenated gasoline has been associated with symptoms of headache, eye irritation, burning of the nose and throat, and cough among adults in Fairbanks, Alaska. Little is known about the effects of long-term, low-level exposures to MTBE.[16]

Pesticides. While high-level, acute poisoning is well understood for most pesticides (see Chapter 20), low-level, chronic, and mixed exposures are poorly studied, particularly in infants and children. Consequently, great uncertainty exists about the significance of contamination of drinking water with pesticides.

PCBs. In the 1980s, epidemiologic studies reported an association between neurologic effects (eg, decrease in visual recognition memory) in infants and young children whose mothers consumed an average of about two meals per month of lake trout or salmon from Lake Michigan prior to and during pregnancy. When these children were studied at age 11 years, a reduction in IQ was found in children whose mothers had higher body burdens of PCBs.[17,18] Similar effects have been reported in infants of women who ate Lake Ontario fish and in other PCB exposure cases. Health officials from the Great Lakes States estimated that a daily dosage of 0.5 µg PCBs per kilogram per day (30 µg PCBs per day for a 60-kg woman) is the lowest observed adverse effects level associated with neurological effects in infants. Long-term health effects are under investigation.

Trichloroethylene. In 1986, a positive association was found between childhood leukemia and drinking water supplied from two municipal wells in Woburn, Mass.[19] The two wells were contaminated with the animal carcinogens trichloroethylene, tetrachloroethylene, and chloroform. Childhood leukemia rates in Woburn reported between 1964 and 1983 were twice the national rates. Several chemical disposal pits, used for several decades, were suspected as the source of these chlorinated products. Although the two affected wells were shut down immediately upon discovery of the contamination, exposure to these carcinogens is believed to have occurred for many years.

Chlorination By-products. Epidemiologic studies show a correlation between THM-containing drinking water and increases in the rates of rectal and bladder cancer.[20] In one study among almost 3000 people with bladder cancer, the rates for those consuming chlorinated surface water for 60 or more years were two times greater than rates of those who had not consumed treated surface water.[12] As a result of extensive testing of the water supplies in the United States, cancer risk analysis of the chemicals found, and suggestive epidemiologic studies in 1981, the US EPA issued a maximum contaminant level for THM in water.

Inorganic Ions

Nitrates

Nitrates themselves are not toxic to humans, but can be converted to more reactive and toxic nitrites by gut bacteria. Nitrates in drinking water above the EPA level of 10 mg/L may cause fatal methemoglobinemia in infants (see Chapter 17).

Radionuclides

Radon

Adult lung cancer has been linked to inhalation of radon. A weak association of radon with gastrointestinal cancer has been suggested in a few epidemiologic studies (see Chapter 22).[22] More evidence is being collected to better assess these risks.

∎ Prevention of Exposure

The public health success of the 20th century in eliminating epidemic cholera and typhoid fever are dramatic evidence of the importance of prevention in managing drinking and recreational water supplies. Historically, water and waste management were local responsibilities. During the environmental movement in the 1970s, Congress enacted laws that unified standards and resulted in the development of high-quality drinking and recreational waters.

Public Water Supplies

The EPA and state agencies require that municipal or commercial water suppliers serving more than 25 people meet all standards developed under the Safe Drinking Water Act of 1974 (see Table 24.2). The Water Pollution Control Act (1972) and the Resource Conservation and Recovery Act (1976) require industrial, commercial, and municipal facilities to meet requirements to prevent contamination of surface and ground waters.

In 1987, increased findings of water supplies contaminated with industrial chemicals led the EPA to promulgate drinking water standards for eight volatile organic compounds, including those most often found in contaminated wells.[23] The EPA and state environmental agencies require municipal water supplies to meet specific standards for pesticides that have been found in ground and surface waters. Restrictions have been placed upon the use of pesticides, which may leach into waters. Drinking water must also meet a standard for THMs of 80 ppb which, as chloroform, is expected to yield no more than one case of cancer per 100 000 persons exposed.

The benefits of chlorinated drinking water in reducing waterborne diseases far outweigh the insignificant risks from traces of THMs in drinking water.

**Table 24.2. National Interim Primary Drinking Water Regulations
(MCL - maximum contaminant levels)**

Contaminant	MCL
Inorganic chemicals	
Arsenic	0.5 (mg/L)
Barium	1
Cadmium	0.010
Chromium	0.05
Fluoride	1.4-2.4
Lead	0.05
Mercury	0.002
Nitrate (as N)	10
Selenium	0.01
Silver	0.05
Organic chemicals	
Chlorinated hydrocarbons	
Endrin	0.0002
Lindane	0.004
Methoxychlor	0.1
Toxaphene	0.005
Chlorophenoxys	
2,4-D	0.1
2,4,5-T, Silvex	0.01
Trihalomethanes	0.1
Turbidity	1 unit
Microbiologic contaminants	1 coliform bacterium per 100 mL as the arithmetic mean of all samples per month
Radioactivity	
Combined radium-226 and radium-228	5 pCi/L
Gross alpha particle activity (including radium-226, but excluding radon and uranium)	15 pCi/L
Average annual concentration of beta particle and photon radioactivity not to produce annual dose equivalent greater than	4 mrem per year
Tritium	20 000 pCi/L
Strontium-90	8 pCi/L

Private Wells

Private wells are not federally regulated. Contamination of well water can occur if the well is shallow, in porous soil, old, poorly maintained, near a leaky septic tank or downhill from agricultural fields or intensive livestock operations. Each state has different testing procedures, sometimes requiring testing only at transfer of land ownership. Testing of private wells is the responsibility of individual homeowners, but in some states may be performed at no cost by the health department if recommended by a health care provider. In rural areas, physicians may provide a valuable public health service by asking patients if their wells have been tested within the last year for coliforms and nitrates by local or county health departments.

In agricultural areas, higher than normal levels of nitrates or coliform bacteria may indicate the presence of pesticides. If so, parents can contact state health and environmental agencies to determine if their well water should be tested for specific pesticides. State agencies may conduct the testing without cost or may recommend private laboratories. Extensive pesticide testing should not be encouraged due to cost and rarity of pesticide contamination.

Home Treatment Systems

Home water filtration and treatment systems that remove lead, chlorine by-products, traces of organic compounds, and bacteria are increasingly popular. These systems, which may attach to the end of a water faucet, generally provide limited health benefits. Most drinking water sources keep contaminants below EPA standards and state criteria. In addition, small, end-of-the-faucet filtration systems are not always highly effective in removing trace substances. If not properly maintained, filters using activated carbon can provide media for the growth of bacteria. Unless the carbon filter is frequently replaced, the first morning draw of tap water can have unacceptable levels of bacteria. In spite of potential drawbacks, some home water systems can be effective in removing lead and other toxic substances. These systems, however, do not remove fluoride.

Home drinking treatment systems or filters are not encouraged unless a chemical problem has been identified. Even then, it is more effective, including from a cost perspective, to have the municipal or commercial water source personnel correct the problem as required by law than to have homeowners assume the responsibility.

Contaminants in Fish

Physicians living in active fishing areas with advisories related to PCBs or mercury should ask women and children if their consumption of fish is in accordance with state-issued fish advisories. Fresh water fish have higher levels of contaminants than saltwater fish.[24,25] Saltwater fish, generally low in contaminants, are the main fish purchased in the marketplace. However, a few saltwater fish may have higher levels of contaminants than fresh water fish. They include swordfish, shark, and tuna, which are long-lived, predatory fish capable of bioaccumulating contaminants.

To reduce hazards from fish consumption, inform parents to:
- eat pan fish rather than predator fish (shark, swordfish, tuna)
- eat small game fish rather than large ones
- eat fewer fatty fish (carp, catfish, lake trout) which accumulate higher levels of chemical toxicants
- trim skin and fatty areas where contaminants such as PCBs and DDT accumulate
- advise women of childbearing age, pregnant women, nursing mothers, and young children to follow fish advisories
- know state fish advisories obtained from state health, environmental, and conservation departments

---

To reduce exposure to PCBs, health scientists in the Great Lakes States, the Agency for Toxic Substances and Disease Registry, and the EPA have recommended a daily dosage of ≤ 0.05 µg PCBs per kilogram per day to protect the developing fetus from neurological effects. This dosage also protects the general public from potential adverse immune system effects and keeps cancer from PCBs within the upper range of acceptable levels (one in 10 000). This dosage can be translated into practical public health advice. For example, fish advisories for Lake Michigan recommend that individuals not eat more than one meal per month of salmon (with an average of 0.7 ppm PCBs), for a maximum of 12 meals per year. Women and children are advised to wait a month before eating another meal of Lake Michigan salmon or any other fish from a restricted category to prevent PCBs from building up in the body. Spacing of meals is less important for other groups, such as adult men. Instructions are also provided to help reduce PCB exposures by cleaning (eg, fat removal) and cooking methods.[24,25]

The EPA has set an acceptable (reference) dose of 0.1 µg/kg per day of mercury to account for variability in the human population.[26,27] Most state health agencies advise limiting intake of fresh water fish having greater than 0.2 ppm of mercury. Other states simply recommend that women and children not eat any large predator fish that tend to concentrate mercury.

■ Frequently Asked Questions

Q *Should I buy bottled water?*
A Unless there are known contamination problems of the drinking water, families should not be encouraged to buy bottled water. Bottled water is not required to meet any higher standards than tap water, and can cost 500 to 1000 times as much.

Q *Should I boil my baby's water or use a home water treatment system?*
A Parents should not boil their infant's drinking water or use a home water treatment system unless the drinking water is contaminated. Drinking water should be boiled only when the water supplier or health or environmental agency issues such instructions. Boiling tap water for 1 minute inactivates or destroys biological agents, but boiling water longer than 1 minute may concentrate contaminants. Unless carefully evaluated and well maintained, home water treatment systems are often ineffective and may even contribute to exposure to waterborne bacteria.

Q *Is it true that federal and state regulations ensure the safety of drinking water?*
A In most cases, regulations provide very safe water. Nonetheless, almost 10% of the population drinks water that does not meet the regulations. Violations are higher where water supply systems serve fewer than 1000 people. Information on drinking water quality and violations can be obtained from the water supplier or state health and environmental agencies. Even water in compliance with all standards may contain harmful contamination.

Q *Should I get my water tested?*
A Under most circumstances, it is not necessary to have drinking water tested. If the local water supply fails to meet a standard, pressure should be exerted on politicians to correct the problem, rather than have people test their own water. As a precaution, people who use private wells less than 50 ft (15 meters) deep and have septic systems should have them tested yearly for coliforms. Quarterly testing for 1 year followed by yearly nitrate testing of private wells is also encouraged in agricultural areas.

Q *Do the benefits of eating fish outweigh the risks from PCBs, mercury, and other contaminants?*
A Fish provide a diet high in protein and low in saturated fats. The consumption of fish may reduce the risk of coronary disease. State and federal health agencies recommend that people who frequently consume fresh water fish follow fish advisories. This permits the consumer to reap the potential benefits of fish consumption and minimize risks due to the intake of PCBs and mercury.

▮ Resources

Agency for Toxic Substances and Disease Registry, Information Center, Division of Toxicology, 1600 Clifton Road, Mail Stop E-57, Atlanta, GA 30333. Internet address: atsdr.cdc.gov

Local and State Health Departments

United States Environmental Protection Agency. Regional offices are listed in the local telephone book. EPA Safe Drinking Water Hotline, 800/426-4791. Internet: http://www.epa.gov/ost/fish/.

US Fish and Wildlife Service, Department of the Interior, Washington, DC 20240

▮ References

1. Okum DA. Water quality management. In: Last JM, Wallace RB, eds. *Public Health and Preventive Medicine.* 13th ed. Norwalk, CT: Appleton & Lange; 1992:619-648

2. Ruttenber AJ. Water: Pollution and availability. In: Blumenthal DS, Ruttenber AJ, eds. *Introduction to Environmental Health*. 2nd ed. New York, NY: Springer Publishing Co, Inc; 1995:221-254

3. Craun GF. The epidemiology of waterborne disease: The importance of drinking water disinfection. In: Talbott EO, Craun GF, ed. *Introduction to Environmental Epidemiology*. Boca Raton, FL: Lewis Publishers; 1995:123-150

4. American Academy of Pediatrics, Committee on Infectious Diseases. Peter G, ed. *1997 Red Book, Report of the Committee on Infectious Diseases*. 24th ed. Elk Grove Village, IL: American Academy of Pediatrics; 1997

5. Landrigan PJ, Carlson JE, Bearer CF, et al. Children's health and the environment: a new agenda for prevention research. *Environ Health Perspect.* 1998;106(suppl 3):787-794

6. Kreiss K. Arsenic toxicity. *Case Studies in Environmental Medicine #5.* Atlanta, GA: US Department of Health and Human Services, Agency for Toxic Substances and Disease Registry. June, 1990

7. US Environmental Protection Agency. *Mercury Study Report to Congress. Vol 1: Executive Summary.* EPA-452/R-96-001a. 1996. Available by contacting 1-800-553-6847

8. Codd GA, Ward CJ, Bell SG. Cyanobacterial toxins: occurrence, modes of action, health effects and exposure routes. *Arch Toxicol Suppl.* 1997;19:399-410

9. Grattan LM, Oldach D, Perl TM, et al. Learning and memory difficulties after environmental exposure to waterways containing toxin-producing *Pfiesteria* or *Pfiesteria*-like dinoflagellates. *Lancet.* 1998;352:532-539

10. Mirkin IR, Anderson HA, Hanrahan L, Hong R, Golubiatnikov R, Belluck D. Changes in T-lymphocyte distribution associated with the ingestion of aldicarb-contaminated drinking water: a follow-up study. *Environ Res.* 1990; 51:35-50

11. Bowen EL, Hu H. Food contaimination due to environmental pollution. In: Chivian E, McCally M, Hu H, Haines A, eds. *Critical Condition: Human Health and the Environment*. Cambridge, MA: MIT Press; 1993

12. Payment P, Richardson L, Siemiatychi J, et al. A randomized trial to evaluate the risk of gastrointestinal disease due to consumption of drinking water meeting current national standards. *Am J Public Health.* 1991;81:703-708

13. Bates MN, Smith AH, Hopenhayn-Rich C. Arsenic ingestion and internal cancers: A review. *Am J Epidemiol.* 1992;135:462-476

14. Harada Y. Congenital (or Fetal) Minamata disease. In: Study Group of Minamata Disease, ed. *Minamata Disease.* Japan: Kumamoto University, 1968;93-117

15. Pouria S, de Andrade A, Barbosa J, et al. Fatal microcystin intoxication in haemolysis unit in Caruaru, Brazil. *Lancet.* 1998;352:21-26

16. Moolenaar RL, Hefflin BJ, Ashley DL, Middaugh JP, Etzel RA. Methyl teritary butyl ether in human blood after exposure to oxygenated fuel in Fairbanks, Alaska. *Arch Environ Health.* 1994;49:402-409

17. Jacobson JL, Jacobson SW. Intellectual impairment in children exposed to polychlorinated biphenyls in utero. *N Engl J Med*. 1996;335:783-789

18. Lonky E, Reihman J, Darvill T, Mather J, Daly H. Neonatal behavioral assessment scale performance in humans influenced by maternal consumption of environmentally contaminated lake Ontario fish. *J GT Lakes Res*. 1996;22:198-212

19. National Research Council. *Environmental Epidemiology: Public Health and Hazardous Wastes*. Washington, DC: National Academy Press; 1991:1

20. Morris RD, Audet AM, Angelillo IF, Chalmers TC, Mostellar F. Chlorination, chlorination by-products, and cancer: a meta-analysis. *Am J Public Health*. 1992; 82:955-963

21. Cantor KP, Hoover R, Hart GEP, et al. Bladder cancer, drinking water source, and tap water consumption: A case-control study. *J Natl Cancer Inst*. 1987;79:1269-1279

22. Bean JA, Isacson P, Hahne RM, Kohler J. Drinking water and cancer incidence in Iowa: II. Radioactivity in drinking water. *Am J Epidemiol*. 1982;116:924-932

23. US Environmental Protection Agency, Office of Water. *Drinking Water Regulations and Health Advisories*. October 1996. Washington, DC: Environmental Protection Agency. 822-R-96-002. October 1996

24. Anderson HA. *Protocol for a Uniform Great Lakes Sport Fish Advisory*. Wisconsin Department of Health and Human Services; 1993; available by writing to the Wisconsin Department of Health and Family Services, Division of Health, 1400 East Washington St, Madison, WI 53703

25. Minnesota Department of Public Health. *Fish and Your Health: Environmental Exposure to PCBs*. June 1993. *An Expectant Mother's Guide*. August 1994. *Mercury in the Environment*. May 1996. Available by contacting 1-800-627-3529 or writing Minnesota Department of Health. Division of Environmental Health, PO Box 64975, St Paul, MN 55164-0975

26. Stern AH. Re-evaluation of the reference dose for methyl mercury and assessment of current exposure levels. *Risk Anal*. 1993;13:355-364

27. Stern AH. Estimation of the interindividual variability in the one-compartment pharmacokinetic model for methyl mercury: implications for the derivation of a reference dose. *Reg Toxicol Pharmacol*. 1997;25:277-288

III
Specific Environments

25 Arts and Crafts

C hildren begin to use and enjoy arts and crafts materials when they are young. Arts and crafts materials abound in homes, child care centers, schools, churches, and park and recreation facilities. Many of these materials contain ingredients that are known to be hazardous. Parents, teachers, and other adults working with children may not be aware of the potential health hazards associated with these common materials.

Dangerous chemicals found in art materials can be divided into metals, solvents, and dusts or fibers.[1] Lead and other toxic metals such as mercury, cadmium, and cobalt are found in paints, pastels, pigments, inks, glazes, enamels, and solder.[2] Legal bans on lead and other metals in paint do not apply to artists' paints, which are used in painting, drawing, ceramics, silk-screening, making stained-glass, and other activities that may be part of art projects involving children or adolescents.[3] Some paper mâché products contain heavy metals from inks found in magazines. Hazardous organic solvents such as turpentine, kerosene, mineral spirits, xylene, benzene, methyl alcohol, and formaldehyde are used in painting, silk-screening, and shellacking, as well as in cleaning tools and preparation of work surfaces.[4] Rubber cement, spray-on enamels, and spray-on fixatives are common art products that also contain organic solvents.[5] Dusts and fibers containing hazardous materials such as asbestos, silica, talc, lead, cadmium, and mercury are generated during reconstitution of powdered pigments, glazes and clay, and the use of pastels.

Physical art hazards result from exposure to noise, dangerous mechanical and power tools, machinery and materials storage, and waste disposal practices. These hazards are most likely to occur in industrial arts settings and are often regulated under Occupational Safety and Health Administration (OSHA) and US Environmental Protection Agency (EPA) rules.[6]

■ Routes of Exposure

The wide variety of arts and crafts activities and materials used by children and adolescents permits the full spectrum of routes of exposure, which depend on the specific activity, materials used, and age of the child.

Inhalation is a major route of exposure for volatile organic solvents, dusts, and fibers. Exposure can occur during normal use, especially if ventilation is inadequate or if necessary personal protective equipment is not available or not properly used. Exposure can also occur through inappropriate exploring of new materials by "sniff testing." Finally, intentional inhalation such as glue sniffing can result in high-level exposure through the lungs.

Accidental ingestion is the route of exposure for many art hazards and may occur when common art materials are improperly stored in unlabeled or empty food containers. Even properly labeled art materials may be ingested by young or developmentally delayed children. Ingestion may also occur through nail biting, thumb sucking or other hand-to-mouth behaviors common in children.

Dermal absorption may occur from improper handling of hazardous art materials, accidental spills, or through contact with cuts or abrasions. Exposure through the conjunctivae may occur from spills, splashes, and rubbing one's eyes.

Physical hazards cause injury in a variety of ways. Noise standards developed to protect adult workers may be exceeded in secondary school industrial arts workshops, exposing children to potential hearing loss. Use of potentially dangerous equipment may result in cuts, crush injuries, fractures, or amputations. Power equipment may cause electrical injury or fires. Techniques requiring repetitive motion may cause tendonitis, carpal tunnel syndrome, or other injuries. Most of these hazards can be minimized through proper industrial hygiene evaluation, engineering measures, and use of personal protective equipment.

∎ Systems Affected and Clinical Effects

Relatively little is known about the effects of chronic low-level exposures to hazardous art materials on children. No case reports of illness in children from low-level exposures to arts and crafts hazards have been described in the literature. Extrapolation from adult experience is questionable, but raises the theoretical possibilities that chronic low-level exposures to hazardous art materials in childhood could exacerbate or cause allergies, hypersensitivity and asthma, central and peripheral nerve damage, psychological and behavioral changes, respiratory damage, skin changes, or cancer.

∎ Diagnostic Methods and Treatment

Diagnosis and treatment are specific to each type of exposure and illness.

∎ Prevention

A variety of preventive measures may greatly reduce exposure to arts and crafts hazards. Toxicity from long-term, low-level childhood exposure has not been documented. Nonetheless, measures designed to prevent exposures that in theory may be harmful are prudent. Some measures apply to all environments in which children use arts and crafts materials; others apply specifically to institutions.

Careful art material selection can eliminate much of the risk from arts and crafts materials. For children, only materials certified to be safe should be selected (see Table 25.1). The Consumer Product Safety Commission (CPSC) considers a child as anyone under the age of 13 years or attending grade school or below. The Center for Safety in the Arts has published a list of safe substitutes, which is available on their World Wide Web site. As children mature, their ability to follow directions, use precautions, and understand risks will allow for careful use of adult art materials and techniques that require precautions to use safely.

Arts and crafts materials are labeled in a variety of ways. The familiar AP or CP (and now the Health Label [no health labeling required]) seals of the Art and Creative Materials Institute (ACMI) certify that an art material can be used without risk of acute or

Table 25.1. Recommendations for Selecting Art Materials for Children Younger Than 13 Years

- read the label and instructions on all arts and craft materials
- buy only products labeled with "Conforms to ASTM D4236" and which bear the AP/CP/Health Label (no health labeling required) seals of the Art and Creative Materials Institute
- do not use materials labeled as "Keep out of Reach of Children" or "Not for Use by Children"
- do not use materials marked with the words "Poison" "Danger," "Warning," or "Caution," or which contain hazard warnings on the label
- do not use donated or found materials unless in the original containers with full labeling

chronic health hazards by everyone, even children and impaired adults. This program covers about 80% of all children's art materials and about 95% of all fine art materials sold in the United States.

In 1983, the American Society for Testing and Materials developed a national voluntary standard, ASTM D4236, *Labeling of Art Materials for Chronic Health Hazards*. This standard requires that art materials must be evaluated by a toxicologist and, if labeling is required, conform to stringent labeling requirements that include the identity of hazardous ingredients, risks associated with use, precautions to take to prevent harm, first aid measures, and sources of further information. All products certified by the ACMI have conformed to this standard since its inception. In 1990 the Labeling for Hazardous Art Materials Act went into effect. This act made the "voluntary" ASTM D4236 standard mandatory for all art materials imported or sold in the United States. This act is administered by the CPSC, which requires that hazardous consumer products, including art materials, have warnings to keep out of reach of children (acute health hazards) or that they should not be used by children (chronic health hazards).

Occasionally art materials available for purchase are improperly labeled. Crayons containing high levels of lead have been labeled "non-toxic." In order to make sure that an art material has been evaluated by a toxicologist, parents should look for the statement, "conforms to ASTM D4236" covering chronic health hazards and an ACMI seal for both acute and chronic health hazards.[7]

Good ventilation in rooms used for arts and crafts activities is always important.

Proper storage and clean-up are also essential. Materials should only be stored in original, fully labeled containers. Appropriate clean-up at the end of an art session includes closing and storing all containers, cleaning all tools, wiping down all used surfaces, and thorough hand washing. Adult art and hobby materials should be similarly labeled and stored out of the reach of children. Half of all artists work in home studios, many of which are in living areas where children also live and may be exposed.

Close supervision of all children during arts and crafts activities can prevent injuries and poisonings, ensure proper use of materials, and allow for the observation of adverse reactions. Eating or drinking should not occur while using art materials. Cuts and abrasions should be covered if they are likely to come in contact with materials being used.

Central ordering at the district or state level in public schools and other large institutions can facilitate the selection of safe art materials. Prevention begins with selection of the safest materials.

Emergency protocols should be in place in case of an injury, poisoning, or allergic reaction. The local poison control center number should be prominently posted. Adequate flushing facilities should be provided in case of spills or eye splashes. Material Safety Data Sheets (MSDS)* should be available on site for all hazardous materials that may be used in high school industrial arts classes. Adult supervisors should have proper first aid and emergency response skills and training.

Art safety education for all supervising adults is desirable. Art activities are common in church schools, child care centers, preschools, elementary and secondary schools, hospitals, chronic care institutions, therapeutic facilities, and at art festivals. Whenever possible, teachers, group leaders, and responsible adults should be trained in art safety. Art teachers should be thoroughly trained in safety for all techniques they use in the classroom. Children with special vulnerabilities should be identified and appropriate measures taken to protect their health. These could include children with

---

* MSDS are information sheets required by law for all industrial products, and available upon request from the manufacturer. They must contain product content information, emergency exposure protocols and emergency telephone numbers for medical personnel treating individuals.

asthma and allergies who might be hypersensitive to normally tolerated exposures. Children with physical, psychological, or learning disabilities may need special assistance in the use of some equipment, or in understanding instructions and following safety techniques.[8]

Industrial arts programs should follow OSHA, EPA, and state guidelines for ventilation, physical plant, fire safety systems, and personal protective equipment. These programs for older children and young adults should have a formal health and safety program.

▌ Frequently Asked Question

Q *Are water-based art supplies always safe?*
A Some water-based, cold-water dyes are sensitizers. Long-term health effects have not been thoroughly studied. In general, water-based supplies are preferable because they avoid the need for organic solvents. Accidental ingestion of even small amounts of organic solvents can be fatal.

▌ Resources

American Association of Poison Control Centers. Internet address: http://www.aapcc.org. Poison control centers are the best resources for medical response to acute exposures. This Web site has listings for state, regional, and Canadian centers including addresses, emergency telephone numbers, fax numbers, and e-mail addresses.

American Industrial Hygiene Association 2700 Prosperity Ave, #250, Fairfax, VA 22031. Telephone: 703/849-8888. Fax: 703/207-3561. e-mail: infonet@aiha.org. Internet address: http://www.aiha.org. This organization gives guidance to institutions designing and managing industrial arts facilities and programs.

Art and Creative Materials Institute (ACMI). 100 Boylston St, Suite 105, Boston MA 02116. 617/426-6400. E-mail: debfanning.acmi @guildassoc.com. Internet address: http:\www.creative-industries. com/acmi

ACMI develops standards for the safety and quality of art materials, manages a certification program to assure the safety of children's art and craft materials and the accuracy of labels of adult art materials that are potentially hazardous, develops and distributes information on the safe use of art and craft materials, provides lists of certified products (both those that are safe for children and adult art materials that may have a hazard potential) to individuals, CPSC, state health agencies, and school authorities, and provides consultations for concerned individuals. ACMI can put you in touch with toxicologists to answer questions about health concerns.

Center for Safety in the Arts. Internet address: http://www.arts wire.org:70/1/csa. Only accessible on the Internet. The Web site includes information on art hazards and children.

US Consumer Product Safety Commission. The CPSC is responsible for developing and managing regulations to support the Labeling for Hazardous Art Materials Act and the Federal Hazardous Substances Act. They instigate actions on mislabeled products and/or misbranded hazardous substances (products whose labels do not conform to these Acts), which may involve confiscations, product recalls, or other legal actions. The CPSC's Web site contains general product safety information and recent press releases. To report a dangerous product or product-related injury or illness, call CPSC's hotline at 800/638-2772 or via e-mail to info@cpsc.gov.

Public Interest Research Group. US PIRG, 218 D Street SE, Washington, DC 20003-1900. Telephone: 202/546-9707. Fax: 202/546-2461. e-mail: uspirg@pirg.org. Internet address: http://www. pirg.org/pirg. Several state PIRGs have conducted surveys of art hazards in schools. Similar methodology was employed by all. Reports may be obtained from individual state groups.

Materials Safety Data Sheets (MSDSs) are available from manufacturers for all products containing hazardous materials. They contain lists of ingredients, emergency procedures for accidents, and hotline numbers for further information.

US Environmental Protection Agency, 401 M St, SW, Washington, DC 20460. Internet address: http://www.epa.gov for Postal Addresses at EPA, or http://www.epa.gov/epahome/postal.htm.

Division of Occupational and Environmental Medicine, Toxicology Program, Duke University Medical Center, Box 5647, Durham, NC 27710. E-mail: stopf001@mc.duke,edu. Internet address: http://occ-env-med.mc.duke.edu/oem/stopford.htm.

The toxicologists offer advice to companies, physicians, poison control centers, and other health care providers concerning risks of art materials. Assessments may be useful for determining the safety and appropriate labeling of specific products or addressing questions of whether a specific job or material may be related to ill health. All arts and crafts materials certified by ACMI are first evaluated by the Duke toxicologists. Individuals with concerns about specific art materials should first contact ACMI.

■ References

1. Amdur MO, Doull J, Klaassen CD, eds. *Casarett and Doull's Toxicology: The Basic Science of Poisons.* ed 4. New York, NY: McGraw Hill; 1991

2. Babin A, Peltz PA, Rossol M. *Children's Art Supplies Can be Toxic.* New York, NY: Center for Safety in the Arts; 1992

3. McCann M. Occupational and environmental hazards in art. *Environ Res.* 1992;59:139-144

4. Lesser SH, Wiess SJ. Art hazards. *Am J Emerg Med.* 1995;13:451-458

5. McCann M. *Artist Beware.* New York, NY: Lyons and Burford Publishers; 1992

6. McCann M. *School safety procedures for art and industrial art programs.* New York, NY: Center for Safety in the Arts, 1994

7. Lu PC. A health hazard assessment in schools arts and crafts. *J Environ Pathol Toxicol and Oncol.* 1992;11:12-17

8. Rossol M. The first art hazards course. *J Environ Pathol Toxicol and Oncol.* 1992;11:28-32

26 Child Care Settings

M ore than half of US children spend some time in child care* away from home. In 1991, more than 7 million US children younger than 5 years whose mothers were employed were cared for by someone other than a parent.[1] More than half of these children were cared for outside the home in either a child care center (32%) or a family child care home (25%).[1] Children receive care outside the home as early as the newborn period, and may spend 50 or more hours per week in child care.[1] Children whose mothers are *not* employed outside the home also spend time in preschool, "mother's time-out" programs, drop-in care, or nursery care during religious services. Regulations regarding age of entry into child care vary by state.

Child care settings are located in single-family homes or buildings specifically designed for child care and within office buildings, schools, churches, malls, health clubs, and other sites. These structures should be designed or modified to meet current national stan-

---

* Common types of child care settings are usually defined as follows: Full-day centers enroll infants, toddlers and preschoolers for at least 4 hours per day, and part-day centers (such as nursery schools, Head Start programs, and preschools) enroll preschool children for less than 4 hours per day. Large family child care homes offer care and education for 7 to 12 children in the home of the caregiver. Small family child care homes offer care for 1 to 6 children in the home of the caregiver. Drop-in facilities offer care for one or more children in a residential or nonresidential setting for less than 10 hours per day, no more than once a week, to any child. (Source: American Public Health Association and American Academy of Pediatrics. *Caring for Our Children: National Health and Safety Performance Standards—Guidelines for Out-of-Home Child Care Programs; 1992).*[2]

dards published by the American Public Health Association and American Academy of Pediatrics in *Caring for Our Children: National Health and Safety Performance Standards—Guidelines for Out-of-Home Child Care Programs*.[2] These standards, which apply to all aspects of child care settings including environmental health aspects, should be met regardless of the setting or whether the care provided is full time or part time.[3]

Regulations relating to the health and safety of children in out-of-home child care programs vary widely among states. Child care centers are usually licensed and regulated by a state agency, whereas family child care homes, hourly drop-off care, and parochial and preschool programs (particularly if they operate part time) may have minimal or no regulatory oversight. Compliance with regulations depends on consensus of providers with the rationale for the regulations as well as the quality and frequency of inspection.[4]

The occurrence of environmental hazards in child care varies widely and is influenced by type of setting, licensing requirements, location and age of the structure, prevalence of hazards in the community, behaviors and practices of adults in the setting, past use of the land or structure, and current use of other parts of the structure. Hazards in a child care setting can adversely affect a group of children. Conversely, children may benefit when hazards are reduced or controlled. Children exposed to environmental tobacco smoke (ETS) or lead paint at home may reduce their exposure by spending time in child care.

■ Data on Environmental Hazards in Child Care

Environmental hazards in child care settings are expected to be similar to those found in other buildings (see Table 26.1). Few studies document environmental hazards in child care, although those few have shown ETS, lead poisoning, and indoor air quality to be a concern (see Chapters 11, 13, and 14).

Environmental Tobacco Smoke

Licensed child care centers usually have policies that restrict smoking among employees. Family child care homes, which are often unregulated, are less likely to have or enforce smoke-free policies. More than 752 000 children in the United States are estimated to be at risk of ETS exposure in licensed child care centers.[5] Only 55% of the centers included in a national survey reported being smoke free both indoors and outdoors.[5] In the other 45% of the centers, smoking was not totally prohibited in the building. Children may be exposed when employees are allowed to smoke when children are not present, or when they smoke in another part of the building that may share a common ventilation system with the center.

While the prevalence of smoking among adults in family child care homes is largely unknown, one study suggests that ETS is an important hazard in this setting. The rate of smoking among caregivers was low for children cared for in child care centers (<1%), but high for children cared for in other homes (26%) or by someone other than a parent in their own homes (26%).[6] These rates contrast with the rate of smoking among mothers who cared for their own children at home (17%). Infants whose mothers smoked were more likely to have a caregiver who smoked. During an infant's first 3 years, approximately one fifth of those with nonsmoking mothers were in a care setting with a caregiver who smoked.

Lead

Few studies have been done about lead hazards in child care. The prevalence of lead in family child care homes is probably similar to the prevalence among homes in the community. A survey of schools, preschools, and child care centers conducted in Washington state found that 62% of 75 facilities built before 1979 contained leaded paint, and 31% contained leaded soil or dust above the levels of concern.[7]

Lead exposure is probably underestimated by routine surveillance systems and inadequate data. When lead paint is identified in the home of a child who has been poisoned by lead, sources away from the home (such as child care settings) are less likely to be quantified because the public health inspector may lack authority or information to evaluate other settings. Two studies of children attending child care centers with leaded paint, dust, or soil,[7,8] found only one child who had a confirmed blood lead level exceeding 10 µg/dL (12 µg/dL).[8] These results, however, cannot be generalized to all child care settings. In both studies, the average age of the participants was about 5 years, and in one study, the rate of participation was low.[7] Children may have been protected from exposure by continual supervision, high frequency of hand washing (averaging once per hour), and standard cleaning practices, including daily wet mopping

Table 26.1. Environmental Hazards Possibly Found in Child Care Settings

Hazard	Likely Sources or Factors Contributing to the Hazards	
	Indoor	Outdoor
Poor air quality	The primary route of exposure is inhalation.	
Environmental tobacco smoke (ETS)	Smoking in the child care area. Smoking in non-child care areas or in other parts of a multiple-use building that are not vented separately from the child care area.	Fresh air intake located near an outside smoking area or an exhaust outlet that emits tobacco smoke.
Carbon monoxide (CO), volatile organic compounds (VOCs), ozone, and other air pollutants	CO from defective or improperly vented stoves, furnaces, or water heaters, dirty or clogged filters; inadequate air exchange in heating/ventilation/air conditioning (HVAC) systems or use of petroleum-fueled space heaters that are intended only for outdoor use. Inadequate ventilation throughout the facility and windows that cannot be opened. VOC emissions from building materials, coverings on floors, walls, ceilings, and cabinet finishes.	Playground located near high-traffic area or near the exhaust outlet of a building. Building emissions may contain ETS, CO, solvents, molds, and other irritants and allergens. Fresh air intake located near a building exhaust outlet or vehicle exhaust. Exposure to air pollutants, such as ozone, industrial emissions, coal, or wood smoke while on the playground or on field trips.
Asbestos	Friable, nonintact asbestos in exposed insulation, ceilings, floors, or duct work. Renovation without appropriate asbestos containment.	
Radon	Cracks and openings in foundations that allow this naturally occurring radioactive gas to leak through the ground into buildings that are inadequately ventilated.	
Heavy metals, hazardous materials	The primary routes of exposure are ingestion, inhalation of aerosols, and skin contact.	

Category		
Lead and other heavy metals	Leaded dust or paint chips, particularly on floors, window sills, and during renovation of pre-1950 structures. Leaded paint on furniture or toys, leaded ceramic dishware, plumbing, remedies and other sources.	Leaded soil, or leaded paint on the building's exterior, fences, sheds, or playground equipment; improperly contained materials from renovations in the vicinity of the setting.
	Arts and crafts supplies, paints; acidic foods or beverages placed in galvanized containers.	Soil contamination at the site from prior industrial use or geological mineral deposits. Toxic clays and play structures, or contents of storage areas accessible to children.
Medications, cosmetics, and chemical products, such as sanitizers, disinfectants, cleaners, solvents, polishes, paints, lawn and garden chemicals, herbicides, pesticides, insecticides, rodenticides, pool chemicals, and petroleum products for outdoor maintenance equipment	Improper storage, labeling, handling, or use of medications or chemical products in any child care area, particularly in the following high risk areas: diaper changing, food preparation and storage, laundry, maintenance and custodial supply rooms, and areas prone to infestation of pests.	Improper storage, labeling, handling, or use of chemical products in any area accessible to children, particularly unsecured storage sheds.
	Infested food preparation and storage areas, bedding, laundry rooms, and spaces under sinks due to preventable problems, such as poor sanitation, water leaks, and unprotected openings to the outside	Infested playgrounds and storage sheds, space under sheds, and debris, and clutter or dense foliage near the foundation.
Physical hazards		
Ultraviolet radiation		Excessive sun exposure because of inadequate shade on the playground, nonrestricted time and duration of outdoor play, and inadequate use of sunscreen.
Noise	Room design or materials that amplify sounds.	Adjacent roadways, airports, or industrial sources of sound.
Other	The primary routes of exposure are inhalation, contact to skin, and ingestion.	
Allergen / asthma triggers	Cockroaches, dust mites, plants, animals, food, mold, VOCs, chemical irritants, toxic building materials, pillows, environmental tobacco smoke, and dust.	Dust, pollen, animals, mold, poor outdoor air quality, and insect venom.

of floors. Therefore, although these results cannot be generalized, there are no data showing that child care settings are a significant source of environmental lead. The risk of exposure may be higher with younger children, poor hygiene and maintenance practices, or when housing renovations occur without appropriate testing and containment measures. The absence of elevated blood lead levels does not necessarily indicate the absence of potential hazards.

Federal regulations address the problem of lead only in the child's home. Federal funding for remediation of lead hazards can be applied to homes, but not to child care settings.

Indoor Air Quality

Crowding may contribute to poor indoor air quality. Levels of CO_2 were measured in 91 child care centers in Quebec. Ninety percent had CO_2 levels that exceeded the office building standard.[9] Increased CO_2 levels were associated with the number of children in a given area. A high CO_2 level reflects poor air quality and serves as a marker for other indoor air pollutants. Although children spend 90% of their time indoors, there are no indoor air standards specified for child care settings (see Chapter 13).

Poisoning

Poisoning may result from incorrect administration of or exposure to medications, arts and crafts materials, toxic plants, cosmetics, chemical products, lawn and garden chemicals, pesticides, pool chemicals, and petroleum products. The incidence of poisoning by these products was higher when children were in their own homes.[10] Children in child care centers may be protected because they are usually supervised by an adult, the facility and equipment are designed for children, and licensing procedures and public health inspections help to eliminate hazards. However, the potential for poisonings is real. In Colorado, health inspectors visiting child care settings 2 weeks after licensing inspections found toxic chemicals accessible to children in 68% of the settings.[11] In Salt Lake City, Utah, misuse of toxic disinfectants to clean mouthing toys and high chair trays was observed during routine inspections.[12] Some products such as pesticides may be used as directed but still are not safe to use in child care settings.[13]

Child care providers are often unsupervised and may not have knowledge about or experience in administering medications. Errors are possible when there are many bottles of medication in the refrigerator or on a shelf.

▌ Characteristics of Child Care That May Exacerbate Hazards

Three characteristics of child care may have an impact on environmental quality. First, staff turnover in child care centers is high, creating a need to continually educate new employees. Second, child care businesses usually operate with a low profit margin. Tuition is often funded by public assistance at fixed dollar amounts, limiting the financing of pest control, lead hazard abatement, or renovation, and discouraging the temporary closing of the center while these activities are under way. When these activities are carried out, public health authorities should provide education to those who operate the center and appropriate oversight to ensure that children are not inadvertently exposed to hazardous conditions. Third, when a child care center is located within a larger facility, such as a church or office building, hazards may arise due to practices that occur in other parts of the facility. For example, an outbreak of contact dermatitis at a child care setting located within a college campus building resulted from exposure to carpet cleaning chemicals.[14] Chemicals appropriate for use in the hallways were not suitable in the child care area where direct skin contact occurs when children play on the floor. In another instance, the director of a child care center located within a building did not have supervisory authority to prevent a maintenance worker from spraying pesticides inappropriately.

▌ Measures to Prevent or Control Environmental Hazards in a Child Care Setting

The National Health and Safety Performance Standards identify numerous control measures.

Primary Prevention

Site Selection
An environmental audit should be conducted prior to selecting a site for a child care facility and before new construction begins or an

older building is renovated. The environmental audit should at least include assessments of (1) historical land use to determine the potential for soil contamination with toxic or hazardous waste; (2) lead and asbestos content in older buildings; (3) potential sources of infestation, noise, air pollution, and toxic exposures; and (4) location of the playground in relation to infested stagnant water, roadways, industrial emissions, and building exhaust outlets. While geological factors may suggest potential radon exposure, there are no reliable methods of testing for radon prior to construction.

Architectural Design and Building Materials

Environmental hazards can be reduced or eliminated with use of appropriate structure designs and selection of building materials.[15] Indoor air quality can be improved by frequent air exchanges and sufficient ventilation of air to the outside; windows that open can safeguard against failure of mechanical ventilation systems; and properly placed fresh-air intakes can prevent exhaust from automobiles and the building systems from reaching hazardous levels inside. Electrostatic air cleaners and high-efficiency filtration systems can be used. Pesticide use and radon exposure can be reduced by design elements. Building materials can be selected to minimize levels of toxic substances (eg, formaldehyde). Appropriate paints should be selected and used as directed.

Plan Review/Construction Remodeling Regulation

Before construction or remodeling is started, environmental health specialists in local health departments should consider reviewing construction or remodeling plans, as is currently done for food service establishments. State or local health departments may need to develop environmental health regulations that specifically address child care facilities.

Monitoring by Public Health Authorities

Child care settings should be monitored by public health officials who visit during construction or remodeling, inspect them prior to opening and routinely during operation, and who investigate complaints. Public health officials must inspect all aspects of the child care setting, not only the food service area, and identify potential environmental hazards so preventive actions can be implemented.[16] Table 26.2 is intended to supplement the important items concerning sanitation, safety, and communicable disease control that are addressed during routine inspection of a child care facility.

Table 26.2. Checklist for Public Health Inspection to Assess Potential Environmental Hazards in a Child Care Setting

- Is smoking permitted in the facility?
- Are medications and chemical products properly labeled, stored in areas inaccessible to children, and in a manner so as not to contaminate food? Are staff members trained in the safe use of chemical products and administration of medications?
- Are arts and crafts supplies free of hazardous substances and labeled in compliance with ASTM (see Chapter 25).
- Are the kitchen and bathroom areas operated in compliance with health department regulations?
- Are hand washing policies followed and monitored? Are soap and clean towels always available?
- Are indoor and outdoor storage closets and sheds locked so their contents are inaccessible to children? All maintenance, lawn care and other hazardous equipment, and all chemical products (such as gasoline, paints, pesticides, and cleaning products) must be inaccessible to children.
- If the building was constructed before 1950, has the building been assessed for lead paint, dust, and soil hazards, and also asbestos hazards? If renovation work is under way, have lead and asbestos hazards been assessed, and have children been protected from the release of these potentially hazardous toxicants?
- If a gas-powered furnace, stove, or other equipment is used in the facility, is there a carbon monoxide detector present in the facility?
- Does the director ensure routine preventive maintenance of the heating systems and gas lines, including routinely changing furnace filters?
- Is there any evidence of mold in the facility? Have flooding or plumbing problems occurred?
- Does the facility appear clean, without areas of peeling and chipping paint?
- Are the rooms adequately ventilated?
- Are wading and swimming pools disinfected according to local health department regulations?

Education

Health departments should have personnel with expertise in environmental hazards, communicable diseases, injury control, sanitation, and safety. Their knowledge can enable child care providers to identify environmental hazards, understand the associated health risks, and recognize acute symptoms of environmental exposure.

To prevent poisonings, directors of child care facilities need to educate all employees, including maintenance personnel, about storing, labeling, and using potentially hazardous products. Janitorial and custodial staff should be regularly monitored to ensure the safest practices. OSHA requires that Material Safety Data Sheets (MSDS) be kept on file to explain health hazards, proper use and storage procedures, and emergency procedures in case of toxic chemical exposure. Staff may also use MSDS to choose nontoxic chemicals.

To avoid having employees of child care centers administer medications to children, pediatricians may consider prescribing formulations that require fewer dosages or altering the time of administration. When medications must be given while a child is in child care, specific written instructions should be either on the bottle or on a separate piece of paper. Instructions are especially important for medications that are used on a prn (as needed) basis. Instructions are needed for prescription and nonprescription medications.

Policies and Procedures

Policies and procedures should be developed to institutionalize safe practices and to ensure appropriate responses to the variety of infrequent but potentially hazardous events. For example, (1) smoking should be prohibited (even among noncaregivers in a family child care home) while children are present and in areas where children may be exposed to ETS; (2) emergency preparedness plans should include procedures for responding to hazardous material incidents; and (3) staff should receive education in administration of medications and use of chemicals.

Secondary Prevention

Some hazardous situations in child care settings may be avoided by educating employees to recognize and appropriately control hazards (eg, by properly storing or using chemicals). Other hazards may require more costly and complex measures. For example, when leaded paint or dust is found, interim control measures may be needed before full abatement is possible. Abatement procedures should meet applicable standards and regulations. When these facilities have limited financial resources, environmental health regulators assure that the health of children is not jeopardized. This may require community collaboration to offset the burden of cost.

Disease in a Child Attending Out-of-Home Child Care
When a child's illness or symptoms may have an environmental etiology, parents, health care personnel, and public health investigators should evaluate potential exposures both in the child's home environment and out-of-home settings. Improvements may have to be made in small increments, over time.

∎ Frequently Asked Questions

Q *Are sandboxes and sand safe for children?*
A Sandboxes are safe if constructed and filled with appropriate materials and then properly maintained. Sandbox frames are sometimes made with inexpensive railroad ties, which may cause splinters and may be saturated with creosote, a carcinogen. Nontoxic landscaping timbers or nonwood containers are preferred.

In 1986, concern was first expressed that some types of commercially available play sand contained tremolite, a fibrous substance found in some crushed limestone and crushed marble (see Chapter 5). It was hypothesized that the long-term effects of exposure to tremolite would be identical to those of asbestos. Despite these concerns, CPSC denied a petition prohibiting marketing of play sand containing significant levels of tremolite. CPSC currently has no standards or labeling requirements regarding the source or content of sand.

Directors of child care facilities and parents may have difficulty determining what sand is safe. They should attempt to buy only natural river, beach, or silica-based materials. They should avoid products that are made from crushed limestone, crushed marble, or those that are obviously dusty. When there is doubt, parents may send a sample of sand to a laboratory for determination of asbestos content. Information about reliable laboratories can be obtained from the US EPA Regional Asbestos Coordinators (see the Resources section in Chapter 5).

Once installed, the sandbox should be covered to prevent contamination with animal feces and parasites. Sand should be raked regularly to remove debris and dry it out. A sand rake does a better job than a garden rake.

Q *Which chemical disinfectants and sanitizers are safe to use in child care settings?*

A To control communicable diseases, it is important to clean and then either disinfect or sanitize objects or surfaces that may become contaminated with food, saliva, feces, or other sources of pathogens. First, objects and surfaces need to be cleaned with detergent and water to remove grease and hardened debris.

Second, contaminated objects and surfaces need to be sanitized or disinfected to reduce the level of harmful pathogens. Mouth and food contact surfaces (such as crib railings, mouthing toys, dishes, high chair trays) should be sanitized. Environmental surfaces (such as doorknobs, counter tops, changing areas, and toilet areas) should be disinfected.

Sanitizing is designed to greatly reduce the number of pathogens and is often necessary after dirt is removed from a surface. Sanitizing refers to the application of heat or a chemical, such as household bleach, on clean surfaces that is sufficient to yield a 99.9% reduction of representative (but not all) disease-causing microorganisms of public health importance. An example of cumulative heat treatment is found in the operation of some household dishwashers. Household dishwashers that effectively sanitize dishes and utensils using hot water may be used to clean and sanitize the outer surfaces of plastic toys. However, dishwashers that utilize a heating element to dry dishes should be used with caution to avoid melting soft plastic toys. Some dishwashers may permit the heating element used for drying to be deactivated while retaining the sanitizing process. Child care staff can consult the manufacturer's user's guide.

Disinfection is more rigorous than sanitizing. It refers to the application of cumulative heat or chemical that results in elimination of almost all microorganisms from inanimate surfaces. Pathogens of public health importance and nearly all other microorganisms are eliminated, but not to the degree achieved by sterilization.

Household bleach (chlorine as sodium hypochlorite) is active against most microorganisms, including bacterial spores, and can be used as a disinfectant or sanitizer depending on its concentration. Bleach is available at various strengths. Household or laundry bleach is a solution of 5.25%, or 52 500 ppm, of sodium hypochlorite. Higher strength industrial bleach solutions are not appropriate to use in child care settings.

Household bleach is effective, economical, convenient, and readily available at grocery stores. It can be corrosive to some metal, rubber, and plastic materials. Bleach must be diluted with water; whether the final mixture is considered a disinfectant or sanitizer depends on the concentration of chlorine. As a disinfectant for environmental surfaces, the recommended dilution is 1/4 cup of household bleach in 1 gallon of water (equivalent to approximately 500 to 800 ppm of available chlorine) or for smaller quantities, 1 tablespoon of household bleach in 1 quart of water. Bleach solutions gradually lose their strength, so fresh solutions must be prepared daily. In child care settings, a bleach solution is typically applied using spray bottles. Spray bottles should be labeled with the name of the solution and the dilution. Contact time is important. What is typically observed in a child care setting is "spray and wipe." Bleach solution should be left on for at least 2 minutes and allowed to dry.

Household bleach can be used to sanitize dishes and eating utensils. The concentration of chlorine used in the process is much less than that used for disinfecting other objects. One rationale for sanitizing dishes and eating utensils is that these objects are typically contaminated by only one person. Other objects are typically contaminated by more than one person, resulting in a potentially greater microbial load and diversity of microorganisms. As a sanitizer for dishes, utensils, mouth toys, and crib railings, the recommended dilution is 1 tablespoon of household bleach in 1 gallon of water (equivalent to approximately 100 ppm of available chlorine). Bleach (the sanitizer) and ammonia (the cleaner) should never be mixed.[17]

"Quats" (quarternary ammonium compounds) are chemicals often used in food service and child care facilities. "Quats" kill vegetative bacteria, fungi, and lipophilic viruses. Unless combined with at least 15% isopropanol, they are not effective against *Mycobacterium tuberculosis*. Therefore, quats without isopropanol is not suitable for use in areas where children are at risk for tuberculosis. Quats do not kill bacterial spores and hydrophilic viruses. Quats should be freshly prepared, used once, and discarded.

It is important to test the concentration of bleach or quats to ensure that the concentration is high enough to function appropriately but low enough to not exceed Food and Drug Administration-approved levels of residue. Test kits can be purchased at restaurant supply stores and should be selected for the specific chemical, either bleach or quats, that is being used.

Before using any chemical other than bleach for disinfecting or sanitizing, the user should consult public health personnel and the manufacturer's MSDS sheets. It is important to read and follow label instructions. Factors to consider when selecting a chemical disinfectant are: Is it inactivated by organic matter? Is it affected by hard water? Does it leave a residue? Is it corrosive by nature? Is it a skin, eye, or respiratory irritant? Is it toxic (by skin absorption, ingestion, or inhalation)? What is its effective shelf life after dilution?

Chemical disinfectants and sanitizers are potentially hazardous to children, particularly if the products are in concentrated form. Products should be stored in their original labeled containers and in places inaccessible to children. Diluted disinfectants and sanitizers in spray bottles must be labeled and stored safely out of the reach of children. Solutions should not be sprayed when children are close by to avoid inhalation and exposure of their skin and eyes.

Table 26.3. Diluting Bleach

Type of Object or Surface	Amount of Household Bleach to Add to Water	Concentration, ppm
To disinfect environmental surfaces, such as: door knobs, counter tops, changing areas, and toilet areas	1/4 cup in 1 gallon of water 1 tablespoon in 1 quart of water	500-800
To sanitize mouth and food contact surfaces, such as: crib railings, mouthing toys, dishes, utensils, and high chair trays	1 tablespoon in 1 gallon of water	100

Q *Should I place my child in child care if a "no smoking" policy is not in place?*

A Children should not be exposed to ETS, and no smoking policies should be written or stated, enforced, and monitored by the director of the center and parents. Children can also be exposed to ETS if persons other than employees are allowed to smoke when children are present, or when the facility has shared ventilation or air spaces that allow ETS to drift (see Chapter 11).

∎ Resources

Child care regulations regarding smoking for every state are posted on the World Wide Web through the federally funded National Resource Center for Health and Safety in Child Care at http://NRC.UCHSC.EDU. This site also has a search engine for accessing specific child care topics by state.

Arizona Safety Information Flip-chart. Emergency and prevention guidelines for early childhood programs, schools and parents. Arizona Department of Health Services, Office of Women's and Children's Health, 1740 W Adams, Phoenix, AZ 85007.

∎ References

1. Children's Defense Fund. *The State of America's Children–Yearbook 1996.* Washington, DC: Children's Defense Fund; 1996

2. American Public Health Association and American Academy of Pediatrics. *Caring for our Children: National Health and Safety Performance Standards–Guidelines for Out-of-Home Child Care Programs.* Washington, DC: American Public Health Association, and Elk Grove Village, IL: American Academy of Pediatrics; 1992

3. American Academy of Pediatrics, Committee on Early Childhood, Adoption, and Dependent Care. The application of health and safety guidelines to out-of-home child care programs. *Pediatrics.* 1994;93:1016-1017

4. Addiss DG, Sacks JJ, Kresnow MJ, O'Neil J, Ryan GW. The compliance of licensed US child care centers with national health and safety performance standards. *Am J Public Health.* 1994;84:1161-1164

5. Nelson DE, Sacks JJ, Addiss DG. Smoking policies in licensed child day-care center in the United States. *Pediatrics.* 1993;91:460-463

6. Holberg CJ, Wright AL, Martinez FD, Morgan WJ, Taussig LM, and Group Health Medical Associates. Child day care, smoking by caregivers, and lower respiratory tract illness in the first 3 years of life. *Pediatrics*. 1993;91:885-892

7. Washington State Department of Health. *Environmental Lead Survey in Public and Private Schools, Preschools and Day Care Centers*. Olympia, Wash: Washington State Department of Health; 1995:1-20

8. Weismann DN, Dusdieker LB, Cherryholmes KL, Hausler WJ, Dungy CI. Elevated environmental lead levels in a day care setting. *Arch Pediatr Adolesc Med*. 1995;149:878-881

9. Daneault S, Beausoleil M, Messing K. Air quality during the winter in Quebec day-care centers. *Am J Public Health*. 1992;82:432-434

10. Gunn WJ, Pinsky PF, Sacks JJ Schonberger LB. Injuries and poisoning in out-of-home child care and home care. *Am J Dis Child*. 1991;145:779-781

11. Aronson SS. Role of the pediatrician in setting and using standards for child care. *Pediatrics*. 1993;91:239-243

12. Corkins D. Personal communication.

13. Fenske RA, Black KG, Elkner KP, et al. Potential exposure and health risks of infants following indoor residential pesticide applications. *Am J Public Health*. 1990;80:689-693

14. Corkins D. Personal communication.

15. Passantino RJ, Bavier RN. Environmental quality of child day-care facilities: an architect's point of view. *Pediatrics*. 1994;94(suppl):1036-1039

16. Brewster RE. *Environmental Health Guidelines for Child Care Facilities*. Denver, Colo: National Environmental Health Association; 1986

17. American Academy of Pediatrics. In: Peter G, ed. *1997 Red Book: Report of the Committee on Infectious Diseases*, 24th ed. Elk Grove Village, IL: American Academy of Pediatrics; 1997:91-92.

27 Workplaces

C urrently, more than 5 million adolescents younger than 18 years are legally employed in the United States, and an additional 1 to 2 million are believed to be employed in violation of wage, hour, or safety regulations.[1] Efforts to improve school-to-work transitions are placing more teenagers into the workplace, and even school-based vocational/technical education that simulates employment conditions may involve hazardous conditions, including chemical exposures. National priorities for volunteer community involvement support increasing participation of adolescents in non-paid activities such as rehabilitation of old housing that may still carry the same risks of exposures as paid employment.[2] While the largest number of employed youth are ages 14 years and older, children who are only 9 or 10 years old may be delivering newspapers or involved in farm work. For more than 80% of high school students, work is a part of their normal schedule during the week. While there are no large-scale studies that describe illness or death resulting from exposures in the workplace among teenagers, studies exist for occupational injuries among working adolescents. They are important because they suggest that there is a problem with teenage exposures to hazardous substances in the workplace. In the past decade, studies have shown that, despite laws intended to protect teenage workers, every year at least 70 children younger than 18 years die from work on the job site.[3] More than 65 000 are injured severely enough to seek care in emergency departments.[4] These studies serve as a marker for concern about occupational exposures, and this is strengthened by the little we do know about exposure-related fatalities.

■ Musculoskeletal Development and Ergonomic Factors

Regulation of Hours and Hazards in Youth Employment
The Fair Labor Standards Act (FLSA) of 1938 remains the major federal law that regulates work for youth younger than 18 years.[5] The law has two parts–the protection of education through regulation of permitted hours of work in a day and in a week, and protection of health and safety through prohibition of work on dangerous machinery or with hazardous chemicals via Hazard orders. Under the FLSA, adolescents younger than 18 years are prohibited from working with hazardous chemicals in nonagricultural jobs.[6] Prohibitions on chemical work in agriculture extend only to age 16 years, and work by children and adolescents on their own family farms is unregulated.[7]

Many states also have laws regulating child labor. Those laws more stringent than federal law apply. Many businesses, particularly small ones, may not be covered by either federal or state law. Recent trends toward increased use of contract workers, especially for newspaper delivery, are problematic because they leave unclear who is responsible for education, supervision, health, and safety.

Another major area of legal exemptions is vocational/technical training. Because such training is assumed to occur with supervision in a safe environment, restrictions based on safety concerns are waived for students in various types of training. No surveillance of exposure resulting in illness or injury has been conducted either in school-based learning sites or on job sites.

Work Permits
In approximately half the states, adolescents must obtain a work permit issued by their school before seeking or starting a job. Some states require the signature of a physician, which offers an opportunity to provide anticipatory guidance.

Enforcement of Child Labor Laws
Child labor laws are enforced by the federal and state Departments of

Labor. Although some illegal child labor is performed by undocumented aliens, most illegal child labor involves US citizens who are employed under conditions that violate the FLSA. Labor inspectors are responsible for enforcing wage, hour, and safety laws for all workers. Thus, most child labor is investigated only when a complaint is made, usually by a parent or occasionally by business personnel. The fines for child labor violations historically have been small compared with the savings from the exploitation of children, although some states have recently increased fines, particularly for repeated violations. Two continuing widespread problems include keeping teenagers at work too late on school nights (an hours violation) or having them clock out at an appropriate time but continue to work without pay.[7]

Perhaps the most critical aspect of child labor law violation relates to safety. Parents should know when their child's work situation violates FLSA standards. If an employer does not abide by wage and hour laws, it may be reasonable to assume that the employer is not following laws to protect the health and safety of the teenager.[8,9]

Exposures of legally employed youth to potentially hazardous materials may occur in job activities that either violate the law or in jobs uncovered by the law because of business size or production. This has been a major issue because of the repeated association between fatalities and conditions that violate safety regulations or the FLSA standards.

■ Routes of Exposure

Dermal
Some chemical exposures involve absorption through the skin or through breaks in the skin. Examples include pesticide exposure in lawn care and agriculture, nicotine exposure while harvesting tobacco, and solvent exposure in auto body shops.[10]

Inhalation
Inhalation injuries result from fumes from metal, such as lead and ammonia. Isocyanates found in auto body paint and some types of shellac are pulmonary sensitizers.

Ingestion
Lead and other heavy metals may be ingested.

■ Clinical Effects

There is no surveillance system in place in the United States for monitoring children's occupational exposures. Information on clinical effects are gathered piecemeal and then fitted together to create usable data. Three major sources of data are: (1) case reports of exposures and acute poisonings from literature and from within adolescent occupational injury studies (many of the latter are based on Workers' Compensation reports); (2) adult occupational medicine literature about exposures that may be extrapolated to adolescents working in similar jobs; and (3) concerns about the safety of various exposures based on a combination of our knowledge of chemical toxicology and of adolescent growth, development, physiology, and anatomy.

Examples of Exposures and Acute Poisonings

A 1989 survey of 50 migrant farmworking adolescents younger than 18 years found that 11% had mixed or applied pesticides, despite child labor laws that prohibit work with hazardous chemicals.[10] No protective equipment was used other than gloves, and it was unclear whether the gloves were impermeable. More than 15% of the youth surveyed reported having had symptoms consistent with organophosphate poisoning, but few had sought medical care. More than 40% had worked in fields wet with pesticides, violating field reentry times suggested by chemical manufacturers, and 40% had been sprayed with pesticides while at work in the fields directly by crop-dusting planes or indirectly by drifting chemicals from planes or tractors.

■ Diagnostic Methods

A thorough history and physical examination are most important. Patients should be screened for specific substances if possible (eg, lead when renovating old houses). Patients should be screened for effects of exposure when the substance cannot be measured (ie, hepatocellular enzymes following solvent exposure).

■ Treatment of Clinical Symptoms

Treatments range from determining and eliminating the source of low-level chronic exposure to advanced cardiac life support in some acute poisonings. It is critical to have knowledge of proper rescue measures to ensure the safety of the rescuer. Specific suggestions for medical treatment may be provided by a local poison control center.

∎ Prevention of Exposure

Prevention through knowledge of substances, routes of exposure, and engineering controls is important.

Patient-Directed Office-Based Strategies

Information can be obtained from industrial hygiene and occupational medicine professionals, occupational medicine acedemics, union or corporate health and safety employees, and local Committee on Occupational Safety and Health groups. State-based Occupational Safety and Health Act program training sections may also be helpful.

Pediatricians should know their state child labor laws. The state Department of Labor provides a one-page poster summarizing work hours, wages, and occupations permitted for adolescents of different ages. This poster must be posted prominently in every workplace. In some states, the office of the US Department of Labor can also provide information.

Pediatricians are encouraged to find out which of their patients work, where they are working, what their job duties are, and the types of chemicals they use in their work. An occupational history should be obtained with a focus on potential hazards (see Table 27.1). Knowledge of job training, including the use of chemicals and first aid, and whether there is an adult supervisor on site is important. Although some workplaces are exempt from FLSA, all workers have the right to know about the chemicals with which they work. Employers are responsible for educating workers about chemical exposures and usage.

Pediatricians should know if adolescent patients are volunteers on projects that involve exposures.

The adolescent's occupation should be considered when diagnosing an illness (eg, chronic fatigue in an adolescent who makes silk screens can be caused by chronic solvent intoxication if he works and/or sleeps in an area with inadequate ventilation).

The adolescent's occupation should be considered in the medical management of known illnesses (eg, asthma that may have been previously under control may flare up when working in the smoking section of a restaurant).

Pediatricians can provide guidance in the choice of occupations for adolescents with chronic disease. Employment opportunities, which may be fewer than those for their peers, are important both for their development and for future adult employment. The potential risks of certain work situations may be addressed by pediatricians with their patients.

Pediatricians should be familiar with Workers' Compensation laws; adolescents may be eligible for compensation for medical expenses and lost wages/lost time due to illnesses from an occupational exposure. Rules governing which industries and workers are covered and when benefits begin differ from state to state.

Pediatricians should be advocates for age-appropriate rehabilitation and follow-up for those injured on the job. Although agricultural-related injuries are often not covered, workers compensation should pay for many cases of rehabilitation resulting from occupational injury/exposure.

▌ Parents Should Make Informed Decisions About the Safety of Their Adolescent

Pediatricians should talk with parents about the potential risks and benefits of having their adolescent employed. Many parents are unaware of injury risk, and may be even less aware of risks associated with chemical exposures. Guidance may help reduce the risks.

Parents should be educated about adolescent growth and development expectations. Youth who are small for their age, especially those who work on farms, are unable to fit into adult-sized protective equipment, resulting in secondary exposures. Youth who are large for their age may be cognitively or emotionally immature; adolescents physically able to perform selected tasks cannot be expected to perform with the judgment of an experienced adult.

While realizing that responsibilities for teenagers should increase within safe limits, parents need support in decisions about safety. Faced with pressure from their children, parents may doubt the wisdom of their decisions. Support for safety is important as families weigh the appropriate limits of teenage independence. Parents should be role models for safety. Parents who are farm workers, for example, can demonstrate and discuss the judicious use, safe handling, safe storage, and safe disposal of chemicals with their adolescent while working together. Parents should be encouraged to discuss exposures to noise and dusts and to share with their adolescents information on protective measures and minimizing exposures.

Table 27.1. Potential Job-Related Exposures

- blood-borne pathogens in nursing homes/hospitals
- cleaning agents in restaurants, nursing homes, and schools
- pesticide exposure in lawn care work, farm work, and when buildings are sprayed
- isocyanate exposure (pulmonary sensitizer) during auto body repair or roofing with newer forms of roofing materials
- potential benzene exposure when pumping gas
- lead exposure from radiators in auto body repair and home renovation
- asbestos exposure in auto brake repair, renovation/demolition of old buildings
- solvent exposure in T-shirt screening
- second-hand smoke in waitstaff jobs
- heat exposure for dishwashers and outdoor workers in the summer or in hot climates
- cold exposure in areas with cold weather and outdoor jobs, potentially exacerbated by wet conditions that contribute to faster heat loss, issue for gas station workers, construction workers, ski area personnel, and whitewater guides
- asthma-producing wood dusts in shop and furniture making
- welding fumes and eye exposures
- cosmetology chemicals and dyes
- tetanus and other biological/infectious hazards in farming (hypersensitivity pneumonitis), veterinary work
- noise-induced hearing loss in farms and factories
- nicotine exposure in harvest of tobacco (Green Tobacco Sickness) in the southeastern United States

▌ Frequently Asked Question

Q *My child has asthma—can I direct him to jobs so that his illness is not exacerbated by the job?*

A Teens need to ask potential employers about the tasks they will be doing, and what types of chemicals they may be exposed to during work. Parents should be concerned about adult supervision, job training, and safety instruction. It is important for parents to visit the workplace. A job that requires personal protective equipment suggests a possible risk that should be explored. Issues of exposure in vocational education and volunteer work need to be considered.

▌ Resources

In addition to the American Academy of Pediatrics, the following is a list of some of the resources available about adolescent occupational exposures.

Department of Labor for your state. Contact for information on child labor laws, wages, hours of work, safety regulations including Hazard orders that prohibit specific types of hazardous exposures, and problems with any of those areas. Some states have health and safety/training offices within their labor departments, which can be especially helpful. In some states, you will be told to call the local office of the US Department of Labor. Telephone numbers are in local phone directories.

Occupational Safety and Health Administration (OSHA), the federal agency that deals with regulatory and enforcement issues. If a teenager has a question about a specific hazard, the teenager or parent (with permission) can call OSHA for assistance. This can be done anonymously, but sometimes an employee may be identifiable. Pediatricians should consider this route especially when concerned about imminent danger to other youth in that workplace. Telephone numbers for OSHA are in local phone directories.

National Institute for Occupational Safety and Health (NIOSH), the federal agency that deals with scientific, research, and educational aspects (800/356-4674). The Division of Safety Research in the Morgantown, WV, NIOSH office has expertise in this area (304/285-5894); work is also currently being done in the NIOSH office in

Cincinnati, OH, concerning exposures in vocational/ technical education settings. In May 1995, NIOSH published "Alert-Request for Assistance in Preventing Deaths and Injuries of Adolescent Workers." This booklet (Department of Health and Human Services Publication No. 95-125, available from NIOSH at the telephone numbers listed above) has background information and a tear-out page to post in the office or to copy for adolescent patients and their parents or for community work.

The NIOSH-funded Educational Resource Centers and academic departments of occupational medicine. These centers educate occupational and environmental medicine physicians and provide continuing education on occupational injury and exposures to many different types of workers.

The COSH groups (community-based Committees on Occupational Safety and Health). Like union health and safety offices, most COSH groups maintain staff capable of answering questions about occupational exposures who have experience in training a wide variety of workers.

Child Labor Coalition, c/o the National Consumers' League, Washington, DC, is a coalition of diverse organizations and individuals (including the AAP, consumer groups, medical professionals, universities, unions, and religious organizations) interested in all aspects of international and US child labor. They have organized conferences, meet monthly, and maintain one of the most up-to-date watches in the nation on federal and state child labor law changes as they evolve (202/835-3323).

National Child Labor Committee, New York, NY, has existed since the 1800s and has historical and legal information. The committee also continues to advocate for the safe employment of youth.

▌ References

1. American Academy of Pediatrics, Committee on Environmental Health. The hazards of child labor. *Pediatrics.* 1995;95:311-313

2. Committee on Injury and Poison Prevention, American Academy of Pediatrics. Injuries in the workplace. In: Widome MD, ed. *Injury Prevention and Control for Children and Youth.* ed 3. Elk Grove Village, IL: AAP; 1997:119-134

3. Centers for Disease Control and Prevention. Work-related injuries and ill-

nesses associated with child labor–United States, 1993. *MMWR Morb Mortal Wkly Rep.* 1996;45:464-468

4. Brooks, DR, Davis LK, Gallagher SS. Work-related injuries among Massachusetts children: a study based on emergency department data. *Am J Industrial Med.* 1993;24:313-324

5. Fair Labor Standards Act of 1938, as amended. Title 29, US Code, Section 201 et seq, 29 CFR 570-580

6. US Dept of Labor. *Child Labor Requirements in Nonagricultural Occupations Under the Fair Labor Standards Act.* Washington DC: Employment Standards Administration, Wage and Hour Division; 1985. Child Labor Bull 101

7. US Dept of Labor. *Child Labor Requirements in Agriculture Under the Fair Labor Standards Act.* Washington DC: Employment Standards Administration, Wage and Hour Division, 1984. Child Labor Bull 102

8. Suruda A, Halperin W. Work-related deaths in children. *Am J Ind Med.* 1991;19:739-745

9. Dunn KA, Runyan CW. Deaths at work among children and adolescents. *Am J Dis Child.* 1993;147:1044-1047

10. Pollack S, McConnell R, Gallelli M, Schmidt J, Obregon R, Landrigan P. *Pesticide Exposure and Working Conditions Among Migrant Farmworker Children in Western New York State.* 1990 American Public Health Association Annual Meeting Abstracts: 317

28 | Schools

S chool-age children spend 35 to 50 hours per week in and around school buildings during school and after-school programs. Younger children spend time in school buildings in kindergarten, preschool, and child care programs. Pediatricians may be called upon to evaluate children who have health concerns relating to possible exposures within school settings.[1]

This chapter discusses possible problems related to school buildings: indoor air quality, radon, asbestos, pesticides, and lead. Additional information can be found in the chapters on each specific topic.

■ Indoor Air Quality

Many school buildings are old and poorly maintained. A recent incident in New York City illustrated the extreme of problems caused by indoor air pollution in a building heated by a coal-fired furnace. In February 1998, 75 children and several adults became ill when carbon monoxide and other fumes were released from the furnace. The cause was attributed to human error and improper functioning of a fan used to force air into the furnace.[2]

Most problems with indoor air quality (IAQ) in schools are less severe and are common to all large buildings. Some IAQ problems are related to school courses, such as materials released into the air from art supplies, from chemistry and biology laboratories, and from wood and metal shops.

Reports by the US Government Accounting Office noted that 20% of primary and secondary schools had IAQ problems; more than half had environmental pollutant or building ventilation problems that could affect air quality.[3] The IAQ may directly influence a child's learning by affecting alertness, attentiveness, and absenteeism and indirectly by affecting the performance and productivity of teachers. Indoor air pollutants can begin within the building or be drawn in from outdoors and may consist of particles, fibers, mists, molds, bacteria, and gases. Levels of air pollutants can vary within the school building or even within a single classroom. Levels can vary with time, such as a weekly increase the day floor stripping is done, or a continuous increase from growth of molds in the heating, ventilation, and air-conditioning (HVAC) systems.

Attributing a child's symptoms to poor IAQ can be difficult to prove. Multiple pollutants may be involved. Signs and symptoms may be nonspecific and similar to those associated with allergies or the common cold.

Symptoms commonly attributed to poor IAQ include:

• headache, fatigue, and shortness of breath

• sinus congestion, coughing, and sneezing

• eye, nose, throat, and skin irritation

• dizziness and nausea

• epistaxis (after exposure to formaldehyde).

Clues to indoor air problems include the following:

• symptoms are widespread within a class or school

• symptoms may diminish or disappear after leaving the school

• onset is sudden after some change at school, such as painting or pesticide application

• children with allergies or asthma have reactions indoors but not outdoors.

■ Specific Air Quality Issues

Sick Building Syndrome
Sick building syndrome (SBS) is a term first used during the 1970s.[4]

In SBS, symptoms can be associated with occupants' presence in that building. A spectrum of complaints is usually involved, all suggesting common ailments. Symptoms may abate when the persons are not in the building.

Poor design, maintenance, and operation of the structure's ventilation systems have been indicated as causes of SBS. Another theory suggests that very low levels of specific pollutants may be present and may act synergistically, or in combination, to cause health problems. Humidity also may be a factor: while high relative humidity may contribute to biological pollutant problems, an unusually low level, less than 20% or 30%, may heighten the effects of mucosal irritants and may itself be irritating.

The prevalence of SBS is unknown. A 1984 World Health Organization report suggested that there may be complaints related to IAQ in as many as 30% of new and remodeled buildings worldwide.[5]

Remedial Action for Sick Building Syndrome

Appropriate persons (eg, school or school district personnel, building investigation specialists, industrial hygienists, and state and local government epidemiologists) should investigate the school, particularly the design and operation of HVAC systems, and correct contributing conditions.

Biological Agents

Biological air pollutants are found to some degree in every school, home, and workplace. Sources include outdoor air, human occupants who shed viruses and bacteria, animal occupants (insects and other arthropods and mammals) that shed allergens, and indoor surfaces and water reservoirs (eg, humidifiers) where mold and bacteria can grow. A number of factors allow biological agents to grow and be released. High relative humidity encourages dust mite multiplication and allows mold growth on damp surfaces. Mite and mold contamination can be caused by flooding, continually damp carpet (which may occur when carpet is installed on damp concrete floors), inadequate exhaust of bathrooms, or kitchen-generated moisture. Appliances such as humidifiers, dehumidifiers, air conditioners, and drip pans under cooling coils (as in refrigerators) may support the growth of bacteria and molds.

Components of mechanical HVAC systems may serve as reservoirs for microbes. These include air intakes near standing water, organic debris or bird droppings, or integral parts of the mechanical system itself, such as humidification systems, cooling coils, or condensate drain pans.

Exposure to conditions conducive to biological contamination (eg, dampness or water damage) has been related to nonspecific upper and lower respiratory tract symptoms. Some episodes of SBS may be related to microbial contamination.

Allergic Reactions

Exposure to biological pollutants may result in allergic reactions, including rhinitis, nasal congestion, conjunctival inflammation, urticaria, and asthma. Notable triggers are allergens derived from house dust mites; cockroaches; pets (cats, dogs, birds, rodents); molds; and protein-containing furnishings (eg, feathers, kapok).

Controlling dust mite infestation is accomplished primarily by maintaining relative humidity lower than 45% to 50%. Vacuum cleaning and use of acaricides (substances that destroy mites) can be effective short-term remedial strategies. Acarocin is an acaricide registered with the US Environmental Protection Agency (EPA) to treat carpets and textile-covered furniture for dust mites. For guidance, school officials can consult EPA and a company experienced in using acaricides.

Mycotoxins

Mycotoxins are fungal metabolites with toxic effects ranging from short-term irritation to immunosuppression and cancer.[6] Most information related to diseases caused by mycotoxins concerns ingestion of contaminated food. However, mycotoxins are contained in some mold spores that can enter the body through the respiratory tract. At least one reported case of neurotoxic symptoms was related to airborne mycotoxin exposure in a heavily contaminated environment.[7] Skin is another potential route of exposure. Toxins of several molds have caused cases of severe dermatosis. In view of the serious nature of the toxic effects reported for mycotoxins, children's exposure to molds and moldy school environments should be minimized.

Biological Agents
Diagnostic Clues
Is the relative humidity in the school consistently higher than 50%?

Are humidifiers or other water-spray systems used? How often are they cleaned? Are they cleaned appropriately?

Have flooding or leaks occurred?

Is there evidence of mold growth (visible growth or musty odors)?

Are organic materials handled in the school?

Is carpet installed on damp or unventilated concrete floors?

Are there pets in the school?

Are there problems with cockroaches or rodents?

Are bacterial odors present (fishy or locker-room smells)?

Is adequate outdoor air provided (sufficient number of air changes per hour)?

Remedial Action for Biological Contaminants

- Provide adequate outdoor air ventilation (15 cubic feet per person per minute).[8]

- Be sure there is no standing water in air conditioners. Maintain humidifiers and dehumidifiers according to manufacturer's instructions.

- Repair leaks and seepage. Thoroughly clean and dry water-damaged carpets and building materials within 24 hours of damage, or remove and replace.

- Keep relative humidity less than 50%. Use exhaust fans in bathrooms and kitchens.

- Control exposure to pets.

- Vacuum carpets regularly. While it is important to keep an area as dust-free as possible, cleaning activities often resuspend fine particles. Sensitive persons should avoid such exposure and have others perform the vacuuming or use a commercially available high-efficiency particulate air (HEPA) filtered vacuum.[9]

Volatile Organic Compounds

Volatile organic compounds (VOCs) are chemicals (eg, formaldehyde, benzene, perchloroethylene) emitted as gases at room temperature.[10,11] Concentrations of many VOCs are consistently higher indoors than outdoors. The VOCs are emitted by thousands of products used in schools including the following:

• building materials and furnishings, especially new pressed wood products (eg, furniture, cabinets) that emit formaldehyde

• office equipment, such as some copiers and printers

• graphics and craft materials, including glues and adhesives, permanent markers, and photographic solutions

• paints and lacquers (and their thinners), paint strippers, pesticides

• cleaning products.

Many of these items carry precautionary labels specifying risks and procedures for safe use; some do not.

Volatile Organic Compounds
Diagnostic Clues
Has the person used art, craft, or photographic materials?
Are chemical cleaners used extensively in the school?
Are new pressed wood products present?
Has remodeling recently been done?
Has the person recently used or been exposed to pesticides, paints, or solvents?

Remedial Action for Volatile Organic Compounds

• Increase ventilation when using products that emit VOCs, and meet or exceed any label precautions. Do not store opened containers of unused paints and similar materials in the school.

• If formaldehyde is the potential cause of the problem, identify, and if possible, remove the source. If not possible, reduce exposure; use polyurethane or other sealants on cabinets, paneling, and other furnishings. To be effective, any such coating must cover all surfaces and edges and remain intact.[12]

∎ Prevention of IAQ Problems

Prevention provides the greatest overall health benefit. As a community leader, the pediatrician can enlist the cooperation of teachers, administrators, and parents in taking preventive actions. A practical yet flexible plan can be found in the Indoor Air Quality Tools for Schools Kit (see the Resources section), designed with the understanding that schools have few monetary and human resources available to address this issue. Six basic methods can be used to lower concentrations of indoor air pollutants.

1. Education of school staff about the sources and effects of pollutants under their control and about the proper operation of the ventilation system can result in reduced exposure.

2. Source management includes source removal, substitution, and encapsulation. The best source management is prevention. When it is practical, the most effective method is never to bring a pollutant into the school. Examples include preventing buses from idling near outdoor air intakes, locating garbage away from HVAC equipment, and eliminating smoking within the school. Source substitution includes selecting less toxic art materials or interior paint. Source encapsulation involves placing a barrier around the source so that fewer pollutants are released into the indoor air.

3. Local exhaust to the outside is very effective in removing pollutants that originate at specific points before they can be dispersed. Well-known examples include exhaust from bathrooms, kitchens, and science laboratory fume hoods. Other examples include science laboratory and housekeeping storage rooms, printing and duplicating rooms, and vocational and industrial areas such as welding booths.

4. Ventilation uses cleaner (ie, outdoor) air to dilute contaminated (ie, indoor) air. Local building codes usually specify the amount of outdoor air that must be continuously supplied to an occupied area. For situations such as painting, pesticide application, or chemical spills, temporarily increasing the ventilation can dilute the indoor concentration of fumes.

5. Exposure control includes knowledge of time of use and location of use. An example of time of use would be to strip and wax floors after school dismissal on Friday, allowing products to release gases over the weekend, thus reducing the level of odors

or contaminants when the school is occupied on Monday. Location of use involves moving the contaminating source as far as possible from occupants or relocating susceptible occupants.

6. Air cleaning primarily involves the filtration of particles as air passes through ventilation equipment. Some gaseous contaminants also can be removed.

▌Radon

The EPA measured radon levels in a randomly selected sample of 927 public schools during the 1990-1991 school year. Short-term screening measurements were made by placing radon detectors in all frequently occupied, ground-contact schoolrooms for 7 days.

Survey results showed that 2.7% of the schoolrooms had short-term radon measurements above the EPA's action level of 4 pCi/L of air.[13]

Schools in some areas of the United States are more likely to have elevated radon levels, but schools with radon problems can be found throughout the United States. Testing the school for radon is the only way to determine whether the school has a radon problem (see Chapter 22).

▌Asbestos

Asbestos was used extensively in schools until the 1970s. In 1980, the EPA estimated that more than 8500 schools contained deteriorating asbestos and more than 3 million students and 250 000 teachers and other adults were at risk of exposure in schools.[14]

To prevent asbestos exposure in schools, the EPA, in compliance with the Asbestos Hazard Emergency Response Act of 1986, developed a systematic strategy for dealing with asbestos in schools and other buildings. The strategy rests on three principles: (1) medical screening of children who have been exposed to asbestos is not recommended because asbestos exposure (except for heavy exposure in industry) does not produce detectable radiographic changes in the lungs until 10 to 30 years after exposure; (2) because no worthwhile medical screening exists, all efforts should focus on prevention of exposure; and (3) visual inspection of walls and ceilings is the key to prevention of exposure.

The asbestos hazard legislation mandates that every room and every surface of every school–public, private, and parochial–must be systematically inspected for the presence of asbestos every 3 years by a trained and certified inspector. Monitoring of levels of asbestos in air in schools is of little value, because release is typically episodic and is usually missed in sampling. If asbestos is found by visual inspection, three options exist for dealing with it—removal, containment, or watchful waiting.

Removal (termed abatement) has been found necessary in only approximately 10% of school buildings. It is mandatory when deteriorating asbestos is readily accessible to children or when renovation of an asbestos-contaminated building is about to occur. While abatement constitutes the definitive treatment, the danger exists that improper abatement can liberate enough asbestos fibers to produce a substantial health hazard. Fibers are so small that ordinary vacuums and containment do not work. Therefore, it is essential that abatement be done only by properly trained and certified workers in a properly sealed situation. A list of certified asbestos removal companies is available through local health departments or the EPA regional office (see the Resources section of Chapter 5). Abatement is a very expensive option.

Containment of asbestos behind drywall, drop ceilings, or other enclosures has proven a useful approach for dealing with asbestos in schools. It has been the strategy most commonly followed. Use of this strategy requires that careful records be kept on the location of enveloped asbestos.

Watchful waiting (termed operations and maintenance) means that nothing is done immediately with asbestos in place, but that its presence, location, and condition are carefully recorded, usually in a computerized log. This approach is permissible when no potential for immediate contact between children and asbestos exists. If renovations are planned or deterioration occurs, the decision must be revisited, and containment or abatement may be required. Any school district that chooses to follow the operations and maintenance option is required by law to re-inspect every 3 years and to maintain detailed records of the location and condition of any asbestos. These inspection records must be available to the public.

Since exposure to asbestos and smoking have a synergistic effect on the development of lung cancer, reduction of the future risk of lung cancer in children who have been exposed to asbestos can be achieved by preventing children from smoking (see Chapter 5).

■ Pesticides

Schools are susceptible to pest problems because they are large, have multiple entrances and exits, prepare and serve food, serve large numbers of children, and are heavily stocked with books and other supplies and equipment that provide habitats for pests. Some school buildings are aging, multilevel, and under severe budgetary constraints, making maintenance and physical plant improvements difficult. Often pest problems are approached in a unimodal fashion involving spraying of pesticides inside and outside the school building. Children may be exposed to high levels of pesticides from "routine" spraying.

Integrated pest management (IPM) is a cost-effective and environmentally sensitive approach to pest management that uses knowledge of pest life cycles and their interactions with the environment in addition to the judicious use of pesticides. An IPM program has been shown to reduce pest problems while decreasing the use of pesticides by using substitutes for chemical treatments and, when chemicals are used, timing treatments to maximize pest destruction based on life cycle characteristics. A hallmark of successful IPM is that it is less expensive and less toxic than the more common practice of routine scheduled pesticide spraying. The Office of Pesticide Programs at the EPA has developed an approach to IPM for schools that offers step-by-step guidance to local school officials for development, implementation, and evaluation of IPM in schools.[15] Because the health effects of pesticide exposure on children are not well studied, an approach that reduces their exposure to these chemicals is desirable (see Chapter 20).

■ Lead

Schools built before the 1970s are likely to contain leaded materials on walls, woodwork, and window casings. Other sources include deteriorating paint, lead pipes, lead-lined water coolers, water fixtures, and lead-containing art supplies. Outside the buildings, playground soil may be contaminated, with higher concentrations found closest to major thoroughfares and in inner-city playgrounds. Children may be exposed to lead if the school is near a point source, such as a smelter or battery manufacturing plant (see Chapter 14).

In contrast to data available on US housing, to our knowledge no studies have comprehensively and systematically assessed the presence of lead in schools and preschools nationwide. There are no comprehensive federal laws pertaining to lead exposure in schools. Schools are indirectly affected by many existing federal regulations.

Paint
Federal legislation pertaining to paint concerns its manufacture only.

Construction and Renovation
No specific legislation concerns school renovations. The 1992 Residential Lead-based Paint Hazard Reduction Act mandates more stringent worker protection, reducing lead contamination during all renovation.

Water
High concentrations of lead can accumulate in water overnight, on weekends, and over school holidays. Schools are not required to meet the 1991 EPA action level of 15 parts per billion (ppb) because EPA regulates only public water systems, not end users. Schools are encouraged to test drinking water and to meet a recommended lead level of 20 ppb or less. The Lead Contamination Control Act of 1988 banned the sale of water coolers that were not lead free and required manufacturers to repair, replace, or recall existing lead-containing water coolers.

Art Supplies
The Labeling of Hazardous Art Materials Act of 1988 requires labeling of art materials such as lead, which contain substances to which exposure constitutes a health hazard (see Chapter 25).

∎ Frequently Asked Questions

Q *Should air ducts be cleaned?*
A Schools considering having heating and air conditioning ducts cleaned should first determine whether contaminated ducts are causing a health problem. Even when contaminants are found in the ducts, the source may be elsewhere, and cleaning the ducts may not permanently solve the problem.

Schools that use cleaning services to clean air ducts should ensure that the service provider protects persons from exposure to dislodged pollutants and chemicals used during the cleaning process. The steps for such protection may include using HEPA filtration on cleaning equipment, providing respiratory protection for workers, and having occupants vacate the premises during duct cleaning.

Q *My child's school is hot and dry. What should I do?*
A Your child may be more comfortable wearing a T-shirt. Normal saline drops will help reduce nasal dryness. Ask the teacher to open a window, if possible.

Q *Asbestos has recently been discovered on the ceiling of my child's school. Should my child have a chest x-ray? Will cancer develop in my child?*
A Asbestos on the ceiling does not by itself constitute a health hazard. The urgent need is to persuade school authorities to determine through visual inspection whether the asbestos is breaking up and whether it is likely liberating fibers into the air. If fibers are being liberated, it is essential that abatement or enclosure be instituted immediately by professionals and that children be evacuated from the affected area until the remedial work is complete. A chest radiograph is not indicated, because asbestos produces no acute changes in the lungs. The risk of lung cancer or of mesothelioma from brief exposure is very unlikely.

If, on the other hand, the asbestos has actively been liberating fibers and this situation has persisted for many weeks or months, it must be properly remediated, and intensified efforts to prevent children from starting to smoke become a particularly high priority.

Q *Our school board has done asbestos inspections as required by federal law, but it will not let parents see the results. Do parents have a right to see this information?*
A Yes. Federal law requires that this information be made available to parents and pediatricians. If the problem persists, you should call the regional office of the EPA and seek guidance from the regional asbestos coordinator.

Q *How do I know if there is a problem with lead in the school?*
A To find out whether your child's school has lead hazards, contact the local school district or the principal of the school to learn whether inspection or testing has been done. Contact your state or local health department to find out what regulations exist for testing the school environment for lead. Find out what the requirements are for remediating any lead hazards.

Remember that even if there is lead in the paint in your child's school, it does not necessarily pose a hazard if the paint is in good shape and inaccessible to your child. However, a hazard may be present if leaded paint or plaster is loose, peeling, or chipping.

∎ Resources

Pediatricians may obtain a free copy of the *Indoor Air Quality Tools for Schools* kit by faxing a request on letterhead to 202/484-1510. The kit includes *Indoor Air Pollutants: An Introduction for Health Professionals,* which contains detailed information on typical indoor air pollutants and provides almost 70 references. For assistance and guidance in dealing with known or suspected adverse effects of indoor air pollution, contact the US Environmental Protection Agency Indoor Air Quality Information Clearinghouse (800/438-4318), EPA regional offices, state and local departments of health and environmental quality, and the local American Lung Association (800/LUNG-USA).

For information on particular product hazards, contact the US Consumer Product Safety Commission (800/638-CPSC). Individual manufacturers, as well as trade associations, also may supply information.

For information about the regulation of specific pollutants, call the EPA Toxic Substances Control Act Assistance Information Service (202/554-1404).

For information on lead, contact the National Lead Information Center (800/LEAD-FYI).

For information on pesticides, contact the National Pesticides Telecommunications Network (800/858-PEST).

For more information about radon, contact the EPA Radon Division, Telephone: 202/233-9425, or contact your state radon program.

∎ References

1. American Academy of Pediatrics, Committee on Environmental Hazards. Asbestos exposure in schools. *Pediatrics.* 1987;79:301-305

2. McFadden RD. Students sickened when fumes from coal furnace seep through school. The *New York Times,* February 3, 1998:B1

3. US Congress, Office of Technology Assessment. *Risks to Students in Schools.* Washington, DC: US Government Printing Office; September 1995. Office of Technology Assessment publication OTA-ENV

4. Gammage RB, Kaye SV. *Indoor Air and Human Health.* Chelsea, Mich: Lewis Publishers, Inc; 1985

5. Turiel I. *Indoor Air Quality and Human Health.* Stanford, Calif: Stanford University Press; 1985

6. Rotter BA, Prelusky DB, Pestka JJ. Toxicology of doxynivalenol (vomitoxin). *J Toxicol Environ Health.* 1996;48:1-34

7. Croft WA, Jarvis BB, Yatawara CS. Airborne outbreak of trichothecene toxicosis. *Atmospheric Environ.* 1986;20:549-552

8. American Thoracic Society. Environmental controls and lung disease. *Am Rev Respir Dis.* 1990;142:915-939

9. Wheeler AE. System selection. *ASHRAE Journal.* Atlanta, GA: American Society of Heating, Refrigerating and Air Conditioning Engineers. June 1998, p 12-16

10. Menzies D, Bourbeau J. Building-related illnesses. *N Engl J Med.* 1997; 337:1524-1531

11. Gold DR. Indoor air pollution. *Clin Chest Med.* 1992;13:215-229

12. Samet JM, Spengler JD, eds. *Indoor Air Pollution: A Health Perspective.* Baltimore, Md: Johns Hopkins University Press; 1991

13. US Environmental Protection Agency Report: *National School Radon Survey.* Research Triangle Park: Research Triangle Institute. August 1992.

14. Support document for proposed rule on friable asbestos-containing materials in school buildings: Health effects and magnitude of exposure. US Environmental Protection Agency (EPA), EPA Report No. 560/12-80-003. Office of Testing and evaluation, Office of Pesticides and Toxic Substances, Government Printing Office, October 1980

15. US Environmental Protection Agency, Office of Pesticide Programs. *Pest Control in the School Environment: Adopting Integrated Pest Management.* Environmental Protection Agency. 735-F-93-012, August 1993

29 Waste Sites

T he potential adverse impact of hazardous waste sites on human health may be a source of concern to families as well as health professionals. The Agency for Toxic Substances and Disease Registry (ATSDR), a component of the US Department of Health and Human Services estimates that 3 to 4 million American children liven within one mile of a hazardous waste site.[1] Uncontrolled hazardous waste sites are prevalent throughout the world. Although accurate worldwide data are lacking, the US Environmental Protection Agency (EPA) in 1995 listed approximately 15 000 sites in the United States in 1996, of which 1371 were listed or proposed for listing on the National Priorities List (NPL), on the basis of a hazard ranking system.[2,3] Each of the 50 states has at least one NPL site; but five states (California, Michigan, New Jersey, New York, and Pennsylvania) contain 37% of all the sites and 30% of the children and youth (from birth through 17 years of age) in the United States.[4] The majority (65% to 70%) of uncontrolled hazardous waste sites in the United States are waste storage/treatment facilities (including landfills) or former industrial properties.[5] Many of these properties have been abandoned, and most have more than one major chemical contaminant. Less common are waste recycling facilities and mining sites, which may be active, inactive, or abandoned. Some of the substances found in uncontrolled hazardous waste sites are heavy metals such as lead, chromium, and arsenic and organic solvents such as trichloroethylene and benzene.[5] An additional group of hazardous waste sites is associated with federal government facilities, in particular military facilities and nuclear energy complexes. The National Research Council has cited 17 482 contaminated sites at 1855 military installations and 3700 sites at 500 nuclear facilities.[6] Some of these sites cover large geographic areas and are contaminated with complex mixtures of wastes.

When the EPA places a site on the NPL, the Superfund Act (passed in 1980* and amended[†] in 1986) provides monies for remediation (cleanup) of the site and an array of public health actions in nearby communities. ATSDR conducts public health assessments to evaluate the potential health hazards faced by communities in proximity to every proposed, listed, or former NPL site and in response to petitions from individuals. In many cases this work is conducted by state health departments under ATSDR sponsorship and review. A site is assigned a hazard category according to the human health hazard it poses on the basis of professional judgment and weight-of-evidence criteria.[5] In the 3-year period from 1993-1995, this process indicated a health hazard at 49% of sites and an urgent hazard at 4% of sites.[5] A site-specific epidemiologic investigation or other type of investigation is needed to establish the actual hazard to health. Of the public health assessments conducted at 1371 sites, 60% to 70% have included recommendations that address the need for intervention to interrupt ongoing exposure pathways.[4] These interventions have included provision of alternate drinking water, issuance of fish consumption advisories, posting of warning notices, restriction of site access, and (rarely) relocation of community residents.

■ Routes of Exposure

Common examples of waste sites include incinerators, landfills, emission stacks, and unsanctioned discharges of wastewater.

Children may be exposed through groundwater, surface water, drinking water, air, surface soil, sediment, or consumable plants or animals.

---

* The Comprehensive Environmental Response, Compensation, and Liability Act of 1980.
† The Superfund Amendment and Reauthorization Act of 1986.

Children, in particular, often find waste sites interesting. They may ignore or fail to notice warning signs, find or create openings in fences, or otherwise gain access to restricted places on or near a site.[7] Often there is considerable variation in exposure depending on climate, season, and time of day.

The effect that exposure to a hazardous substance(s) has on an infant's or child's health is related to the nature of the pollutant dose received, the toxicity of the substance, and the individual's susceptibility.

∎ Clinical Effects

The overall impact of hazardous waste sites on national health is difficult to assess because of conflicting information from epidemiologic studies and limitations of the methodologies used.[8] Many studies have been interpreted as "negative," meaning that no statistically significant increase in adverse health effects was found. These observations may reflect the true absence of adverse effects or the inability to detect such effects due to inadequacies in study design or sample size. Likewise, studies interpreted as "positive" may reflect a true effect or other types of study design flaws, such as misclassification of exposure or inappropriate choice of comparison groups. Most studies to date have not shown adverse effects from waste sites.

Adverse health effects have been reported in a small number of investigations of communities around hazardous waste sites.[8] These effects have ranged from nonspecific symptoms such as headache, fatigue, and irritative symptoms, to specific conditions such as low birth weight,[9] congenital heart defects,[10] and a constellation of neurobehavioral deficits.[11] Most investigations have included some children in the study population, but only a few have focused primarily on health effects in infants and children. The following are examples of findings considered "positive":

- Children exposed to trichloroethylene in drinking water supplies at 15 different sites in 5 states had increased reporting of speech and hearing impairments.[12]

- Children exposed to lead from a smelter showed poor neurobehavioral function and peripheral nerve function 15 to 20 years later, when tested as young adults.[13]

- Children living near a municipal waste incinerator had a threefold increase in risk of lower respiratory tract illnesses.[14]

▌ Diagnostic Methods

An exposed infant or child can remain asymptomatic, develop nonspecific symptoms, or develop signs and symptoms frequently associated with common medical conditions. Because of this range of outcomes, a history of exposure should be obtained when evaluating the etiology of unexplained symptoms. A standard exposure history is available.[15]

Individual Evaluation

As in other aspects of medicine, the history guides laboratory testing. Blood or urine tests may be indicated when a child is symptomatic and there is a recent history of a specific exposure (eg, when a child has climbed over a fence and played in a site known to be contaminated with a specific toxicant). Generally, laboratory tests to document exposure are not recommended in the absence of signs or symptoms.

Community Studies

In formal epidemiologic studies, laboratory biological tests may be useful to determine if there is an association between exposure and any adverse health effects.

A biomarker of exposure provides a reasonable measure of the internal body level of a substance over a period of time that depends on the pharmacokinetics of that substance. Testing may be performed on blood (for lead), urine (for metallic mercury, arsenic), breast milk (for PCBs), or other tissue. Analytical methods and human reference ranges are available for many of the substances found most commonly at hazardous waste sites. In some cases, age-specific reference ranges are available to facilitate interpretation of levels found in infants and children. It may be difficult to interpret the results, however, when reference ranges for children are not available.

Highly sensitive standardized medical test batteries are available for use in epidemiologic studies to evaluate subclinical and clinical organ damage or dysfunction related to noncancer health conditions, such as immune function disorders,[16] kidney dysfunction,[17] lung and respiratory diseases,[18] and neurotoxic disorders.[11] Because of their low specificity, these test batteries are not useful outside the context of a formal study.

▌ Treatment

Treatment of acute exposure to one or more substances from a hazardous waste site depends on the substance; the route, dose, and duration of exposure; and the presence of any symptoms or ill effects.[19]

∎ Prevention of Exposure

In the United States, the EPA is responsible for cleaning up waste sites under the Superfund Act.

Prevention of Exposure
Engineering Controls

Destruction of contaminants by incineration or other chemical or biological reactions.

Removal of the contaminants to a safer location.

Disruption of the exposure pathway (for example, an alternate water supply or perimeter fence).

Dust control and other measures to protect workers and neighbors during the cleanup process.

Engineering solutions to eliminate relatively small, acute problems (removal actions). They can also be complicated "remedial actions" that involve complex planning to permanently solve a complicated waste site problem.

Administrative Controls

Temporary or permanent relocation of residents.

Deed restrictions (for example, to prevent future use of the land for residential or child care purposes).

Ordinances to control future land use.

Health advisories (warnings about eating fish or swimming in certain waters).

Personal Preventive Actions

- Compliance with advisories mentioned in previous section.
- Connection to a safer water supply.
- Fencing of children's play areas to avoid exposure to soil contaminants.

∎ **Frequently Asked Questions**

Q *I am confused by the conflicting information I hear about the risks to my children from waste sites. Can you clarify this?*

A The risks depend on the amount, type, and duration of exposure and the types of chemicals involved. However, it is difficult to know the exact details of a child's exposure, so it is difficult to know the risk precisely. In addition, for many chemicals, the effects of exposure in childhood are not well known and can only be estimated from the toxic effects found in experiments with animals.

Q *Did exposure from a waste site cause my child's illness? or, One of my children has an illness that is linked to the waste site. Will my other children become ill also?*

A It is difficult to prove that one child's illness was caused by exposure to one particular waste site. Most of the illnesses that can be caused by exposure to toxic chemicals have more than one possible cause. Also, not every child who is so exposed becomes ill. If several children (or adults) become ill at about the same time, the same place, or following the same exposure, a linkage is more likely.

Q *My child was exposed to a hazardous waste site for a short time and did not get sick (or got sick and has recovered). I am worried about long-term illness from this exposure.*

A If there are no immediate symptoms, most likely there will be no long-term effects. Most chemical exposures without immediate symptoms do not cause delayed effects. Most experts believe that diseases such as cancer are unlikely unless there has been a prolonged period of exposure.

Q *Will my child get cancer from exposure to a waste site?*

A Although a number of chemicals found at waste sites are carcinogens (known or predicted to cause cancer), the chances of getting cancer from exposure to a waste site is thought to be small. If the child was exposed to one or more carcinogens, the amount and duration of the exposure are important risk factors. Most experts believe that development of cancer is unlikely unless there has been exposure for many years.

Q *Is my child's learning disability (or attention-deficit disorder) caused by exposure to a waste site?*

A A number of chemicals found at waste sites may affect the nervous system. They include heavy metals (such as lead and mercury), organic solvents (such as toluene), and certain types of pesticides (such as carbamates and organophosphates). The risk to the child depends on how long the child was exposed, the child's age at exposure, the degree of exposure, and the child's susceptibility.

Q *How can I protect my child from future exposure to hazardous waste sites?*

A It is best to avoid areas where soil is contaminated by hazardous waste. Explain to children the meaning and importance of posted warning signs, and strongly advise children to stay out of restricted areas. Do not let children swim in streams or other bodies of water that are known to be contaminated. Such conditions are usually posted, but if there is doubt, the local health department should be contacted. Know the source of your household drinking water and if uncertain about contaminants, have it tested. Children, pregnant women, and others should not eat certain fish caught from contaminated waters. Fishing license brochures available locally list advisories on which fish are safe to eat. If a parent or other caregiver works at a hazardous waste site, soiled work clothes should not be brought into the home. Dust can be a source of exposure for children.

∎ Resources

Information Available 24 hours/day

ATSDR/CDC Fax on-demand system: 404/322-4565

ATSDR Child Health Web Site: http://atsdr1.atsdr.cdc.gov:8080/child

ATSDR Toll Free Access: 888/42-ATSDR (888/422-8737)

ATSDR Chemical emergencies and accidental releases: 404/639-6360

Chemical poisoning emergencies (see local telephone directory)

Hazardous waste sites: 202/260-0056

Poison control centers (see local telephone directory)

Additional Information

ATSDR Educational materials: 404/639-6204

ATSDR Medical management of acute toxicity: 404/639-6360

Association of Occupational and Environmental Clinics: 202/347-4976

ATSDR Toxicity information for individual chemicals: 404/639-6300

ATSDR Toxicological Profiles: 404/639-6300

State health department: Consult telephone book blue pages

Local health department: Consult telephone book blue pages

ATSDR and EPA Regional Offices:

I. Boston (CT, MA, ME, NH, RI, VT): 617/223-5590

II. New York (NJ, NY, Puerto Rico, Virgin Islands): 212/637-4307

III. Philadelphia (DC, DE, MD, PA, VA, WV): 215/814-3139

IV. Atlanta (AL, GA, FL, KY, MS, NC, SC, TN): 404/562-1782

V. Chicago (IL, IN, MI, MN, OH, WI); 312/886-0840

VI. Dallas (AR, LA, NM, OK, TX): 214/665-8361

VII. Kansas City (IA, KS, MO, NE): 913/551-7692

VIII. Denver (CO, MT, ND, SD, UT, WY): 303/312-7010

IX. San Francisco (AZ, CA, HI, NV, Guam, Samoa): 415/744-2194

X. Seattle (AK, ID, OR, WA); 206/553-2113

EPA Hazardous Waste/Community Right to Know Hotline: 800/535-0202

Superfund Records of Decision: 703/920-9810

■ References

1. Agency for Toxic Substances and Disease Registry. *Promoting Children's Health: Progress Report of the Child Health Workgroup, Board of Scientific Counselors.* Atlanta, GA: US Department of Health and Human Services, Public Health Service, Agency for Toxic Substances and Disease Registry; April 30, 1998

2. US Environmental Protection Agency. National Priorities List for hazardous waste sites: proposed rule. *Federal Register.* 1996;61:67678-67682

3. US Environmental Protection Agency. National Priorities List for uncontrolled hazardous waste sites: final rule. *Federal Register.* 1996;61:67655-67677

4. Agency for Toxic Substances and Disease Registry. *Hazardous Substances Release/Health Effects Database (HazDat).* Atlanta, GA: US Department of Health and Human Services, Public Health Service, Agency for Toxic Substances and Disease Registry; 1999

5. Agency for Toxic Substances and Disease Registry. *Report to Congress, 1993, 1994, 1995.* Atlanta, GA: US Department of Health and Human Services, Public Health Service, Agency for Toxic Substances and Disease Registry; 1996

6. National Research Council. *Ranking hazardous-waste sites for remedial action.* Washington, DC: National Academy Press; 1994;29;37

7. Agency for Toxic Substances and Disease Registry. *Healthy Children–Toxic Environments: Acting on the Unique Vulnerability of Children Who Dwell Near Hazardous Waste Sites. Report of the Child Health Workgroup, Board of Scientific Counselors.* Atlanta, GA: US Department of Health and Human Services, Public Health Service, Agency for Toxic Substances and Disease Registry; April 28, 1997

8. Johnson BL. *Impact of Hazardous Waste on Human Health.* Chelsea, MI: Ann Arbor Press; April 28, 1999

9. Amler RW. Assessment of reproductive disorders and birth defects in communities near hazardous chemical sites: Introduction. *Reprod Toxicol.* 1997;11: 221-222

10. Savitz DA, Bornschein RL, Amler RW, Bove FI, Edmonds LD, Hanson JW, et al. Assessment of reproductive disorders and birth defects in communities near hazardous chemical sites. I. Birth defects and developmental disorders. *Reprod Toxicol.* 1997;11:223-230

11. Amler RW, Gibertinin M, editors. *Pediatric environmental neurobehavioral test battery.* Atlanta, GA: US Department of Health and Human Services, Public Health Service, Agency for Toxic Substances and Disease Registry; September 1996

12. Agency for Toxic Substances and Disease Registry. *National Exposure Registry Trichloroethylene (TCE) Subregistry Baseline Technical Report (Revised).* Atlanta, GA: US Department of Health and Human Services, Public Health Service, Agency for Toxic Substances and Disease Registry; December 1994

13. Agency for Toxic Substances and Disease Registry. *A Cohort Study of Current and Previous Residents of the Silver Valley: Assessment of Lead Exposure and Health Outcomes.* Atlanta, GA: US Department of Health and Human Services, Public Health Service, Agency for Toxic Substances and Disease Registry; August 1997

14. Agency for Toxic Substances and Disease Registry. *Study of Effect of Residential Proximity to Waste Incinerators on Lower Respiratory Illness in Children.* Atlanta, GA: US Department of Health and Human Services, Public Health Service, Agency for Toxic Substances and Disease Registry; April 1995

15. Agency for Toxic Substances and Disease Registry/National Institute for Occupational Safety and Health. *Case Studies in Environmental Medicine: Taking an Exposure History.* Atlanta, GA: US Department of Health and Human Services, Public Health Service, Agency for Toxic Substances and Disease Registry; 1992

16. Straight JM, Kipen HM, Vogt RF, Amler RW. *Immune Function Test Batteries for Use in Environmental Health Field Studies.* Atlanta, GA: US Department of Health and Human Services, Public Health Service, Agency for Toxic Substances and Disease Registry; August 1994

17. Amler RW, Mueller PW, Schultz MG. *Biomarkers of Kidney Function for Environmental Health Field Studies.* Atlanta, GA: US Department of Health and Human Services, Public Health Service, Agency for Toxic Substances and Disease Registry; April 1998

18. Metcalf SW, Samet J, Hanrahan J, Schwartz D, Hunninghake G. *A Standardized Test Battery for Lungs and Respiratory Diseases for Use in Environmental Health Field Studies.* Atlanta, GA: US Department of Health and Human Services, Public Health Service, Agency for Toxic Substances and Disease Registry; September 1994

19. Agency for Toxic Substances and Disease Registry. *Managing Hazardous Materials Incidents: Medical Management Guidelines for Acute Chemical Exposures.* Three volumes. Atlanta, GA: US Department of Health and Human Services, Public Health Service, Agency for Toxic Substances and Disease Registry; 1992-1994

IV
Complex Situations

30 | Cancer

E nvironmental carcinogens refer to external causes of cancer in humans. Many chemical agents discussed in this chapter also are discussed elsewhere in this manual.

Human carcinogens usually have been first recognized by clinicians who observed clusters of cases and traced them to their causes. The latent period must be relatively short for the exposure to result in childhood cancer. It is more likely that because of long latent periods, exposures during childhood will lead to cancers in adulthood. Diethylstilbestrol, ionizing radiation, and chemotherapy, however, have short latent periods for exposures that enable cancer to develop in childhood. About 60 chemical or physical agents are known to cause cancer in humans.[1] The carcinogenicity of environmental agents may be enhanced or diminished by interaction with one another or by genetic influences.

■ Routes of Exposure

Carcinogens such as radiation may be ingested, injected (radioisotopes), or inhaled (radon decay products). Similarly, chemical and biological carcinogens may be inhaled, ingested, or absorbed through the skin. These carcinogens occur in pollutants, tobacco products, naturally in the diet, or in medications. Occasionally, what is considered a therapeutic advance has proved to have deleterious effects, including cancer, so practitioners must remain vigilant to all therapeutic innovations and their potential hazards.

▌Biological Processes and Clinical Effects

The effects of environmental carcinogens, whether chemical or physical, have been attributed to the damage they do to DNA. Oncogenes are one class of latent cancer genes. When activated, they transform normal cells to cancer cells. Tumor suppressor genes are the other main class of cancer genes. Normally they regulate development (eg, of the eye or kidney). When these genes are inactivated (mutated), they no longer regulate growth of the organ, and cancer develops (eg, retinoblastoma or Wilms' tumor). Substances that are immunosuppressants of all types act by diminishing immunosurveillance and destruction of the earliest neoplastic cells. These cells appear throughout life but usually are eliminated, a defense that lessens with age.

The carcinogenic effect of a chemical is detectable when the dose is high or chronic, as in medicinal, occupational, or large accidental exposures. Note that if an effect has been sought but not found after high exposures, it is unlikely to be found at lower ones.

▌Physical Agents

Solar radiation: A substantial proportion of all cancers in humans involves the skin; skin cancers may be induced by ultraviolet (UV) light.[2] Because of the long latent period, skin cancers rarely occur in childhood, except when there is markedly heightened sensitivity, as in xeroderma pigmentosum, which has an inherent DNA repair defect, or in albinism due to lack of pigment in the skin that protects against UV damage. In the general population, the darker the complexion, the lower the frequency of skin cancer. Maps that show cancer mortality disclose that mortality due to malignant melanoma is significantly higher in the southern United States than in the northern United States. The incidence of melanoma has increased more rapidly than that of most cancers, and children who experience repeated sunburns are at risk[3] (see Chapter 23).

Ionizing radiation: Children are more susceptible than adults to radiation-induced leukemia, especially of the acute lymphocytic type. The peak incidence occurs 5 years after exposure, and some excess persists for 25 years. The excess of radiogenic thyroid cancer begins at 10 years of age and persists for decades. Breast cancer was induced by childhood exposure to the atomic bomb in Japan, with diagnosis at about 25 years of age; the risk was greater when exposure occurred to persons younger than 20 years. The lowest dose at which excesses of these three cancers were detected in atomic bomb survivors was 0.20 to 0.49 Gy (20 to 49 rad)[4] (see Chapter 22).

The carcinogenic effects of intrauterine exposure to radiation also have been studied. Diagnostic *in utero* exposures have been associated with various cancers in children younger than 10 years, but recent studies show a significant excess only of childhood leukemia.[5] Atomic bomb exposure of children younger than 15 years did not increase the frequency of lymphoma, brain cancer, or embryonal cancers (which are among the commonest cancers of childhood). This observation leads to doubt that in utero exposures can induce these specific cancers.

Radiotherapy is associated with an increased risk of second primary cancers; treatment for Hodgkin's disease, for example, has been associated with an excess of osteosarcoma, soft-tissue sarcoma, leukemia, skin cancer, and breast cancer.[6] In some genetic disorders, such as hereditary retinoblastoma and the nevoid basal cell carcinoma syndrome, there is increased susceptibility to radiogenic cancers.

Exposure to radon decay products (also known as radon daughters or radon progeny), which come from uranium—ubiquitous in rocks and soil—is associated with an increased risk of lung cancer in adults. Whether children are more susceptible than adults to the carcinogenic effects of radon exposure is unknown.

The threat of accidental release of radiation from nuclear reactors was largely theoretical until 1979. Then, in Pennsylvania at Three Mile Island, an equipment failure resulted in radiation exposure to neighboring communities. The doses of radiation received by the general population nearby were too small to produce increases in cancer rates, mutations, or teratogenic effects. To protect the thyroid, potassium iodide therapy was recommended, but was difficult to administer.

In 1986, a partial meltdown at a nuclear reactor in Chernobyl, Ukraine, occurred. Substantial amounts of radioactive isotopes were released into the atmosphere. Fallout occurred primarily in Ukraine and Belarus, in neighboring countries, and, to a lesser extent throughout the world. Twenty-nine heavily exposed workers at the reactor died. Near the plant 135 000 people were evacuated. Twenty-five thousand people who lived 3 to 15 km from the plant were estimated to have received 350 to 550 mSv (35 to 55 rem) from external irradiation. This amount is 7 to 11 times the annual dose-limit for radiation workers. Additional exposures occurred from the ingestion of radioisotopes (fallout) which contaminated food and water. Surprisingly, thyroid cancer developed in hundreds of children after a latent period of only 3 years.[7] Other such nuclear accidents may be expected to occur as a result of natural catastrophes, human error, or deterioration of nuclear facilities.

Asbestos: Exposure to asbestos fibers increases the frequency of lung cancer, especially in smokers, and, after a latent period as long as 40 years, can cause mesothelioma. During the 1950s, school-room ceilings were routinely sprayed with asbestos, which deteriorated with time. As a result of recent public health initiatives, the asbestos has been removed or walled off, but it is conceivable that mesothelioma may develop in adults exposed as school children, and those who smoke may have an increased risk of lung cancer (see Chapter 5).

▌ Biological Agents

Tobacco: Active smoking is a well-established cause of cancer. Studies on the health effects of passive smoking indicate an increase in the frequency of adult lung cancer among nonsmokers chronically exposed to the cigarette smoke of others. This effect is biologically plausible given the known carcinogens in tobacco smoke. The risk of lung cancer is increased after exposure in childhood to environmental tobacco smoke from smoking parents[8] (see Chapter 11).

Smokeless tobacco causes oral cancer in young adults.[9] The habit of chewing tobacco has grown among high school students who are using professional athletes as role models. In 1985, a Consensus Development Panel of the National Institutes of Health estimated that at least 10 million persons in the United States used smokeless tobacco and concluded that strong evidence exists that it causes cancer of the mouth.[9] The Council on Scientific Affairs of the American

Medical Association concurred and urged that restrictions applied to advertising cigarettes be applied to the advertising of snuff and chewing tobacco. Pediatricians have an opportunity and responsibility to prevent tobacco-related cancers by educating their patients.

Diet: A variety of natural chemicals in food may be carcinogenic in people. Among them are aflatoxins, sassafras, cycasin, and bracken (their natural constituents are carcinogens), which can be found in peanuts, peanut butter, and many other foods, as well as protein pyrolysates produced when certain foods are cooked. Some food constituents protect against cancer in experimental animals. Among these anticarcinogens are carotenoids and dietary fiber.[10]

It has been difficult to derive strong evidence that individual components of the diet are carcinogenic in humans because of the long latent periods, the role of metabolic conversion, and possibly interactions that may potentiate or inhibit carcinogenesis.

Laboratory experimentation and human correlational studies suggest that overeating contributes to cancer of the endometrium, and fats in particular contribute to cancer of the breast and colon.[10] The composition of the diet is believed to affect the bacterial flora of the intestines, which in turn produce carcinogenic metabolites through degradation of bile acids and cholesterol. In addition, high fiber content is believed to diminish the frequency of colon cancer by speeding transit time and thus diminishing contact between dietary carcinogens and intestinal mucosa.

Data from epidemiologic studies, clinical observations, and animal experimentation are insufficient for strong recommendations to be made about specific dietary factors, but no harm would be done and other health benefits might result from following the recommendations that several medical organizations have issued about diet and cancer: reduce fat consumption from 40% to 30% of calories; include whole-grain cereals, citrus fruits, and green or yellow vegetables in the daily diet; limit consumption of salt-cured and smoke-cured foods and alcoholic beverages; and maintain optimal body weight.[10]

▮ What to Do When Clusters Are Observed

Occasionally a cluster of cancers occurs within a neighborhood or school district, often by chance. Clusters of cancers occasionally may be environmentally induced (ie, the histories of the affected persons reveal a large exposure in common, usually a drug or occupational chemical).[11] In the office practice, the pediatrician can make novel observations about environmental or inherent causes of specific types of childhood cancers. A single case may draw attention to the suspected carcinogen, as in respiratory cancers induced by war-time exposure to mustard gas during its manufacture in Japan or liver neoplasia due to oral contraceptives that was noted in Michigan.[11]

When a cluster is observed, the pediatrician should determine whether the cancers are of the same or related types. Cancers of the same type are more likely than diverse types to be induced by an environmental carcinogen. Diagnosis by cell type and primary anatomic site should be verified. Cases should be excluded if the latent period is too short or if the neoplasm was present before the child resided, attended school, or was otherwise exposed in the area. If the exclusions do not dispel the clusters, an environmental epidemiologist from the state department of health should be consulted.

The association between two events need not be causal. Establishing causality is enhanced by showing (1) a logical time sequence (ie, the presumed causal event preceded the effect); (2) specificity of the effect (ie, one type rather than multiple types of cancer caused by a given exposure); (3) a dose-response relationship; (4) biologic plausibility (ie, the new information is consistent with previous knowledge); (5) consistency with other observations about cause and effect (eg, determining whether the relationship of fat consumption to colon cancer rates is the same throughout the world); (6) the exclusion of concomitant variables (alternative explanations) in the analysis; and (7) disappearance of the effect when the cause is removed. Not all of these elements can be evaluated or will hold true for even the most fully studied effects of an environmental exposure. The pediatrician's job is not to establish causality but to work with the department of health in evaluating the situation.

▌ Searching for Clues to Cancer Causes

In searching for clues to cancer causes, a few questions can produce a wealth of new information. Family history ranks first. Ideally, each medical record for patients with cancer should include a recent pedigree showing illnesses in each first-degree relative (parents, siblings, and children of the index case), as well as information about other relatives with cancer or other potentially related diseases, such as immunologic disorders, blood dyscrasias, or congenital malformations. Second, physicians should inquire about the parents' occupational and other exposures during pregnancy (including smoking) and about the child's exposures to environmental tobacco smoke, chemicals, radiation, and unusual infections. Other findings may be important to determining the cause: coexistent disease, such as multiple congenital malformations; multifocal or bilateral cancer in paired organs (a possible clue to hereditary transmission); cancer of an unusual histologic type; cancer at an unusual age (eg, adult-type cancers in childhood); cancer at an unusual site; or marked overreaction to conventional cancer therapy (eg, acute reaction to radiotherapy for lymphoma in ataxia-telangiectasia). From such occurrences, new understanding of the origins of childhood cancer may be derived in the future, as they have been in the past.

▌ Frequently Asked Questions

Q *What steps can I take to prevent cancer in my child?*
A The causes of most childhood cancers are unknown. Most cases of cancer occur in adulthood, and we still do not know the steps to decrease the chances of the development of certain types of cancer in adulthood. Children should be encouraged not to smoke or use smokeless tobacco products. Adults should not be allowed to smoke when children are present. Children should not sunburn and should be encouraged to wear sunscreen when outdoors. Important preventive measures for parents include testing their home for radon and making sure no friable asbestos exists in the home.

Q *Why did neuroblastoma develop in my 3-month-old child?*
A Almost all childhood cancer in the United States occurs at random. In one study, 500 children were studied, and no cause of neuroblastoma could be found. We know that damage to DNA occurs at a specific location in chromosome 1 in neuroblastoma, but rarely do we know what causes the mutation in this or other childhood cancers. We know, for example, that Japanese atomic bomb survivors had an excess of leukemia, among other cancers. The mutation may occur during normal reshuffling of genetic materi-

al. Usually the damage is repaired, and cancer does not develop, but unfortunately this defense is sometimes breached.

Q *The cat's been sick. Could the cat have caused my child's leukemia?*

A Cats develop a similar disease due to a virus, which they can transmit to other cats but not to humans. The same is true of chickens and cattle, in which a leukemia-like disease is virally induced. There is no evidence that pets transmit cancer to humans.

Q *Several children in our neighborhood have cancer. Could it be due to the same cause?*

A Most causes of cancer in humans have been first recognized by the occurrence of a cluster of cases. Such discoveries are infrequent and generally involve rare cancers due to heavy exposures to a carcinogen. The many types of cancer (more than 80) give rise to thousands of random clusters each year in the United States, in neighborhoods, schools, social clubs, sports teams, and other groups of people. By drawing boundaries on a scatter map near the cases, random clustering can appear to be unusual. In any event, more evidence than a cluster is needed, including a dose-response effect (the bigger the dose the more frequent the effect) and biologic plausibility considering other knowledge about cancer. In most clusters there are many different types of cancers and many different causes, rather than a single cause.

Q *Will my child with cancer give my other children cancer?*

A Cancer is not transmitted from one child to another. Occasionally, a predisposition to specific cancers is transmitted through the ova or sperm cells of the parent. For example, retinoblastoma runs in families. Usually signs of predisposition to hereditary cancer can be detected in the histories of families with genetic disorders. For children at risk, early detection and treatment can improve survival and well-being. Thus, few children die of retinoblastoma today.

Q *A member of our household smokes. Could that be the cause of my child's cancer?*

A There is no evidence that childhood cancer has been induced by exposure to environmental tobacco smoke. Cancers in children younger than 15 years are generally of a different microscopic category (nonepithelial) from cigarette-induced cancers (epithelial), and no evidence currently exists that the childhood types are inducible by environmental tobacco smoke. On the other hand, adult cancers, such as lung cancer, leukemia, and lymphoma, have been associated with exposure to maternal smoking which occurs before the child reaches age 10.

Q *Is it possible that the drugs I took during pregnancy started my child's cancer?*
A Drugs commonly used during pregnancy have not been shown to be carcinogenic in the offspring.

Q *I have heard that peanut butter may cause cancer. Is this true?*
A It is true that peanuts may become contaminated with molds producing aflatoxin, a carcinogen. The US Food and Drug Administration regulates the amount of aflatoxin permitted in foods such as peanut butter.

Q *Is childhood cancer increasing?*
A Yes, the incidence of childhood cancer is increasing at approximately 1% per year. Despite this, childhood cancer is rare. Childhood cancers represent only 2% of the total cancer cases in the United States during a year. There are no definitive answers about why cancer in children is increasing. One possibility is that changes in the diagnostic classification of disease may affect the incidence rates. Such changes could result in apparent increases in cancer incidence. Another possibility is that we have better diagnostic tools now.[12] The potential role of environmental factors has not been fully evaluated.

■ Resource

National Cancer Institute: 800/4-CANCER

■ References

1. Tomatis L, Kaldor JM, Bartsch H. Experimental studies in the assessment of human risk. In: Schottenfeld D, Fraumeni JF Jr, eds. *Cancer Epidemiology and*

Prevention. 2nd ed. New York, NY: Oxford University Press; 1996:11-27

2. Council on Scientific Affairs. Harmful effects of ultraviolet radiation. *JAMA*. 1989;262:380-384

3. American Academy of Pediatrics, Committee on Environmental Health. Ultraviolet light: a hazard to children. *Pediatrics*. 1999;104:328-333.

4. Miller RW, Delayed effects of external radiation exposure: a brief history. *Radiat Res*. 1995;144:160-169

5. Miller RW, Boice JD Jr. Cancer after intrauterine exposure to the atomic bomb. *Radiat Res*. 1997;147:396-397

6. Bhatia S, Robison LL, Oberlin O, et al. Breast cancer and other second neoplasms after childhood Hodgkin's disease. *N Engl J Med*. 1996;334:745-751

7. Williams D. Thyroid cancer and the Chernobyl accident. *J Clin Endocrinol Metab*. 1996;81:6-8

8. Committee on Passive Smoking. Board on Environmental Studies and Toxicology. National Research Council. *Environmental Tobacco Smoke. Measuring Exposures and Assessing Health Effects*. Washington, DC: National Academy Press; 1986

9. Consensus Development Panel. National Institutes of Health. Health applications of smokeless tobacco use. *JAMA*. 1986;255:1045-1048

10. Willett WC. Diet and health: what should we eat? *Science*. 1994;264:532-537

11. Miller RW. The discovery of human teratogens, carcinogens and mutagens: lessons for the future. In: Hollaender A, de Serres FJ, eds. *Chemical Mutagens: Principles and Methods for Their Detection*. Vol 5. New York, NY: Plenum Publishing Corp; 1978:101-126

12. Linet MS, Ries, LA, Smith MA, Tarone RE, Devesa SS. Cnacer Surveillance Series: recent trends in childhood cancer incidence and mortality in the United States. *J Natl Cancer Inst*. 1999;91:1051-1058

31 Environmental Disparities

C ertain communities, especially those with low income or minority residents, may be disproportionately exposed to pollution. Children may have greater exposure than adults to environmental pollutants in air, water, and food. The likely confluence of these two trends is that children in low income or minority communities may be the population most exposed, and least protected, from environmental health threats.

▋ Disparities in Mortality and Morbidity

Racial and ethnic differences in infant mortality and the prevalence and severity of many childhood diseases are well-recognized. Representative diseases will be discussed in this chapter. Environmental factors may account for some of the differences in morbidity and mortality among race/ethnic groups, but this has not been well clarified.

Infant mortality

Since the early 1900s, the infant mortality rate in the United States has always been higher for nonwhite infants than for white infants.[1] The reasons for the racial disparities are not fully understood. Sudden infant death syndrome (SIDS) is a major contributor to excess infant mortality in nonwhites. The rate of deaths from SIDS is higher among Alaskan Natives, American Indians, and African Americans.[2,3] In addition to race/ethnicity, important environmental risk factors for SIDS include prone sleep position, maternal smoking during pregnancy, postnatal exposure to environmental tobacco smoke, and (possibly) exposure to outdoor air pollution.[4-6] Recently, dramatic decreases have been noted in the infant mortality rate and the rate of SIDS among Alaskan Natives and American Indians living in the Pacific Northwest.[7] The reason or reasons for the decreases are not fully understood.[8]

Asthma
Puerto Rican, African American, and Cuban American children in the US have a higher prevalence of asthma than white children.[9-16] African American children are nearly twice as likely to have asthma as white children. African Americans younger than 24 years are 3 to 4 times more likely to be hospitalized for asthma. Much of this increase is thought to be due to poverty rather than to race.[17,18] Children of Hispanic mothers have a rate of asthma 2.5 times higher than that of whites and a rate more than 1.5 times higher than that of African Americans.[19] Within the Hispanic population, the highest prevalence of asthma among children occurred in Puerto Ricans (11.2%), followed by Cuban Americans (5.2%) and Mexican Americans (2.7%). These data are in contrast to the incidence of asthma in non-Hispanic blacks (5.9%) and non-Hispanic whites (3.3%).[19]

Infant Pulmonary Hemorrhage
Clusters of cases of acute pulmonary hemorrhage have been reported among infants in Cleveland, Chicago, and Detroit.[20-22] The majority of infants in these clusters have been African American. It is not known whether race is a risk factor for infant pulmonary hemorrhage, or whether race is associated with socioeconomic status or with the prevalence of other specific risk factors, for which race may be a marker.[21]

■ Disparities in Exposure

Air Pollution Exposure
Minority children may experience greater exposure to polluted indoor and outdoor air. Indoors, they may have greater exposures to dust

mites, molds, and cockroaches.[23] They may also live in neighborhoods with substandard outdoor air quality. For instance, 52% of all whites in the United States live in counties with high ozone concentrations. For African Americans the figure is 62% and for Hispanics 71%. Higher percentages of African Americans and Hispanics than whites reside in counties with higher levels of carbon monoxide, sulfur dioxide, nitrogen dioxide, lead, and particulate matter.[24]

Food Exposure
Ethnic minorities may be exposed to certain chemical contaminants in the food supply due to dietary habits. Native Americans and subsistence fishing communities may be at much greater health risk from contaminants in fish. For example, the Penobscot Indian Nation has a fish consumption rate nearly twice the national average (see Chapter 24).

Lead Exposure
Despite recent large declines in blood lead levels, young children of low-income, urban minority families may have blood lead levels above 10 µg/dL. In 1991-1994, an estimated 11.2% of African American, 4% of Hispanic American, and 2.3% of white non-Hispanic children younger than 6 years had blood lead levels above 10 µg/dL.[25] Eight percent of low income children had blood lead levels above 10 µg/dL, compared with 1% of children from high-income families (see Table 31.1).

Pesticide Exposure
Nearly 3 decades ago, several surveys reported that levels of dichlorodiphenyltrichloroethane (DDT) and its metabolites (in fat or blood) were higher in African Americans than in whites.[26] In a community in Florida, DDT and DDE levels in blood were significantly lower in the affluent groups than in the low-income groups, in both African Americans and whites. However, in comparable income groups, African Americans had higher DDT levels than whites.[26]

Children of farm workers may accompany their parents to the fields, live in housing contaminated by direct pesticide spray or drift from nearby fields, and work in the fields themselves.[27] A recent California Department of Health Services pilot project suggests a potential for higher residential exposure to some pesticides for children of farm workers as opposed to children of non-farm workers.

Table 31.1. Percentage of Children Aged 1-5 Years With Blood Lead Levels (BLLs) ≥ 10 µg/dL by Year Housing Built and Selected Characteristics, and Weighted Geometric Mean (GM) BLLs, by Selected Characteristics

| Characteristic | Year Housing Built | | | Total | |
	Before 1946 %	During 1946-1973 %	After 1973 %	%	GM BLL (µg/dL)
Race/Ethnicity					
Black/non-Hispanic	21.9	13.7	3.4	11.2	4.3
Mexican American	13.0	2.3	1.6	4.0	3.1
White, non-Hispanic	5.6	1.4	1.5	2.3	2.3
Income					
Low	16.4	7.3	4.3	8.0	3.8
Middle	4.1	2.0	0.4	1.9	2.3
High	0.9	2.7	0.0	1.0	1.9
Urban status Population ≥1 million	11.5	5.8	0.8	5.4	2.8
Population < 1 million	5.8	3.1	2.5	3.3	2.7
Total	8.6	4.6	1.6	4.4	2.7

Source: Reference 25.

Dust samples were obtained from homes within one-quarter mile of agricultural fields where approximately 50 agricultural pesticides were used. A total of 10 different pesticides were detected.[28] Half of the homes had at least one resident who was a farm worker. The pesticides diazinon and chlorpyrifos were detected only in the homes of farm workers. In the homes of two farm workers, risk estimates for diazinon ingestion suggested that the toddlers' exposure to house dust may exceed the Environmental Protection Agency's chronic oral reference dose. The study did not look at the ethnicity of the residents in these homes; however, the vast majority of farm workers are people of color.

Rituals

In certain ethnic groups, rituals may be a potential route of exposure to environmental contaminants. For example, some Hispanic Americans who practice Santeria may sprinkle elemental mercury in the house, possibly resulting in elevated levels of mercury in the indoor air (see Chapter 15).

Water Exposure

Many small, rural, or low-income neighborhoods do not have access to safe and affordable drinking water supplies. Some water contamination problems may affect certain populations disproportionately. There are situations where certain racial and socioeconomic populations are exposed to higher levels of contaminants in water than in the general population.[29]

Waste Sites

The siting of hazardous waste sites may disproportionately occur in minority neighborhoods. A report by the United Church of Christ's Commission for Racial Justice revealed that three of the five largest hazardous waste landfills in the United States are in African American or Hispanic neighborhoods and that the mean percentage of minority residents in areas with toxic waste sites is twice that of areas without toxic waste sites.[30] In 1994, in recognition of the disproportionate impact of environmental hazards on low income communities, President Clinton issued an Executive Order seeking to achieve environmental justice.[31]

Children in poverty face an array of formidable challenges in their lives. Pediatricians must work together to protect all children, especially children in low income or minority communities, from environmental threats to their health.

■ References

1. MacDorman MF, Atkinson JO. Infant mortality statistics from the 1996 period linked birth/infant death data set. *Monthly Vital Stat* Rep. 1998;46(12)

2. Irwin KL, Mannino S, Daling J. Sudden infant death syndrome in Washington state: why are Native American infants at greater risk than white

infants? *J Pediatr.* 1992;121:242-247

3. Oyen N, Bulterys M, Welty TK, Kraus JF. Sudden unexplained infant deaths among American Indians and whites in North and South Dakota. *Paediatr Perinat Epidemiol.* 1990;4:175-183

4. American Academy of Pediatrics, Task Force on Infant Positioning and SIDS. Positioning and SIDS. *Pediatrics.* 1992;89:1120-1126

5. MacDorman MF, Cnattingius S, Hoffman HJ, Kramer MS, Haglund B. Sudden infant death syndrome and smoking in the United States and Sweden. *Am J Epidemiol.* 1997;146:249-257

6. Woodruff TJ, Grillo J, Schoendorf KC. The relationship between selected causes of post neonatal infant mortality and particulate air pollution in the US. *Environ Health Perspect.* 1997;105:608-612

7. Centers for Disease Control and Prevention. Decrease in infant mortality and sudden infant death syndrome among Northwest American Indians and Alaskan Natives–Pacific Northwest, 1985-1996. *MMWR Morb Mortal Wkly Rep.* 1999;48:181-184

8. Centers for Disease Control and Prevention. Guidelines for death scene investigation of sudden, unexplained infant deaths: recommendations of the Interagency Panel on Sudden Infant Death Syndrome. *MMWR Morb Mortal Wkly Rep.* 1996; 45(No.RR-10):1-22

9. Gergen PJ, Mullally DI, Evans R. National survey of prevalence of asthma among children in the United States, 1976 to 1980. *Pediatrics.* 1988;81:1-7

10. Schwartz J, Gold D, Dockery DW, Weiss ST, Speizer FE. Predictions of asthma and persistent wheeze in a national sample of children in the United States. *Am Rev Respir Dis.* 1990;142:555-562

11. Weitzman M, Gortmaker S, Sobol A. Racial, social, and environmental risks for childhood asthma. *Am J Dis Child.* 1990;144:1189-1194

12. Weitzman M, Gortmaker SL, Sobol AM, Perrin JM. Recent trends in the prevalence and severity of childhood asthma. *JAMA.* 1992;268:2673-2677

13. Cunningham J, Dockery DW, Speizer FE. Race, asthma and persistent wheeze in Philadelphia school children. *Am J Public Health.* 1996;86:1406-1409

14. Centers for Disease Control and Prevention. Asthma mortality and hospitalization among children and young adults—United States, 1980-1983. *MMWR Morb Mortal Wkly Rep.* 1996;45:350-353

15. Ray NF, Thamer M, Fadillioglu B, Gergen PJ. Race, income, urbanicity, and asthma hospitalizations in California. *Chest.* 1998;113:1277-1284

16. Gergen PJ, Weiss KB, Changing patterns of asthma hospitalization among children: 1979 to 1987. *JAMA.* 1990;264:1688-1692

17. Wissow LS, Gittelsohn AM, Szklo M, Starfield B, Mussman M. Poverty, race, and hospitalization for childhood asthma. *Am J Public Health.* 1988;78:777-782

18. Crain EF, Weiss KB, Bijur PE, Hersh M, Westbrook L, Stein RE. An estimate of the prevalence of asthma and wheezing among inner-city children. *Pediatrics.* 1994;94:356-362

19. Beckett WS, Belanger K, Gent, JF, Holford TR, Leaderer BP. Asthma among Puerto Rican Hispanics: a multi-ethnic comparison study of risk factors. *Am J Respir Crit Care Med.* 1996;154;894-899

20. Centers for Disease Control and Prevention. Acute pulmonary hemorrhage/hemosiderosis among infants—Cleveland, January 1993–November 1994. *MMWR Morb Mortal Wkly Rep.* 1994;43:881-883

21. Centers for Disease Control and Prevention. Acute pulmonary hemorrhage among infants—Chicago, April 1992–November 1994. *MMWR, Morb Mortal Wkly Rep.* 1995;44:67-74

22. Pappas MD, Sarniak AP, Meert KL, Hasan RA, Leih-Lai MW. Idiopathic pulmonary hemorrhage in infancy: clinical features and management with high frequency ventilation. *Chest.* 1996;110:553-555

23. Sarpong SB, Hamilton RG, Eggleston PA, Adkinson NF. Socioeconomic status and race as risk factors for cockroach allergen exposure and sensitization in children with asthma. *J Allergy Clin Immunol.* 1996;97:1393-1401

24. Wennette DR, Nieves LA. Breathing polluted air. *EPA J.* March/April 1992

25. Centers for Disease Control and Prevention. Update: blood lead levels—United States; 1991-1994. *MMWR Morb Mortal Wkly Rep.* 1997;46:141-146

26. Davies JE, Edmundson WF, Raffonelli A, Cassady JC, Morgade C. The role of social class in human pesticide pollution. *Am J Epidemiol.* 1972;5:96:334-341

27. Zahm SH, Devesa S. Childhood cancer: overview of incidence trends and environmental carcinogens. *Environ Health Perspec.* September 1995;103(suppl 6):177-184

28. Bradman MA, Harnly ME, Draper W, et al. Pesticide exposures to children from California's Central Valley: results of a pilot study. *J Expo Anal Environ Epidemiol.* 1997;7:217-234

29. Calderon RL, Johnson CC Jr, Craun GF, et al. Health risks from contaminated water: do class and race matter? *Toxicol Industrial Health.* 1993;9:879-900

30. Commission for Racial Justice, United Church of Christ. *Toxic Wastes and Race in the United States: A National Study of the Racial and Socioeconomic Characteristics of Communities with Hazardous Waste Sites*; 1987

31. Presidential Executive Order on Environmental Justice. EO. 12898. *Federal Register.* February 11, 1994

32 Questions About Multiple Chemical Sensitivities

Pediatricians might be dismayed when asked to evaluate a child for the complaint of multiple chemical sensitivity (MCS). Also termed "environmental illness," "20th century syndrome," and "idiopathic environmental intolerance," MCS is a highly controversial condition based on patient attribution of symptoms with no objective physical or laboratory correlates. In addition, because of the firm beliefs held by patients and physicians about MCS, objective investigation and discussion of this problem is difficult. Although the complaint of MCS is most commonly seen in middle-aged women, conditions attributed to MCS are occasionally reported to occur in children. Attention-deficit disorder and hyperactivity are two conditions that are increasingly being attributed to sick schools and low-level chemical exposures. To answer parental concerns about MCS, pediatricians should be familiar with the condition.[1-3]

People with MCS complain of a myriad of symptoms when exposed to low levels of a wide variety of chemically-unrelated substances. Adults with MCS often can recall an initial sensitizing exposure to an overpowering chemical. Their symptoms involve most organ systems and commonly include headache, fatigue, confusion, memory loss, gastrointestinal problems, joint and muscle pains, irritability, depression, skin problems, and upper respiratory tract problems. In children, learning disorders and behavioral problems also have been ascribed to MCS. Advocates for the disorder claim that many additional people, including children, have the disease but have not yet discovered the role of chemicals. Symptoms are attributed to chemical exposures at levels well below those known to cause toxicologic effects. Over time, a person's sensitivity increases and decreases; sensitivity also expands from a single chemical to a wide variety of unrelated substances. Pesticides, perfumes, cigarette smoke, formaldehyde, and gases released from new carpets are substances commonly implicated in MCS. Reportedly, symptoms also can migrate from one target organ system to another over time; this phenomenon is called switching. The severity of disability in adults with MCS ranges from those who continue with their usual lifestyle after making some modifications to those who completely withdraw from "normal" life to avoid chemical exposure.

Odor may be or often seems to be a prominent factor in precipitating the symptoms of MCS and also is an important protective reflex in the presence of toxic exposures. The olfactory nerve mediates odor perception, while branches of the trigeminal nerve perceive irritation and pungency for taste and smell; these two nerves innervate different areas of the brain. Most investigators agree that an explanation of the role of odor is a necessary component of any model of the causes of MCS.

■ Historical Background

The late Theron Randolph, an allergist from Chicago, Ill, first described MCS during the 1950s.[4] He believed that traditional allergists defined "sensitivity" too narrowly by limiting it exclusively to antibody-antigen reactions. In contrast, Randolph hypothesized that foods and chemicals might cause other derangements of the immune system. He postulated that increasing exposure to petroleum products, pesticides, synthetic textiles, and food additives in modern life were responsible for his patients' health problems, which included mental and behavioral disturbances, as well as rhinitis, headache, and asthma. A group of physicians who supported Dr Randolph's concept of environmental illness, often called clinical ecologists, eventually founded the American Academy of Environmental Medicine.

In several position papers, traditional medical organizations have questioned the scientific basis of MCS. The subspecialty of allergy for example, as represented by the American Academy of Allergy and Immunology, asserted that there were no adequate studies to support the theories of the clinical ecologists and, in 1986, issued a position statement stating that the diagnostic and therapeutic principles of clinical ecology were based on unproven and experimental methods.[5] Similarly, the American College of Physicians in 1989 and the American Medical Association in 1992 criticized clinical ecology.[6,7]

▌ Proposed Causative Mechanisms

A number of different models have been proposed to explain MCS. They can be roughly grouped into three categories: physiologic, psychogenic, and limbic-olfactory; a discussion of each follows. The phenomena currently described as MCS might, in fact, represent several different conditions mistakenly given one descriptive label. If this were true, there would necessarily be a specific causative mechanism for each condition. The models discussed herein consider MCS as a single entity.

The immunologic model is an example of a physiologic explanation for MCS phenomenology. This model postulates that chemicals may damage the immune system so that it no longer functions normally. However, no clinical laboratory, other than those associated with clinical ecologists, has found consistent immunologic abnormalities in patients with MCS. Even for proponents of MCS, the immunologic theory does not provide a satisfactory construct for explaining MCS and is now mainly of historical interest.

Investigators also have proposed a classic conditioned response to odor as an explanation for MCS. After an initial traumatic exposure to a strong-smelling odor, subsequent exposure may cause a conditioned response of the same symptoms to much lower concentrations of the chemical. This conditioned response may be accompanied by varying degrees of "stimulus generalization" the development of symptoms in response to other strong odors. Some researchers have suggested that an extreme form of this response be called an "odor-triggered panic attack."[8]

Disorders of porphyrin metabolism also have been postulated to explain symptoms. Persons given a diagnosis of neuropathic porphyria can have episodes of neurologic and psychiatric symptoms that seem similar to those of MCS. Also, a large number of chemicals and drugs can cause transient disturbances of the heme-forming system. However, the results of laboratory evaluations of persons with MCS are not typical of those seen in confirmed porphyrias, and any relationship between the two conditions is highly speculative.[9]

Psychogenic mechanisms also have been suggested as having a role in the occurrence of MCS. Affective disorders, somatoform disorders, and anxiety are the most frequent psychological conditions used to explain MCS. Some studies have shown that persons in whom environmental illness develops have a high degree of preexisting psychiatric morbidity and a tendency toward somatization.[10,11] These findings suggest that psychologic factors, although not necessarily causative, seem to predispose some people to the development of a generalized chemical sensitivity.

The limbic-olfactory model of MCS provides a speculative biological explanation for the affective and cognitive symptoms. The model depends on the anatomic links between the olfactory nerve, the limbic system, and other regions of the brain. Some have hypothesized that subconvulsive kindling (the ability of a subthreshold electrical or chemical stimulus to cause a response) and time-dependent sensitization are central nervous system constructs that provide a mechanism by which low-level chemical exposures can be amplified and produce symptoms referable to multiple organ systems.[12] Proponents of this hypothesis draw analogies to animal studies to support the model; opponents point out that the studies using animals have included chemicals at pharmacological doses much larger than those usually encountered in an environmental setting. No known data obtained from studies in humans support this theory.

Basic descriptive epidemiologic data about MCS have not been collected. One major difficulty is the lack of a case definition for MCS. MCS is a symptom-based condition with no objective signs or documentable end-organ damage; there has been no consensus case definition in the medical community. Another problem is that most reports about MCS have consisted of case series or the clinical experiences of referral practices. The only population-based prevalence data on MCS come from several questions about chemical sensitivities included in the 1995 California Behavioral Risk Factors Surveillance telephone survey of 4000 randomly selected California residents. Of the general population contacted in the survey, 16% reported sensitivities to everyday chemicals (12% to more than one chemical), and 6% claimed to have been diagnosed with MCS by a physician.[13] This survey included only adults older than 18 years; no prevalence figures were available for the pediatric age group.

∎ Clinical Evaluation of a Child Believed to Have Chemical Sensitivity

The pediatrician should approach the evaluation of a child whose parents believe that the environment is the cause of the child's symptoms in the same manner as any other problem: with an open mind, a willingness to listen, and a methodical workup.

The pediatrician should consider the child's clinical presentation. By using the patient history and selecting appropriate clinical tests, the pediatrician should rule out conditions that are part of the differential diagnosis and determine the most likely diagnosis.[14] The diagnosis of the problem directs the treatment, which the pediatrician modifies for the child's particular circumstances. Often, the diagnosis may not be apparent. Symptomatic treatment can be useful while the pediatrician observes the child's condition over time.

Upper respiratory tract symptoms often are encountered, and the possibility that the child has allergies should be considered. Although rhinorrhea, nasal obstruction, and sneezing are the most obvious allergic symptoms, atopic children also present with fatigue and irritability due to chronic upper respiratory tract problems and lack of sleep. Headache and dizziness, common complaints in MCS, can be manifestations of chronic sinus disease. Allergic stigmata found on physical examination will suggest a diagnosis of allergy, that can be supported with appropriate skin testing. A response to drug treatment or environmental interventions will confirm the diagnosis. Other diseases to consider in the differential diagnosis are diseases with symptoms that are nonspecific and inconstant, including Lyme disease, Munchausen by proxy, or psychosocial problems such as school phobia.

∎ Diagnostic Methods

No laboratory tests are diagnostic for MCS, and none is recommended for its evaluation. When appropriate, laboratory testing to rule out other diagnoses or underlying medical conditions should be performed. Testing should be done only at laboratories that adhere to the guidelines for quality control established through the Clinical Laboratory Improvement Act. These laboratories are inspected to ensure good practice and have demonstrated their proficiency.

A number of unproven tests and treatments have been proposed for the diagnosis and treatment of MCS. For example, the use of positron emission tomography and single-photon emission-computed tomography scans has been suggested. However, they are not recommended. The method for these techniques is not sufficiently standardized or validated. The treatment approaches for MCS have included rotation diets, sublingual or intradermal provocation-neutralization, and the use of saunas for chemical detoxification; none has been proven to be effective in double-blinded studies.[15]

Examining a child with alleged MCS is a challenge for the pediatrician who is faced with treating the child's health as it fits into the family's belief system. Exploring the basis for the beliefs and keeping an open mind to the different values that underlie them will allow effective and compassionate use of the pediatrician's medical knowledge and skills. In the absence of clear alternative explanations for the child's complaint, the pediatrician who supports the parent's or patient's attribution of symptoms to environmental chemicals may validate untested and unproven notions that lead to inappropriate beliefs and behaviors.[16]

❚ Frequently Asked Questions

Q *I have been told that my child has a short attention span and that he is frequently inattentive in class. The teacher has suggested psychological testing. My child is fine at home. Could these problems be related to chemical exposure at school?*

A A thorough evaluation of the child's difficulty and appropriate testing are initial steps in dealing with this problem. Parental anxieties about learning and behavior problems have often focused on concern about chemical exposure in the schools. Sources of potential environmental contamination cited in schools include cleaning agents, art supplies (glues, markers, and aerosol sprays), pesticides, and diesel exhaust fumes from school buses. Dust and molds also are sources of pollution. There is an unproven assertion in the lay press that approximately two thirds of the cases of attention-deficit/hyperactivity disorder are caused by environmental illnesses, food sensitivity, or both. The peer-reviewed literature does not support an association between chemical exposures in schools and learning problems.

Q *My child is being made sick by the chemicals that she is exposed to in school. Can you, as my pediatrician, intervene and help me decrease my child's exposure to chemicals in the school?*

A Parents often ask pediatricians to write a letter supporting the child's withdrawal from some activity or area in the school. In these instances, the pediatrician should be open-minded but careful about fostering negative associations between the child and the child's environment.

Another issue raised by this question is less obvious but of crucial importance in considering the problem of chemical sensitivity: the patient's causal attribution of symptoms to a chemical exposure. At present, MCS is defined in terms of the patient's report of a temporal relationship between perceived exposures to chemicals and the appearance of symptoms. In the case of children, the situation is complicated because it is usually the parent who attributes the child's symptoms to chemical exposure. While there might be a temporal relationship between the exposure and symptoms, few data exist to support a causal relationship.

Q *What do I need to do to my home to prevent my child from being exposed to chemicals that might be toxic?*

A It is important for parents to understand that their child's exposure to chemicals is cumulative: the sum of inhalation, ingestion, and dermal exposures. Parents should be encouraged to consider all activities and situations in which their child might be exposed. The home inventory is designed to alert parents to potentially toxic exposures in the home (see Chapter 3). The school environment may be a source of additional exposures to chemicals (see Chapter 28).

▌ Resources

Pediatricians who have expertise in environmental health are valuable resources for advice about MCS. Another good resource about environmental medicine is the Web page and mailing list of the Department of Occupational and Environmental Medicine at Duke University. It can be accessed at http://occ-env-med.mc. duke.edu/eom/. Besides having a large repository of environmental information, the page has links to many other environmental sources on the World Wide Web.

Another resource is the National Foundation for the Chemically Hypersensitive, 1158 N Huron, Linwood, MI 48634; 517/697-3989.

∎ References

1. Sparks PJ, Daniell W, Black DW, et al. Multiple chemical sensitivity syndrome: a clinical perspective. *J Occup Med.* 1994;36:718-730

2. Hileman B. Multiple chemical sensitivity. *Chem Eng News.* 1991;69:26-42

3. Twombly R. MCS: a sensitive issue. *Environ Health Perspect.* 1994; 102: 746-750

4. Randolph TG. Sensitivity to petroleum including its derivatives and antecedents. *J Lab Clin Med.* 1952;40:931-932

5. American Academy of Allergy and Immunology, Executive Committee. Clinical ecology. *J Allergy Clin Immunol.* 1986;78:269-271

6. American College of Physicians. Clinical ecology. *Ann Intern Med.* 1989;111:168-178

7. Council on Scientif Affairs, American Medical Association. Clinical ecology. *JAMA.* 1992; 268:3465-3467

8. Shusterman D, Dager SR. Prevention of psychological disability after occupational respiratory exposure. *Occup Med State Art Rev.* 1991;6:11-28

9. Ellefson RD, Ford RE. The porphyrias: characteristics and laboratory tests. *Regul Toxicol Pharmacol.* 1996;24:S119-S125

10. Simon GE, Daniell W, Stockbridge H, Claypoole K, Rosenstock L. Immunologic, psychological, and neuropsychological factors in multiple chemical sensitivity: a controlled study. *Ann Intern Med.* 1993;119:97-103

11. Black DW, Rathe A, Goldstein RB. Environmental illness: A controlled study of 26 subjects with "20th century disease." *JAMA.* 1990; 264:3166-3170

12. Bell, IR, Miller CS, Schwartz GE. An olfactory-limbic model of multiple chemical sensitivity syndrome: possible relationships to kindling and affective spectrum disorders. *Biol Psychiatry.* 1992;32:218-242

13. Kreutzer R, Neutra R. *Evaluating Individuals Reporting Sensitivities to Multiple Chemicals.* Atlanta, Ga: Agency for Toxic Substances and Disease Registry; June 1996

14. Plioplys AV. Chronic fatigue syndrome should not be diagnosed in children. *Pediatrics.* 1997;100:270-271

15. Ziem GE. Multiple chemical sensitivity: treatment and follow up with avoidance and control of chemical exposures. *Toxicol Ind Health.* 1992;8:73-86

16. Wolraich ML, Wilson DB, White JW. The effect of sugar on behavior or cognition in children: a meta-analysis. *JAMA.* 1996;274:1617-1621

33 | Communicating About Risk

P hysicians and professional health organizations are among the most trusted and credible sources for information on environmental issues.[1] Pediatricians who are skilled in communicating environmental health risks are better able to obtain complete patient histories and accurately assess situations that may involve environmental health risks. Failure to deal appropriately with environmental health risk and communication issues may lead to unnecessary stress for pediatricians, patients, and parents; loss of credibility and trust in the pediatrician; incorrect diagnosis; and/or inappropriate or inadequate medical interventions. Effective two-way communication is necessary to come to a mutual understanding of the nature and extent of the health risk and to select appropriate management options. Utilizing the basic concepts of risk communication may assist the pediatrician, patient, and/or parent to select appropriate ways of understanding and controlling the health risk related to environmental exposures.

Communicating about environmental health risks involves a number of factors, some involving complex information: differing levels of science background between the pediatrician and the parent; public phobias about science, medicine, and technology and the parents' ability to understand or control; lack of data; uncertainty about what data might mean in terms of long-term impact on health; lack of trust and credible information sources; lack of clear prevention steps; implications of bad parenting because parents have allowed exposure; misleading or conflicting information from different sources; perceptions of risk; concerns about health, economics, the environment and conservation, governmental process, safety, racism, fairness and equity; legal implications or ongoing litigation; and fear of social ostracism or reprisals, such as losing jobs, if local industries/employers are involved.

■ The Basics of Environmental Health Risk Communication

Health risk communication can be defined as the purposeful exchange of information about the existence, nature, form, severity, or acceptability of risks.[2] Having access to a variety of sources of information will assist pediatricians with answering parents' questions, addressing their concerns, and reducing environmental risks to children's health (see Appendix D).

Dimensions of Risk Perception

A 1990 Roper Poll described a major discrepancy in the ranking of environmental health threats between scientists and the public.[3] Each sector defined "risk" differently. Scientists tend to see risk objectively, based on hazards affecting a large population, and think of risk in statistical terms. Members of the public see risk more subjectively—naturally, parents are concerned with the implications of risk factors for their own community and family. The public perception of risk includes many factors.[4] The following variables may make a hazard seem more threatening or riskier:

- Trust. Risk information that comes from trustworthy sources is more readily believed.

- Familiarity. Familiar risks are less likely to cause outrage. For example, living in an area where lead has been mined for 90 years may make one less likely to be concerned about lead exposure than someone who has not lived in a mining area.

- Control. Most people feel safer when potential risks are under their control; eg, they feel safer driving a vehicle themselves than being a passenger. People generally feel less at risk when they make their own choices.

- Fairness. A person who feels trapped with the risk from a situation while others derive the benefit will find the risk unfair and, therefore, more serious and more unacceptable.

- Catastrophe. Situations that bring to mind environmental disasters, such as those that occurred in Bhopal or Chernobyl, are more likely to be feared as health risks.

- Naturalness. A risk that is natural or seen as humanly unavoidable is less likely to provoke outrage than one that is seen as caused by people, industry, or government.

- Children. Situations in which children may be affected are more likely to be perceived as a risk.

In 1988, Covello and Allen developed seven cardinal rules for the US Environmental Protection Agency (EPA) that have since been widely used by various governmental agencies to guide their risk communication practices.[5]

Cardinal Rules of Risk Communication

Involve the parent in identifying and solving the problem.

Have a communication plan and a clear message.

Listen to the parent's story.

Be honest, frank, and open.

Work with credible sources.

Provide access to information.

Speak clearly and with compassion—or refer the person to someone who can.

Striking a Balance

The effective risk communicator wants to raise concern when it is warranted to ensure that appropriate action steps are taken to protect health and to reassure those who may be anxious unnecessarily. These can be difficult tasks. Two possible ways to communicate effectively include explaining how health standards are set and using risk comparisons.

Using Standards

Parents may need to understand how standards are set—how numbers that relate to risk are derived —before they can begin to understand what these numbers may mean in terms of their child's health risks. Although threshold exposure limits and air and drinking water standards exist for some toxic substances, many of these standards for chemical exposure have been created to protect the health of adults in occupational settings. In 1995, the US Environmental Protection Agency announced the first policy on assessing health risks to children from environmental hazards.[6] To assess the risk of exposure to a child in an environmental setting, it may be necessary to understand how and why the standard was set and the data on which the standard was based. In the case of pesticides, tolerances have been set on the basis of (1) levels resulting from "good" agricultural practice; (2) limits of methods for analysis; (3) available acute and chronic toxicology data; (4) estimated dietary intake; and (5) estimated impact of regulation on the food supply.

Using Risk Comparisons

Hypothetical risks can be difficult to communicate. In explaining risk information, it is tempting to use risk comparisons. It may seem helpful to compare the quantitative or qualitative risks of various exposures and/or behaviors. Risk comparisons can sometimes help parents put risk information in the context of their own situation. Comparisons, however, may backfire because parents may find them inappropriate, irrelevant, or offensive. Irrelevant or misleading comparisons harm trust and the credibility of the pediatrician.

Pediatricians should keep the patient and parent backgrounds and concerns in mind when comparisons are used to discuss risk. The factors that people use in their perception of risk should be considered.

Some Guidelines for Risk Comparisons

The most acceptable comparisons match the same risk at two different times or can be related to a recognized standard (eg, "Now that the radon problem in your house has been remediated, your family's lung cancer risk from exposure to radon has been reduced by 85%"). The pediatrician may also compare different estimates of the same risk (eg, the worst case scenario with the most likely estimate of risk). Comparisons of risks that are related may be helpful to parents. For example, a relevant comparison may be with other risks from the same source (eg, "Over her lifetime, your daughter's medical and dental x-rays produce less risk of lung cancer than her exposure to naturally occurring radon in our neighborhood"). Comparisons of risks that are perceived as unrelated should be avoided (eg, comparing the risk of environmental exposures to the risk of smoking, driving a car, or being hit by lightning).

▌ Answering Tough Questions

Are the PCBs in the water responsible for my child's poor perform-ance in school?

My daughter has asthma. We have lived near a dump all her life. Is her asthma caused by our proximity to the dump?

My baby was born with birth defects. I was exposed to pesticides from crop dusting during my pregnancy. Did they cause my baby's birth defects?

These types of questions are difficult to answer because of the lack of specific data about exposure levels and gaps in toxicology data. In discussing such concerns with parents, listen to and understand their concerns and give appropriate feedback. Answer questions as specif-ically as possible—if the question cannot be answered, explain why and discuss the type of information that would be needed to provide an answer. Describe what the parents or patient can do to reduce their risks or what can be done by others.

▌ Planning by Pediatricians for Risk Communication

Understand the patient's and parents' concerns. Identify their per-ceptions of risk as well. Consider their cultural background, employ-ment, language barriers, and environmental disparity issues when these may be parental concerns.

Determine the goal of the message. What do the patient and par-ents need and want to know? Do they need to take an action or change or adopt a new behavior? Determine the information that needs to be obtained and communicated. If possible, focus on no more than three key pieces of information. Use simple, clear lan-guage. Emphasize any action-oriented messages: what can or should be done to protect the patient's health?

Other physicians, local businessmen, local health officials, local elected officials, or the media may need to be contacted to identify or prevent additional exposures or disease.

Understand the factors that affect risk communication. Credibility is maintained best by not offering unrealistic reassurance to the patient or parents.

Select a variety of communication channels and consistently reinforce the message(s) over time. Try to ensure that office staff and other health care professionals present a consistent message to the patient and parents. It may be helpful to provide printed information that the patient and parents can take home to read and refer to.

Implement and evaluate the communication effort. Practice delivering the message if necessary. Prepare in advance for the tough questions that can be anticipated. Make sure the patient and/or parents know how to reach the office if they have questions later.

■ References

1 . McCallum D, Hammond SL, Morris LA. *Public Knowledge and Perceptions of Chemical Risks in Six Communities: Analysis of a Baseline Survey.* Washington, DC: US Environmental Protection Agency; 1990

2. Tinker TL. Recommendations to improve health risk communication: Lessons learned from the US Public Health Service. *J Health Commun.* 1996; 1:197-217

3. Covello V. *Tools and Techniques for Effective Risk Communication.* Atlanta, Ga: Agency for Toxic Substances and Disease Registry; 1994

4. Hance BJ, Chess C, Sandman PM. *Improving Dialogue With Communities: A Risk Communication Manual for Government.* New Jersey Department of Environmental Protection, Division of Science and Research; 1989

5. Covello VT, Allen FW. *Seven Cardinal Rules of Risk Communication.* Washington, DC: US Environmental Protection Agency, Office of Policy Analysis; 1988

6. Environmental Protection Agency. *Environmental Health Threats to Children.* Washington, DC: Environmental Protection Agency, Office of the Administrator; September 1996

V
Appendices

AAP Policy Statements From the Committee on Environmental Health

Current

Thimerosal in Vaccines—An Interim Report to Clinicians
PEDIATRICS, Vol 104, No 3, September 1999

Ultraviolet Light: A Hazard to Children
PEDIATRICS, Vol 104, No 2, August 1999

Screening for Elevated Blood Lead Levels
PEDIATRICS, Vol 101, No 6, June 1998

Toxic Effects of Indoor Molds
PEDIATRICS, Vol 101, No 4, April 1998

Risk of Ionizing Radiation Exposure to Children
PEDIATRICS, Vol 101, No 4, April 1998

Noise: A Hazard to the Fetus and Newborn
PEDIATRICS, Vol 100, No 4, October 1997

Environmental Tobacco Smoke: A Hazard to Children
PEDIATRICS, Vol 99, No 4, April 1997

The Hazards of Child Labor
PEDIATRICS, Vol 95, No 2, February 1995

PCBs in Breast Milk
PEDIATRICS, Vol 94, No 1, July 1994

Use of Chloral Hydrate for Sedation in Children
PEDIATRICS, Vol 92, No 3, September 1993
AAP News, Vol 9, No 5, May 1993 Policy Summary

Ambient Air Pollution: Respiratory Hazards to Children
PEDIATRICS, Vol 91, No 6, June 1993
AAP News, Vol 9, No 5, May 1993 Policy Summary

Radon Exposure: A Hazard to Children
PEDIATRICS, Vol 83, No 5, May 1989

Asbestos Exposure in Schools
PEDIATRICS, Vol 79, No 2, February 1987

Smokeless Tobacco - A Carcinogenic Hazard to Children
PEDIATRICS, Vol 76, No 6, December 1985

Retired Statements

Lead Poisoning: From Screening to Primary Prevention
PEDIATRICS, Vol 92, No 1, July 1993
AAP News, Vol 9, No 4, April 1993 Policy Summary
Retired 6/98

Statement on Childhood Lead Poisoning (Joint with COIPP)
PEDIATRICS, Vol 79, No 3, March 1987
Retired 10/93

Involuntary Smoking: A Hazard to Children
PEDIATRICS, Vol 77, No 5, May 1986
Retired 4/97

Special Susceptibility of Children to Radiation Effects
PEDIATRICS, Vol 72, No 6, December 1983
Retired 4/98

**The Environmental Consequences of Tobacco Smoking:
Implications for Public Policies that Affect the Health of
Children**
PEDIATRICS, Vol 70, No 2, August 1982
Retired 2/87

PCBs in Breast Milk
PEDIATRICS, Vol 62, No 3, September 1978
Retired 9/94

National Standard for Airborne Lead
PEDIATRICS, Vol 62, No 6, December 1978
Retired 2/87

Infant Radiant Warmers
PEDIATRICS, Vol 61, No 1, January 1978
Retired 6/95

Hyperthermia from Malfunctioning Radiant Heaters
PEDIATRICS, Vol 59, No 6, June 1977
Retired 2/87

Carcinogens in Drinking Water
PEDIATRICS, Vol 57, No 4, April 1976
Retired 2/87

Effects of Cigarette Smoking on the Fetus and Child
PEDIATRICS, Vol 57, No 3, March 1976
Retired 9/94

Noise Pollution: Neonatal Aspects
PEDIATRICS, Vol 54, No 4, October 1974
Retired 10/97

Animal Feedlots
PEDIATRICS, Vol 51, No 3, March 1973
Retired 9/94

Pediatric Problems Related to Deteriorated Housing
Newsletter, Vol 23, No 2, January 15, 1972
Retired 2/87

Lead Content of Paint Applied to Surfaces Accessible to Young Children
PEDIATRICS, Vol 49, No 6, June 1972
. Retired 2/87

Earthenware Containers: A Potential Source of Acute Lead Poisoning
Newsletter, Vol 22, No 13, August 15, 1971
Retired 2/87

Neurotoxicity from Hexachlorophene
Newsletter, Vol 22, No 7, May 1971
Retired 2/87

Acute and Chronic Childhood Lead Poisoning
PEDIATRICS, Vol 47, No 5, May 1971
Retired 11/86

Pediatric Aspects of Air Pollution
PEDIATRICS, Vol 46, No 4, October 1970
Retired 2/87

More on Radioactive Fallout
Newsletter Supplement, Vol 21, No 8, April 15, 1970
Retired 2/87

Smoking and Children: A Pediatric Viewpoint
PEDIATRICS, Vol 44, No 5, Part 1, November 1969
Retired 2/87

Present Status of Water Pollution Control
PEDIATRICS, Vol 34, No 3, September 1964
Retired 2/87

Hazards of Radioactive Fallout
Newsletter, Vol 13, No 4, April 1962
Retired 2/95

Statement on the Use of Diagnostic X-Ray
PEDIATRICS, Vol 28, No 4, October 1961
Retired 2/87

Radiation Hazards and Epidemiology of Malformations on Diagnostic Use of X-Ray
Newsletter, Vol 12, No 6, June 1, 1961
Retired

Pediatrics Supplements

The Susceptibility of the Fetus and Child to Chemical Pollutants
Supplement to PEDIATRICS, Vol 53, No 5, Part II, May 1974

Conference on the Pediatric Significance of Peacetime Radioactive Fallout
Supplement to PEDIATRICS, Vol 41, No 1, Part II, January 1968

B Common Abbreviations

AChE	acetylcholinesterase
ASTM D4236	American Society for Testing and Materials Standard (art materials)
AT	ataxia-telangiectasia
BAL	dimercaprol
BLL	blood lead level
dBA	decibels weighted by the A scale
DDE	dichlorodiphenyldichloroethane
DDT	dichlorodiphenyltrichloroethane
DEET	diethyltoluamide
DHEA	dehydroepiandrosterone
DMSA	dimercaptosuccinic acid (succimer)
EMF	electromagnetic fields
ETS	environmental tobacco smoke
eV	electron volts
Gy	Gray
HEPA	high-efficiency particulate air
HBO	hyberbaric oxygen
HVAC	heating, ventilation, and air conditioning
HVOD	hepatic veno-occlusive disease
IAQ	indoor air quality
IPM	integrated pest management
KI	potassium iodide

LOAEL	lowest observable adverse effect level
MCS	Multiple chemical sensitivities
mG	milligauss
mR	milliroentgen
MSDS	material safety data sheets
MTBE	methyl tertiary butyl ether
NAAQS	National Ambient Air Quality Standards
NMSC	nonmelanoma skin cancer
NOAEL	no observable adverse effect level
NPL	National Priorities List
Pa	pascals
PBB	polybrominated biphenyl
PCB	polychlorinated biphenyl
PCDD	polychlorinated dibenzodioxin
PCDF	polychlorinated dibenzofuran
pCi	picocuries
PDCB	p-dichlorobenzene
PM_{10}	particles smaller than 10 µm
PM_{25}	particles smaller than 2.5 µm
PO_2	partial pressure of oxygen
ppb	parts per billion
ppm	parts per million
ppt	parts per trillion
PSI	pollutant standards index
Quats	quanternary ammonium compounds
R	roentgen
RBE	relative biological effectiveness
SBS	Sick Building Syndrome
Sv	Sievert
TCDD	2,3,7,8 tetrachlorodibenzo-p-dioxin
THM	trihalomethane
TSCA	Toxic Substances Control Act
UVR	ultraviolet radiation
VOC	volatile organic compound

C Curricula for Environmental Education in Schools

Environmental education is defined as "an active process that increases awareness, knowledge, and skills that result in understanding, commitment, informed decisions, and constructive action that ensure stewardship of all interdependent parts of the earth's environment" (North Carolina Environmental Education Plan, April 1995) Environmental education should begin early and continue through high school. Children who receive environmental education may be able to prevent environmental illness both through personal health choices and through community involvement. As adults, these children should be well prepared to participate in the political process as informed and environmentally literate citizens.

A number of excellent environmental education curricula have been developed over the past two decades. Environmental health education curricula are also emerging. The most successful environmental education programs result from combining excellent curricula with the efforts of enthusiastic individuals at the local school level.

Health professionals can stimulate environmental health education efforts in the schools through volunteerism in the classroom, school health programs, and technical partnerships with local school boards and state departments of education. Direct classroom volunteerism can take the form of assisting teachers in designing and executing hands-on environmental science and environmental health activities that actively link human health to the state of the physical environment. Within the tradition of school health is the concept of the "healthy school environment." Enthusiastic clinicians can help local schools identify ways in which the school environment can be made more healthy. A specific agent or toxicant should be selected for such work. Examples could be developing a plan for the school to reduce pesticide use or working with students and faculty to assure that the school is in compliance with state and federal health and safety regulations. They can participate in PTA activities and teacher training on environmental health issues pertinent to their community, drawing examples from their practices. Finally, they can work at the district or state department of education level to introduce environmental health education systemically. Increasingly, states are creating offices of environmental education within departments of education to stimulate pre-service and in-service teacher training as well as inclusion of environmental sciences in K-12 curricula. Health professionals can add valuable insight and expertise to this process by stimulating discussion of the links between the environment and human health.

▌Environmental Education Curricula

General Environmental Education

1. Project Learning Tree, 111 19th Street NW Suite 780, Washington DC 20036, or look at their World Wide Web site at http://eelink.umich.edu/plt.html. Telephone: 202/463-2700.

Project Learning Tree uses the forest and trees as a "window on the world" for the purpose of increasing students' understanding of our complex environment; to stimulate critical and creative thinking; to develop the ability to make informed decisions on environmental issues; and to instill the confidence and commitment to take responsible action on behalf of the environment (K-12).

2. Project WILD, 201 Culbertson Hall, Montana State University, Bozeman, MT 59717-0057, or look at the World Wide Web site at http://eelink.umich.edu/wild/wildhome.html. Telephone: 301/493-5447.

The Project WILD K-12 Activity Guide focuses on wildlife and habitat, while the Project WILD Aquatic Education Activity Guide emphasizes aquatic wildlife and aquatic ecosystems. The guides are organized thematically and are designed for integration into existing courses of study.

3. Project WET, 201 Culbertson Hall, Montana State University, Bozeman, MT 59717-0057, or look at the World Wide Web site at http://eelink.umich.edu/wet1/html. Telephone: 406/994-5392.

The goal of Project WET is to promote awareness, appreciation, knowledge, and stewardship of water resources through the development and dissemination of classroom-ready teaching aids, and the establishment of state and internationally sponsored programs (K-12).

4. Environmental Education Link: Environmental Education on the Internet. A project of the National Consortium for Environmental Education and Training, a major environmental education professional group, with support from the United States Environmental Protection Agency. http://www.nceet.snre.umich.edu.

5. California Department of Education, Office of Environmental Education, 721 Capitol Mall, PO Box 944272, Sacramento, CA. 94244-2720.

This office has reviewed and rated hundreds of environmental education curricula, K-12, and published them in a series of compendia.

Environmental Health Education

1. National Institute of Environmental Health Sciences, Marian Johnson-Thomason, Director of NIEHS Office of Institutional Development, PO Box 12233, Research Triangle Park, NC 27709. Telephone: 919/541-1919.

NIEHS sponsors demonstration projects around the country for the purpose of developing environmental health curricula for K-12.

2. Environmental and Occupational Health Sciences Institute, Brenda Steinberg, Director of Resource Program, 170 Frelinghuysen Rd, Piscataway, NJ 08854. Telephone: 732/445-0110.

EOSHI is jointly sponsored by the University of Medicine and Dentistry of New Jersey, Robert Wood Johnson Medical School and Rutgers, the State University of New Jersey. They have developed and widely disseminated environmental health curricula for K-12 throughout New Jersey and other states.

The Toxicology, Risk Assessment and Pollution (ToxRAP™) curriculum series includes three modules: Early elementary/K-3,

Intermediate Elementary/4-6, and Middle School/6-9. The Early Elementary Module (*The Case of the Green Feathers*) focuses on pollen and other air pollutants that can cause allergic reactions in children. The Intermediate Elementary Module (*What is Wrong with the Johnson Family?*) discusses indoor air polution, with special attention to carbon monoxide. The Middle School Module (*Mystery Illness Strikes the Sanchez Household*) investigates air contaminants that include dust from lead-based paint.

3. Baylor College of Medicine Division of School-Based Programs. Nancy Moreno, PhD, *My Health, My World* Project Director. 1709 Dryden, Suite 545, Houston, TX 77030. Telephone: 800/798-8244.

The *My Health, My World* project has developed teaching units on current environmental issues for students in grades K-4. Each unit weaves physical, earth, and life sciences together to promote understanding of environmental processes and how they affect health and well-being. Three units are available. *My World Indoors* creatively explores air quality in the home, school, and work. *Water and My World* provides a perspective on water and why it is important to health and well-being. *My Home, My Planet* looks at changes in the upper atmosphere, such as global warming, and how the changes may affect human health.

Environmental Health Resources

Disclaimer: *The Academy does not review or endorse the information provided by these organizations.*

National Associations and Organizations

Alliance to End Childhood Lead Poisoning
227 Massachusetts Ave, NE, Suite 200
Washington, DC 20002
202/543-1147; Fax: 202/543-4466
E-mail: aeclp@aeclp.org
http://www.aeclp.org

American Association of Poison Control Centers
3201 New Mexico Ave, NW, Suite 310
Washington, DC 20016
202/362-7217
http://www.aapcc.org

American Cancer Society
1599 Clifton Rd, NE
Atlanta, GA 30329
404/320-3333 or 800/ACS-2345; Fax: 404/329-7530
http://www.cancer.org

American Lung Association
432 Park Ave S, 8th Floor
New York, NY 10016
800/LUNG-USA
http://www.lungusa.org

American Public Health Association
800 I St, NW
Washington, DC 20001
202/777-2742

Asthma and Allergy Foundation of America
1125 15th St, NW, Suite 502
Washington, DC 20005
202/466-7643; Fax: 202/466-8940
http://www.aafa.org

Asthma Information Center
Journal of the American Medical Association
http://www.ama-assn.org/special/asthma

Center for Children's Health and the Environment
Mount Sinai School of Medicine
One Gustave L. Levy Place
Box 1043
New York, NY 10029-6574
212/241-8689; Fax: 212/360-6965
http://www.mssm.edu/cpm

Center for Safety in the Arts, Inc
http://www.artswire.org:70/1/csa

Children's Environmental Health Center
Haborview Medical Center
m/s 359739
Seattle, WA 98104-2499
206/526-2121; Fax: 206/731-8247
http://www.weber.u.washington.edu/~oempwww/pehsu

Children's Environmental Health Network
5900 Hollis St, Suite R3
Emeryville, CA 94608
510/597-1393; Fax: 510/597-1399
E-mail: cehn@cehn.org
http://www.cehn.org

Children's Health Environmental Coalition
PO Box 846
Malibu, CA 90265
310/589-2233; Fax: 310/589-5856
E-mail: chec@igc.apc.org
http://www.checnet.org

CCHW Center for Health, Environment and Justice
150 S Washington, Suite 300
PO Box 6806
Falls Church, VA 22040
703/237-2249
http://www.essential.org/cchw

Coalition for America's Children
1634 Eye St, NW, 11th Floor
Washington, DC 20006
202/638-5770; Fax: 202/638-5771
http://www.benton.org

Energy Efficiency and Renewable Energy Clearinghouse
PO Box 3048
Merrifield, VA 22116
800/363-3732 Fax: 703/893-0400
http://www.eren.doe.gov/consumerinfo

Environmental Defense Fund
257 Park Ave S
New York, NY 10010
212/505-2100; Fax: 212/505-2375
http://www.edf.org

Environmental Health Coalition
1717 Kettner Blvd, Suite 100
San Diego, CA 92101
619/235-0281; Fax: 619/232-3670
http://www.environmentalhealth.org

Environmental Justice Resource Center
223 James P. Brawley Dr, SW
Atlanta, GA 30314
404/880-6911; Fax: 404/880-6909
http://www.ejrc.cau.edu

Healthy Mothers, Healthy Babies
121 N Washington St
Alexandria, VA 22314
703/836-6110; Fax: 703/836-2470

Healthy Schools Network, Inc.
96 S Swan St
Albany, NY 12210
518/462-0632; Fax: 518/462-0433
http://www.hsnet.org

Midwest University Radon/Indoor Air Quality Project
University of Minnesota
266 McNeal Hall
1985 Buford Ave
St Paul, MN 55108-6136
612/624-8747; Fax: 612/625-3113
E-mail: rniaq@chez.che.umn.edu
http://www.dehs.umn.edu/schooliaq.html

Institute for Children's Environmental Health
PO Box 757
463 First St
Langley, WA 98260
360/221-7995; Fax: 360/221-7993
E-mail: ELISE@WHIDBEY.com

Learning Disabilities Association of America
4156 Library Rd
Pittsburgh, PA 15234-1349
412/341-1515; 412/341-8077; Fax: 412/344-0224
http://www.ldanatl.org

March of Dimes Birth Defects Foundation
1275 Mamaroneck Ave
White Plains, NY 10605
914/428-7100; Fax: 914/428-8203
http://www.modimes.org

Mothers of Asthmatics, Inc
2751 Prosperity Ave, Suite 150
Fairfax, VA 22031
800/878-4403; Fax: 703/573-7794
http://www.aanma.org

National Association of Physicians for the Environment (NAPE)
6410 Rockledge Dr, Suite 412
Bethesda, MD 20817-1809
301/571-9790; Fax: 301/530-8910
http://www.napenet.org

National Environmental Education and Training Foundation
734 15th St, NW, Suite 420
Washington, DC 20005
202/628-8200; Fax: 202/628-8204
E-mail: west@neetf.org

National Environmental Health Association
720 South Colorado Blvd, Suite 970, South Tower
Denver, CO 80246-1925
303/756-9090; Fax: 303/691-9490
E-mail: staff@neha.org
http://www.neha.org

Natural Resources Defense Council
71 Stevenson St, Suite 1825
San Francisco, CA 94105
415/777-0220; Fax: 415/495-5996
http://www.nrdc.org

National Safety Council, Environmental Health Center
1025 Connecticut Ave, NW; Suite 1200
Washington, DC 20036
202/293-2270; Fax: 202/293-0032
http://www.nsc.org

Pew Environmental Health Commission
Johns Hopkins School of Public Health
111 Market Pl, Suite 850
Baltimore, MD 21202
410/659-2690; Fax: 410/659-2699

Physicians for Social Responsibility
1101 14th St, NW, Suite 700
Washington, DC 20005
202/898-0150; Fax: 202/898-0172
http://www.psr.org

Teratology Society
1767 Business Center Dr, Suite 302
Reston, VA 20190-5332
703/438-3104
http://www.teratology.org

Government Agencies
Agency for Toxic Substances and Disease Registry (ATSDR)
1600 Clifton Rd, NE; Mail Stop E-28
Atlanta, GA 30333
404/639-6360 (Information Center Clearinghouse)
Fax: 404/639-0744
http://atsdr1.atsdr.cdc.gov:8080/child

> Emergency Response Branch: 404/639-0615
> Hazardous Waste Sites Hotline: 800/424-9346

Methyl Parathion Hotline: 601/762-1202
Toxicological Profiles: 800/858-7378

Centers for Disease Control and Prevention
National Center for Environmental Health
4770 Buford Hwy, NE; Mail Stop F-28
Atlanta, GA 30341-3724
770/488-7300; Fax: 770/488-7310

Consumer Product Safety Commission
4340 East West Hwy
Bethesda, MD 20814
800/638-2772; Fax: 301/504-0124
http://www.cpsc.gov

Department of Health and Human Services
Office of Disease Prevention and Health Promotion
PO Box 1133
Washington, DC 20013-1133
800/336-4797; Fax: 301/984-4256
http://www.odphp.osophs.dhhs.gov

US Environmental Protection Agency
401 M St, SW
Washington, DC 20460
202/260-2090
For regional EPA office information, see chapters 5 and 22.
http://www.epa.gov

Chemical Spills Emergency Hotline: 800/424-8802
Hazardous Waste/Community Right to Know
Hotline: 800/424-9346
Indoor Air Quality Information Clearinghouse:
800/438-4318; http://www.epa.gov/iaq
Office of Child Health Protection: 202/260-7778
Office of Pesticide Programs: 703/305-5017
National Pesticides Hotline: 800/535-PEST
http://www.epa.gov/pesticides
Safe Drinking Water Hotline: 800/426-4791
Toxic Substances Control Act (TSCA) Information Line:
202/554-1404

Food and Drug Administration
Office of Public Affairs
5600 Fishers Ln
Rockville, MD 20857
301/827-3666; Fax: 301/443-4915
http://www.cfsan.fda.gov

Food Safety and Inspection Service
Food Safety Education Office
1400 Independence Ave, SW
Washington, DC 20250
202/720-7943; Fax: 202/720-1843
E-mail: fsis.webmaster@usda.gov
http://www.fsis.usda.gov

Health Resources and Services Administration
Maternal and Child Health Bureau
Parklawn Bldg, Room 1445
5600 Fishers Ln
Rockville, MD 20857
301/443-3376; Fax: 301/443-1989

National Cancer Institute
National Institutes of Health
9000 Rockville Pike
Bethesda, MD 20892
800/4CANCER
http://www.nci.nih.gov

National Institute for Occupational Safety and Health
200 Independence Ave, SW
Washington, DC 20201
800/356-4674

> Project EPOCH-Envi
> NIOSH, Division of Training and Manpower Development
> Curriculum Development Branch
> Robert Taft Laboratories
> 4676 Columbia Pkwy
> Cincinnati, OH 45226-1998
> 800/356-4674

National Institute of Environmental Health Sciences (NIEHS)
PO Box 12233
Research Triangle Park, NC 27709
919/541-1919; Fax: 919/541-3592

Environmental/Occupational Medicine Academic Awards
　　Chief, Environmental Health Resources Branch
　　Division of Extramural Research and Training
　　NIEHS　PO Box 12233
　　Research Triangle Park, NC 27709
　　919/541-7825

National Lead Information Center
8601 Georgia Ave, Suite 700
Silver Spring, MD 20910
800/424-LEAD
800/LEAD-FYI
http://www.epa.gov/lead

Occupational Safety and Health Administration
Office of Administrative Services
200 Constitution Ave, NW, Room N-310
Washington, DC 20210
202/693-1999
http://www.osha.gov

Chairs of the AAP Committee on Environmental Health

Committee on Radiation Hazards and Epidemiology of Malformations
Robert A. Aldrich, MD, 1957-1961

In 1961, the Committee was split in two: a short-lived Committee on Malformations and the Committee on Environmental Hazards.

Committee on Environmental Hazards
Lee E. Farr, MD, 1961-1967
Paul F. Wehrle, MD, 1967-1973
Robert W. Miller, MD, PhD, 1973-1979
Laurence Finberg, MD, 1979-1980

In 1979, the Academy established the Committee on Genetics with Charles Scriver as chair. In 1980, the Academy combined this Committee with the Committee on Environmental Hazards to form the:

Committee on Genetics & Environmental Hazards
Laurence Finberg, MD, Co-Chair, 1980-1983
Charles Scriver, MD, Co-Chair, 1980-1983

In 1983, the two committees were separated again.

Committee on Environmental Hazards
Philip J. Landrigan, MD, MSc, 1983-1987
Richard J. Jackson, MD, 1987-1991

In 1991, the Committee was renamed the Committee on Environmental Health.

Committee on Environmental Health
J. Routt Reigart, MD, 1991-1995
Ruth A. Etzel, MD, PhD, 1995-1999
Sophie J. Balk, MD, 1999-

AAP Patient Education Materials Related to Environmental Health Issues

Following is a list of patient education materials from the American Academy of Pediatrics relating to environmental health issues. To obtain pricing information or to order the materials, contact the AAP Department of Marketing and Publications at 847/228-5005.

HE0106   *Allergies in Children*

HE0236   *Anemia and Your Young Child*

HE0193   *Ear Infections and Young Children*

HE0168   *Environmental Tobacco Smoke: A Danger to Children*

HE0181   *Fun in the Sun: Keep Your Baby Safe*

HE0177   *How to Help Your Child with Asthma*

HE0251   *Lead Poisoning: Prevention and Screening*

HE0180   *Middle Ear Fluid in Young Children*

HE0065   *The Risks of Tobacco Use: A Message to Parents and Teens*

HE0189   *Smokeless Tobacco (Guidelines for teens)*

HE0088   *Smoking: Straight Talk for Teens*

HE0218   *Your Child and the Environment*

Index

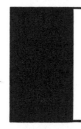

Index